ALLE ZEIT WACH 1842

Neurobiology and Behavior of Honeybees

Edited by

Randolf Menzel · Alison Mercer

With 128 Figures

Springer-Verlag
Berlin Heidelberg New York
London Paris Tokyo

Prof. Dr. RANDOLF MENZEL
Institute of Animal Physiology
Free University of Berlin
Königin-Luise-Straße 28–30
1000 Berlin 33
FRG

Dr. ALISON MERCER
University of Otago
Department of Zoology
Dunedin
New Zealand

Cover Illustration: The waggle dance, redrawn from Fig. 44 in K. von Frisch's book, „Tanzsprache und Orientierung der Bienen" (1965), by P. Adam.

ISBN-13: 978-3-642-71498-6 e-ISBN-13: 978-3-642-71496-2
DOI: 10.1007/978-3-642-71496-2

Library of Congress Cataloging-in-Publication Data. Neurology and behavior of honeybees. Includes bibliographies and index. 1. Honeybee–Physiology. 2. Honeybee–Behavior. 3. Nervous system–Insects. 4. Insects–Physiology. 5. Insects–Behavior. I. Menzel, Randolf, 1940- . II. Mercer, Alison, 1954- . QL568.A6N48 1987 595.79'9
87-9496

Softcover reprint of the hardcover 1st edition 1987

2131/3130-543210

Preface

The honeybee Apis mellifera has become a model system par excellence for neuroethological research. No other insect species is so well known with respect to individual and social behavior, sensory capacity, orientation, communication, stereotyped and plastic behavior. In science and in history, the honeybee occupies a unique position in the relationship between man and animals. More than 10, 000 years ago, stone-age man already knew of the delights of honey, and was wary enough of the bee's aggressive behavior that he protected himself with smoke, as can be seen in the impressive cave paintings of Arana near Bicorp (Valencia, Spain). The Ancient Greeks and Egyptians also knew many details about the social and individual behavior of the honeybee, and often built special hives to enable easier access to the honey e. g. fired clay tubes in the case of the Egyptians. Aristotle (1) observed that nectar and pollen collecting bees worked particularly effectively by continuing to search at the same plant species: "On every journey out of the hive, the bee never lands on different varieties of flowers, but always on the same type of flower flying, for example, from violet to violet before flying back to the hive. As soon as she is back in the hive, she shakes free her (pollen) load whilst being followed by three or four other bees. What these other bees receive from her is difficult to see". Here, Aristotle was describing the bee (waggle) dance - perhaps the first citation of this extraordinary behavior. 400 years later, around 50 A. D., Plinius described in "Naturalis historia" (Vol. 11, Part 16 and 49) the use of observation hives with horn windows, these enabling the first observations to be made on the social life of the bee colony.

The beginning of scientific research into the behavior of bees was marked by the discoveries of Christian Konrad Sprengel, who was a botanist and school teacher living in Berlin. In 1793 he published a book entitled "The discovered secret of Nature with respect to the construction and fertilization of flowers" (8). The discovered secret was that flowers developed distinct characteristics that enabled insects, especially bees, to distinguish between the various species of flower. Therefore, it was necessary that the bees recognized and also learned the color, form, odor, and structural characteristics of the flowers. He wrote: "When the crown of a flower is colored at a particular place, then it is so because it serves to guide the insect more easily to the nectar. Furthermore, this enables the insect to recognize its food source whilst flying in the air". Charles Darwin, who knew of Sprengel's work, expressed this situation in different terms: "That insects should visit the flowers of the same species for as long as they can is of great significance to the plant, as it favours cross-fertilization of distinct individuals of the same species; but no-one will suppose that insects act in this manner for the good of the plant. The cause probably lies in insects being thus enabled to work quicker; they have just learned how to stand in the best position of the flower, and how far and in what direction to insert their proboscides.........Memory also comes into play for, as already remarked, bees know the position of each clump of flowers in a garden" (4, p. 417).

Whilst Darwin and other well-known entomologists such as Bethe (2), Buttel-Reepen (3), Forel (5), and Lubbock (7) experienced no difficulties in describing such activities as orientation to landmarks, color vision, scent perception, learning and memory, the rigorous scientific work required to substantiate such observations was first undertaken by Karl von Frisch (6). Over a period of 80 years of intensive work, von Frisch and his students quantitatively analyzed the visual, olfactory and mechanical senses, as well as many aspects of social communication within the colony such as the waggle dance. Furthermore, von Frisch and his co-worker Lindauer were also the first to describe hitherto unknown perceptual capacities such the bee's ability to orientate to polarized light and the magnetic field of the earth. Perhaps the most important discovery made by von Frisch was that bees are easily trained. This observation and the methods used to train the bees has provided the key to a treasure chest of scientific discoveries. The rapid learning ability of the bee, and its long lasting memory and large degree of choice motivation, has been the source of many new insights and discoveries over the last 8 decades.

Today, research is directed not only towards analysis of the behavioral, perceptual and learning capabilities of the bee, but also towards an understanding of the neuronal mechanisms involved. The work of Karl von Frisch and his students provides a stable foundation for all future studies of the neurobiology and behavior of bees. The neuroethological approach introduced by him brings together the diverse aspects of behavioral, sensory physiological and neurobiological research on bees, many of which are considered in this book. Hopefully, bee researchers will continue to collectively learn from their much treasured experimental subjects in the sense expressed by Francis Bacon in 1620:

"Those who have treated of the sciences have been either empirics or dogmatical. The former like ants only heap up and use their store, the latter like spiders spin out their own webs. The bee a mean between both, extracts matter from the flowers of the garden and the field, but works and fashions it by its own efforts. The true labor of philosophy resembles hers, for it neither relies entirely or principally on the powers of the mind, nor yet lays up in the memory the matter afforded by the experiments of natural history and mechanics in its raw state, but changes and works it in the understanding. We have good reason, therefore, to derive hope from a closer and purer alliance of these faculties (the experimental and rational) that has yet been attempted". (Novum Organon, XCV Aphorism).

We are grateful to the contributors of this book for their enthusiasm to present and share their ideas and data. The help of Ms Loretta Doemland-Smith, Frau Sybille Schaare and Mr Mirko Whitfield in preparing the camera-ready manuscript is greatly appreciated.

This book is dedicated to Karl von Frisch on the occasion of his 100th birthday.

Randolf Menzel, Berlin
Alison Mercer, Dunedin

REFERENCES

(1) Aristoteles. 1949. Tierkunde, Ed. P Gohlke, Paderborn, IX.

(2) Bethe, A. 1898. Dürfen wir Ameisen und Bienen psychische Qualitäten zuschreiben? Arch. ges. Physiol. 70: 1- 45.

(3) Buttel-Reepen, H. v.. 1900. Sind Bienen Reflexmaschinen? Biol. Zbl. 20, 97-304.

(4) Darwin, C. 1876. Cross and self-fertilization in the vegetable kingdom. London, Murray.

(5) Forel, A. 1910. Das Sinnesleben der Insekten. München, Reinhardt.

(6) Frisch, K. v.. 1965. Tanzsprache und Orientierung der Bienen. Berlin-Heidelberg-New York, Springer Verlag.

(7) Lubbock, J. 1882. Ants, bees, wasps. London.

(8) Sprengel, Chr. K. 1793. Das entdeckte Geheimnis der Natur im Bau und in der Befruchtung der Blumen. Berlin. (reprint 1894 W. Engelmann, Leipzig).

Contents

Introduction
M. Lindauer 1

EVOLUTION AND GENETICS

The Evolution of Honeybees
F. Ruttner (With 8 Figures) 8

Behavior Genetics of Honeybees (Apis mellifera L.)
R. F. A. Moritz and C. Brandes (With 5 Figures) 21

THE FORAGING HONEYBEE

Social Foraging by Honeybees: How a Colony Tracks Rich Sources of Nectar
T. D. Seeley and R. A. Levien (With 7 Figures) 38

New Perspectives on the Dance Orientation of the Asian Honeybees
F. C. Dyer (With 4 Figures) 54

Perception of Foraging Costs and Intakes, and Foraging Decisions
K. D. Waddington (With 2 Figures) 66

The Bee's E-Vector Compass
S. Rossel and R. Wehner (With 11 Figures) 76

PHYSIOLOGICAL ASPECTS OF BEHAVIOR

Texture Sensitivity in the Life of Honeybees
P. G. Kevan 96

Thermoregulation by Individual Honeybees
B. Heinrich 102

Sleep Research on Honeybees: Neurophysiology and Behavior
W. Kaiser and J. Steiner-Kaiser (With 3 Figures) 112

Behavioral and Pharmacological Analysis of the Stinging Response in Africanized and Italian Bees
N. Balderrama, M. Díaz, A. Sequeda, J. Núnez, H. Maldonado (With 4 Figures) 121

VISUAL SYSTEM

The Structural Basis of Information Processing in the Visual System of the Bee
W. A. Ribi (With 4 Figures) 130

Processing of Visual Information in the Honeybee Brain
H. Hertel and U. Maronde (With 10 Figures) 141

Motion Sensitive Descending Interneurons, Ocellar L_D Neurons and Neck Motoneurons in the Bee: A Neural Substrate for Visual Course Control in Apis mellifera
L. J. Goodman, W. A. Fletcher, R. G. Guy, P. G. Mobbs (With 8 Figures) 158

Color Vision in Honeybees: Metric, Dimensions, Constancy, and Ecological Aspects
W. Backhaus, A. Werner and R. Menzel (With 7 Figures) 172

The Ocellar System of the Honeybee
J. J. Milde (With 9 Figures) 191

NEUROANATOMY AND SIGNAL PROCESSING IN THE BRAIN

Chemical Neuroanatomy of the Honeybee Brain
G. Bicker, S. Schäfer, V. Rehder (With 7 Figures) 202

Synaptic Connectivity in the Mushroom Bodies of the Honeybee Brain: Electron Microscopy and Immunocytochemistry of Neuroactive Compounds
F.-W. Schürmann and K. Elekes (With 3 Figures)........ 225

Immunohistochemical Localization of a Gastrin / CCK-like Peptide in the Brain of the Honeybee
M. J. Noble and L. J. Goodman (With 3 Figures)........ 235

Biogenic Amines and the Bee Brain
A. Mercer (With 4 Figures)........ 244

Neural Signal Processing in the Median Protocerebrum of the Bee
J. Erber and U. Homberg (With 6 Figures)........ 253

DEVELOPMENT

Hormonal Regulation of Age Polyethism in the Honeybee, Apis mellifera
G. E. Robinson (With 4 Figures)........ 266

Organization and Plasticity of the Olfactory System of the Honeybee, Apis mellifera
C. Masson and G. Arnold (With 5 Figures)........ 280

LEARNING AND MEMORY

Flower-shape, Landmark, and Locale Memory in Honeybees
J. L. Gould (With 6 Figures)........ 298

Memory Traces in Honeybees
R. Menzel (With 8 Figures)........ 310

SUBJECT INDEX........ 327

Introduction

Martin Lindauer
Röntgenring 10, 8700 Würzburg, FRG

KARL VON FRISCH, A PIONEER IN SENSORY PHYSIOLOGY AND EXPERIMENTAL SOCIOBIOLOGY

We human beings roam across vales and hills, meadows and woods, and delight in the fragant carpet of flowers in their colorful magnificance, and in the chirping of crickets and the song of birds. Who would entertain the idea that our experience is only a tiny fraction of the real environment? The physicist has shown, however, that the electromagnetic spectrum extends from the long wavelengths of radio waves via infra-red and ultra-violet to the short wavelengths of x-rays and gamma rays. The human eye perceives the minute section from 400-800 nm -approxiametely a billionth part of the spectrum! We know today that in the field of ultrasound, there exists important information for other animals to which our ear is deaf. The biochemist has analyzed the structure of countless molecules to which many animals are attracted, or from which they shy away, but to which our nose is not sensitive in any way. It was a major achievement in this century when Karl von Frisch, the pioneer of modern sensory physiology and behavioral research, presented to us the means for the discovery of such unknown worlds. It is easier to understand the work of this dedicated biologist, if one looks into the initimate circumstances of his family life, where his love of nature was already fostered from an early age. Born in the Josephstädter Strasse, a corner protected from the metropolitan noise of Vienna, his room was already turned into a menagerie during his early grammar school days. His diary lists as companions: 9 different kinds of mammals, 16 species of birds, 26 different reptiles and amphibians, 27 kinds of fish, and 45 species of invertebrates. He later wrote, "I shall never forget my mother's patient tolerance towards those sometimes obnoxious companions".

From earliest childhood he showed the curiosity characteristic of the future zoologist, in that he not only described the morphology and behavior of an animal, but also asked questions concerning casual relationships i.e. the function of the vital processes. His sharp powers of observation are testified in a letter written to his mother when he was nine years old:

"Dear Mamma,

just consider, my salamanders which I brought back from Kolta, laid 30 eggs yesterday afternoon, and from last night till today 31 eggs, each one distinctly separated on a different leaf of a water plant, which they later put together in this way: (A drawing is included).

Many regards from

Your Karl".

Decisive new ideas and encouragement for his later profession as a dedicated researcher in the field of comparative animal physiology came from his uncle Sigmund Exner, Professor of Physiology at the University of Vienna. After his doctoral thesis on color change in fish, v. Frisch turned to sensory physiology and became the pioneer of this new discipline in zoology.

In 1912, a colony of bees was acquired for the summer residence of the von Frisch family, which was situated in Brunnwinkel, near to St. Gilgen in the Salzkammergut. The colony had been obtained for the purpose of challenging the thesis of the famous ophthalmologist C. von Hess (of Munich), who had stated that all invertebrates were completely colorblind. V. Frisch asked himself why the colorful patterns of meadows existed, if it were not to act as "Wirtshausschilder", or "inn-signs", to lead the bees to the sources of nectar. Using food training experiments, v. Frisch began to test the bees' sensory perception, and especially the problem of how bees take their bearings in their environment and how they communicate with one another.

With the simplest of equipment, he tested the bees in a series of well considered experiments. A dish of sugar water was offered to attract foraging bees to a table, the dish being placed on a piece of blue cardboard so that the bees saw the color blue as they approached the table and fed from the sugar water. With a fine brush and shellac paint, the bees were individually marked as they sucked the sugar water, so that the behavior of the forager bees could be observed behind the glass panes of an "observation hive" after their return. It is the simplicity of this methodical approach that characterizes the genius behind many of v. Frisch's experiments. Despite this simplicity, v. Frisch was always very critical of his experimentation, as a personal remark he once made to me during my Dr. Thesis illustrates: "Denken Sie immer, um Ihren Futtertisch stehen 5 Beobachter, die versuchen, alles zu kritisieren, was Sie mit Ihren Bienen tun". (Always imagine that there are 5 observers standing around your experimental table, and that they are trying to criticize everything you do with your bees.) It is well known among bee researchers the particular caution he showed in his color sense experiments. To ensure that the bees could distinguish color, and not simply differentiate between various shades of grey, the blue cardboard he used was surrounded by pieces of card of the same size ranging in color from white through various shades of grey to black. The position of the card was constantly changed to avoid the possibility that the bees were being trained to the card location. Close attention was required to avoid traces of scent being deposited on the blue cardboard when the bees alighted, and thus new, clean cardboard was always used. Well founded and convincing results only came after much painstaking and detailed work, as is illustrated by the researcher's own words:" The fruits I could reap were sparesly placed between many great disappointments". With success, came of course great joy. This was highlighted by an event in 1914, at the congress of zoologists in Freiburg, when v. Frisch presented "A demonstration of experiments to prove color perception in totally color blind animals". The color training of the bees was demonstrated in the open air, and it was reported that during the experiment, the bees alighted obediently on the empty blue cardboard. When they found it empty, one bee searched in the near vicinity and landed on the blue tie of one of the onlookers! This was enough to convince the congress members that bees were indeed capable of color perception.

I should like to point out here a particular strategy of all of v. Frisch's experimental work: he used all of his discoveries, especially those concerning the bee dance, as a building block for new ideas and experimental designs. Only in this way was he able to bridge ecological problems. Furthermore, looking back at his research work we can now say that it comprised the basis of a new discipline which we now call etho-ecology. His experiments testing the color sense of bees demonstrates this in an impressive way. It was initially discovered that the bee's eye is insensitive to the color red, and that red is in fact seen as a shade of grey. Since the visible spectrum of the bee is shifted further into the short wavelength domain, ultraviolet also becomes an important color. This provoked the question of how far this perception of UV light was connected with the biology of the bee. Forty years later, the problem was solved by a student of v. Frisch - K. Daumer. Now we know that the "apparently" white and yellow blossoms of flowers are seen by the bee as an impressive UV pattern that shows the way to the nectar-guide. This UV combined with yellow gives the brilliant "color" bee purple on the flower petals. Every lover of nature must surely feel a sense of amazement when he or she realizes the close relationship between the characteristics of the bee eye and the color of flowers, and that this relationship is a "symbiosis" that has evolved over many millions of years.

Over a period of time more complicated and involved questions began to be asked with regards to the bee's perception of forms, recognition of patterns etc, and each time a new wealth of information was discovered. Today much of this knowledge fills the text books and conference reports in the fields of sensory physiology, neurobiology, and ecology - an astonishing fact when one realises that the ground work for all this knowledge on the bee was performed only 74 years ago in Brunnwinkl on the Wolfgangsee.

Much progress has also been made in other fields of sensory physiology. At that time, it was not clear where the bee's sense organs for smell were located. An American scientist had put forward the theory that the whole chitin shell was interspersed with olfactory cells, but v. Frisch established beyond all reasonable doubt that the antennae were in fact the base of the sense of smell. He was fascinated with the idea that the tactile sensory system of the antennae, together with the olfactory system, would enable the bee to have a "spatial sense of smell", or "Räumliches Riechen" as he called it. This concept has achieved high priority in the field of neurobiology with regards to the "multi-modal" processing of information. Associated with this work, were the later advances made in the field of chemo-receptors, especially by Schneider and Boeckh who discovered receptors that were "specialists" for cetain scents to which our human noses were completely insensitive. Among these scents there were certain catagories of special importance to bees e.g. the scent of Nasanoff glands (Sterezelduft), which attracts the returning bees to the hive, or the scent of the queen's mandibular gland through which she commmunicates with the drones on her nuptial flight. This research has partially contributed to the fundamental basic knowledge behind biological pest control, which today gives us hope of successfully counteracting dangerous pests of fruits, cereals, and woods.

The end of World War II and the difficult years of the Nazi regime, when v. Frisch was under the threat of dismissal from employment, also witnessed the highlight of v. Frisch's life. Although his first communication concerning the language of bees was published as early as 1920, it was to be another 25 years before the total information content of the bee's dance could be fully explained. It was already known that a successful forager bee returning to the hive with a full honey stomach, performed a "round dance" on the honey comb with excited mincing steps, and that the dance announced the presence of food in the nearby vicinity. The scent of flowers carried home in the nectar and on the body hairs gave information regarding the species of flower that had been visited. The fact of one bee communicating with other foraging bees, and giving precise information as to the whereabouts of a food source was certainly exciting enough. However, further investigations carried out in Brunnwinkl in 1945, led v. Frisch to believe that the dance of the bee also carried additional information concerning the direction and distance of the food source from the hive. The first surprise encountered was that the "round dance" changed to a "tail-wagging dance" if the food table in his experiments was gradually moved to more than 50 m from the hive. He concluded that the rhythm of the dance was related to distance, and that an increase in the distance between the food source and the hive resulted in a slower tail-wagging in the dance. This discovery again provoked the question of how the forager bee understood this dance. For a food source 100 m from the hive, v. Frisch recorded 10 tailwagging runs 1/4 minute, for 200 m this was reduced to 8 per 1/4 minute, for 500 m 6 per 1/4 minute, whilst for 1000 m only 4 runs per 1/4 minute were recorded. These results were obtained only after several tedious years of work, and were often interrupted by changes in the weather, which resulted in forager bees failing to show up, or by interference from strange bees. As well as being able to indicate distance, the bees were also able to accurately indicate the direction of the food source. The question obviously arose as to how the bees were able to inform one another about the presence of a small target that was 8 km from the hive. If the food source remained constant, it was observed that the direction of the tail-wagging run on a vertically placed honey comb changed from hour to hour, and in such a way that it was directly proportional to the changing position of the sun as it moved across the sky. In other words, on its flight the bee memorizes the angle between the actual position of the sun and the course of her flight, this angle then being expressed as vectors of the gravitational field during the dance in the dark hive. This is an astonishing achievement of the bee's brain, since the dance angle to be communicated has to be transferred from an optical sense to that of a gravitational sense. The information represented in the dance on the comb has been shown to be equally valid for all bee species studied to date. For example, a tail-wagging run straight up means "you must fly directly towards the sun", whilst a tail-wagging run straight down means "the food source is directly opposite to the sun", and a run which is 60° to the left of the straight up position indicates that the food source is directly 60° to the left of the sun. It is quite clear, therefore, that the angle between the flight course and the sun is directly proportional to the field of gravity.

This remarkable discovery also highlighted further problems which had previously been unconsidered. The biggest surprise was that bees continued to use the sun as a reference point during their dances even when the sun was hidden behind clouds or large structures such as a rock. It was later determined that as long as there is a small patch of blue sky visible, then the bees are able to utilize the pattern of polarized light to fix the position of the sun. Indeed, I was fortunate enough to witness the crucial experiment that established this fact. When a polaroid sheet was held above the head of a dancing bee and then rotated in various directions, the angle of the tail-wagging also changed by the same amount. After this had been established, there followed a hurried search for the part of the eye that was able to detect polarized light. It has now been established that the molecules of the optical pigment are orientated in parallel in the microvilli of the optical cells, and that this arrangement is the basis of "dichroitic absorption".

Using the sun as a compass does of course present the bee with a major problem. Unlike a magnetic compass, which constantly indicates one direction, the bee must account for the changing position of the sun in the sky during each day and throughout the year. It was already known that bees have an excellent sense of time, but an effective explanation of the bee's ability to account for the changes in the position of the sun was still not forthcoming. A blue print for such an "experiment crucis" had lain in v. Frisch's desk for many years, but he constantly hesitated in putting this experiment into effect. "People will think we have gone crazy if we attempt to ascribe such a complicated system of orientation to the bees". Only after continuous encouragement did we undertake such an experiment. It started, when a bee hive was transferred from its native habitat to that of a strange locality, and when we began one afternoon to train a small group of bees to a food source 200 m south of the hive. We expected that the bees would memorize many distinctive features of the environment on their way to the target, and that they would also take note of the position of the sun i.e. that they would fly to the left of the sun to reach their destination. During the night, the hive and the south-trained bees were transferred to a non-familiar environment. The next morning four feeding tables were set up, one at each point of the magnetic compass and each one 200 m from the mother hive. The question that was being put to the test was would the bees fly southward (as they had been trained), or would they choose the eastern feeding site i.e. the feeding site which was at the same angle to the sun as the station at which they had found food the day before. To be quite honest, we were afraid that the bees would return to the hive the moment that they had left the flight hole and noticed a strange environment.

However, the south-trained bees flew directly to the true south and thus proved that the sun was indeed the perfect point of orientation. Today, it is well known that many other groups of animals e.g. ants , crabs, birds, fish, salamanders, tortoise etc use this sun orientation system.

I was priviliged to spend 15 summers with Karl von Frisch conducting these and many other experiments. Throughout this time, there constantly arose new questions such as how do bees circumnavigate a projecting rock? or how does a bee deal with a wind that is blowing at an oblique angle to the direction of flight? is there a special code in the bee dance to indicate whether the target is located up- or downwards? how relevant are the features of the landscape compared with the sun compass? One point in those early days was still unclear. During the dance routines, the bees made small mistakes which were not accidental, but which followed a regular sequence throughout the day. I continued to investigate this problem with my colleague H. Martin during the next 10 years, and we finally arrived at the conclusion that the Earth's magnetic field influenced the indication of the direction of the flight. Nowadays, bio-magnetism is a very up-to-date field of research. It is now well known that many animals use the Earth's magnetic field to orientate themselves in their environment, and that the diurnal fluctuations in the magnetic field are also used as a time cue. Nothing is still known, however, about the reception mechanisms involved. New problems are still arising, and thus I would like to conclude this chapter with an analogy quoted from Karl von Frisch.

"The life of the bee is like a magic well,
The more you draw from it,
The more there is to draw."

Evolution and Genetics

The Evolution of Honeybees

Friedrich Ruttner

Institut für Bienenkunde Oberursel (Polytechnische Gesellschaft), Universität Frankfurt, 6000 Frankfurt, FRG

Abstract. The common gene pool of the main subfamilies of Apidae is "Electrapis" of the Eocene, a rather vague group comprised of individuals with a varying mosaic of meliponoid, bomboid and apinoid characters. The subfamilies evolved in different directions and radiated during different epochs as shown by the rank of taxonomic units: Meliponinae -18 genera (300 species), Bombini - 3 genera (290 species), Apinae - 1 genus (4 species). True honeybees are found in early and middle Miocene, Synapis ssp. and Apis armbrusteri (25 and 12 mill. yrs.), both very similar or almost identical to the recent tropical A. dorsata. The two young (Pleistocenic) species A. mellifera and A. cerana show substantial evolutionary changes especially in behavior, an expansion to different climatic zones and a taxonomic radiation. A quantitative estimation of time-related evolution, based on changes in 16 angles of wing venation suggests two steps: 1) In the middle Caenozoic, the true "Apis-type" of wing venation and other body structures appeared, presumably together with Apis-specific highly social organisation; a long-lasting evolutionary stagnation followed, up to the recent open-air nesting Apis species. 2) The second step started at the end of the Caenozoic, including such revolutionary behavioral changes as multi-comb cavity nesting and perfect thermohomeostasis with wintering ability. It resulted in colonization of large new ecological zones extending across 30° latitude and immigration into the Ethiopean region. This two-step hypothesis is compatible with all available data derived from the fossil record, the peculiar taxonomic structure of the genus and the recent distribution and ecological adaptations of the species.

EVOLUTION OF THE MAIN SUBFAMILIES OF APIDAE

Recent honeybees can be traced to polymorphic bees of the Baltic amber (Eocene), originally named Electrapis Cock., although they have nothing to do with the present genus Apis. They combine meliponoid, bomboid and apinoid characters in various ways (22). Three subgenera, Electrapis s.str., Protobombus and Roussyana were established due to the similarity to Apinae, Bombinae and Meliponinea, respectively (23). Some species of Trigona, but no true Apinae or Bombinae, were found in the Eocene (23).

Each of the three eusocial subfamilies are well characterized by their general structure and adapted in a peculiar way to different environments. The predominantly small Meliponinae with more or less large perennial colonies in sophisticated nests is strictly pantropical; the large, sturdy pubescent Bombini with relatively small seasonal colonies in cool (even arctic and alpine) climate; the generally large slender Apini which succeeded in attaining remarkable independence from environmental conditions by a very high level of social organization (homeothermy).

Subfamily-specific, too, is the epoch of major taxonomic radiation: early Caenozoic in Meliponinae (20); late Caenozoic in Bombini (21); end of Caenozoic-Pleistocene in Apini, as will be demonstrated later. This time difference of evolution is reflected by rank differences of the taxa: Meliponinae - 18 genera, more than 300 species; Bombini - 3 genera, about 290 species; Apini - 1 genus, 4 species (partly with many subspecies).

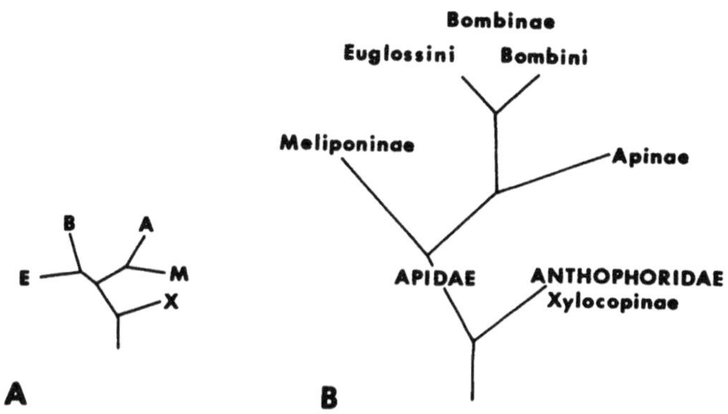

Fig. 1 - Phylogenetic diagram of Apidae. A from (11), B from (21).

In spite of this clear characterization of the subfamilies, the deduction of a plausible phylogenesis is not easily achieved. The reason for this is a seemingly irregular distribution of original apoid and derived characteristics among subfamilies and tribes. Listing the characteristics given by Winston and Michener and adding a few others, a rather even distribution of derived characters among the following three groups is found: Apis, Apis+Bombini, and Apis+Meliponinae. The conventional cladistic tree (11) is shown in Fig. 1a. It was modified with convincing evidence (22) by shifting Apini from the neighborhood of Meliponinae to Bombinae. Whatever the similarity, the main fact remains that the close relationship of all subfamilies of Apidae is probably best represented by the idea of a descent from a common gene pool in the Eocene, with Meliponinae being a little ahead.

EVOLUTION WITHIN APINAE

The fossil record

The true Apis-type is first found in the lower Miocene (Rhenian browncoal of Rott near Bonn, 25 mill. yrs. ago). It was named Synapis henshawi by Cockerell 1907, later classified as subgenus of Apis (23) with the three species henshawi, dormiens and kaschkei. From the

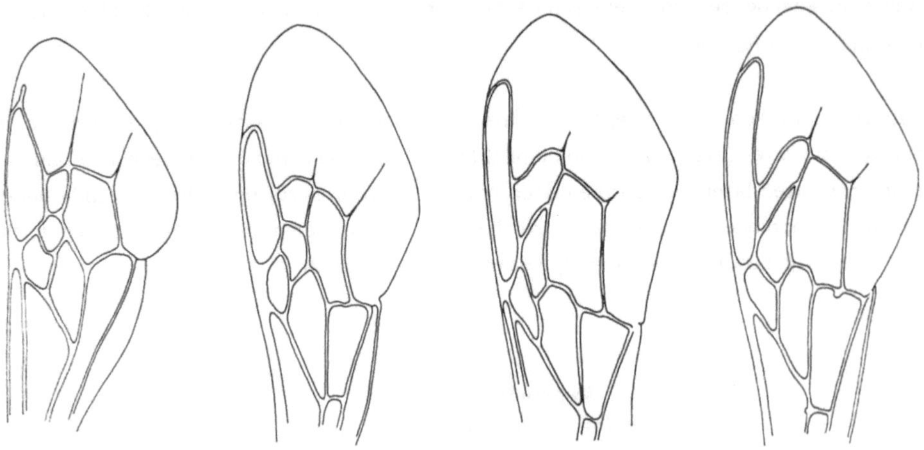

Fig. 2 - Fore wing venation pattern of fossil and recent Apidae.

upper Miocene (Sarmatian, 12 mill. yrs. ago) are the fossil bees of the Randecker Maar and of Böttingen (SW Germany), both classified as Apis armbrusteri (23). Quite a few well preserved specimens of both Synapis and A. armbrusteri are available.

A clear trend in changes of wing venation is observed from Electrapis to Apis mellifera (Fig. 2): 1) Stretching of venation in the length axis of wing; 2) Migration of the third cubital vein along the radialis in the direction of wing basis. In consequence, the venation pattern becomes definitely more slender. In order to estimate the changes in wing pattern numerically, methods of morphometric honeybee taxonomy (16) were applied by joint factor analysis of fossil and recent Apidae using data of 16 wing venation angles. The honeybee wing venation proved to be a rich source for genetic and taxonomic analyses: it can be measured exactly, it is of high heritability and independent of body size, and shows significant geographic variation; that means, it reacts sensitively to processes of evolution even at the subspecies level.

Results: Four compound clusters are visible in the graphic representation of factor 1 and 2 (Fig. 3): a) Bombus, b) Synapis + Apis armbrusteri + A. dorsata, c) A. florea, and d) A. cerana + A. mellifera. In general, the single species are well separated within these groups. Electrapis has an isolated position near Bombus. The common cluster Synapis + A. dorsata shows that wing venation has not changed much since the early Miocene. The partial clusters A. armbusteri - A. dorsata (time difference 12 mill. yrs.) are completely overlapping. This stagnation of tropical (and subtropical) Apis species since the Miocene is astonishing, especially compared to changes in other Caenozoic animals. Ample evidence exists that in honeybees changes in ecological adaptations or geographic isolation are soon followed by changes in wing venation. Therefore, it may be concluded that the evolutionary inertia in

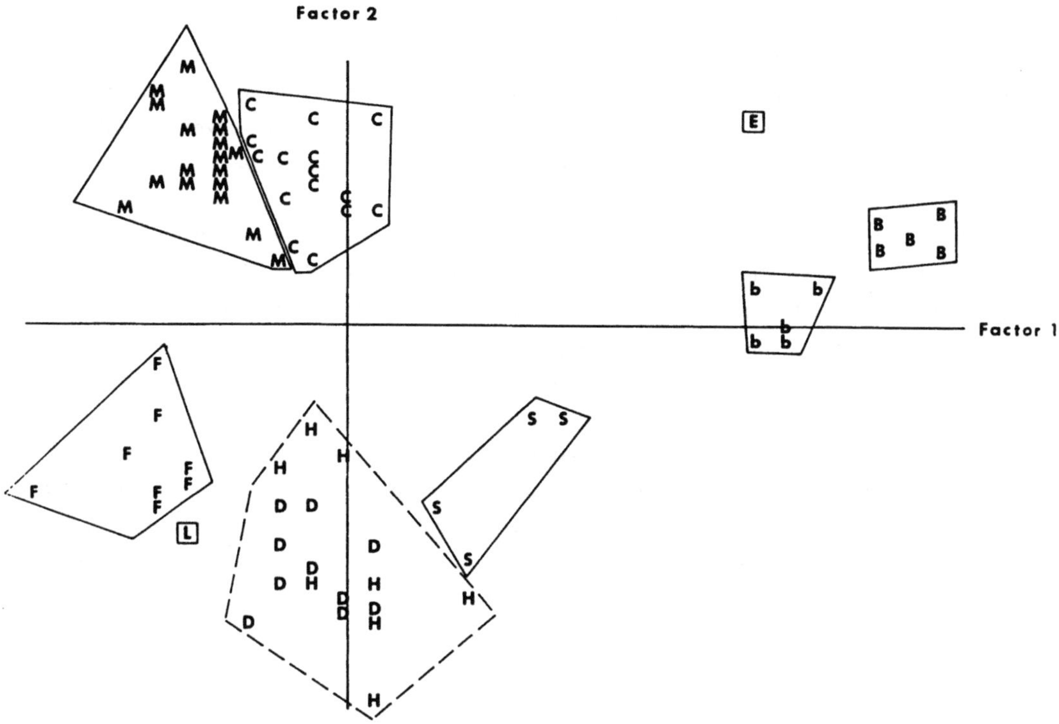

Fig. 3 - Factor analysis of 16 wing venation angles of various Apidae. B = Bombus hortorum;b = Bombus hortorum; C = A. cerana; D = A. dorsata; E = Electrapis; F = A. florea; H = A. armbrusteri; M = A. mellifera; S = Synapis.

wing venation is an expression of biological stability: it is likely that Synapis and A. armbrusteri were similar in their ethological characteristics to the present open-air nesting A. dorsata. Climatic conditions of the European Miocene with its predominately Indo-Malayan elements are in agreement with this assumption. It is a general experience "that the origin of new types, the origin of new morphological and biological characteristics and the origin of the higher taxa are three problems that cannot be separated from each other" (10).

The assumption of Caenozoic open-air nesting Apis species in Europe gives the key for explaining the odd fact that the colonization of the African continent occurred very late, and then only by A. mellifera. Land bridges existed during different epochs, but open-air nesting species are evidently limited in their migration ability across unfavorable zones.

The same analysis (Fig. 3) shows an eruptive evolution of the two temperate zones species, A. cerana and A. mellifera. The statistical distance of these species to A. armbrusteri is distinctly larger than the difference between the two Miocenic species Synapis and A. armbrusteri - in spite of the greater time difference. This change in wing venation pattern coincides with the evolution of the first insect with perfect thermo-homeostasis.

The clusters of A. cerana and A. mellifera are very close, but not overlapping. The genetic isolation of the two species did not take place before one to two million years ago at most (during or at the beginning of the Pleistocene) as can be seen by the immature stage of speciation of cerana-mellifera (15). Isolation of taxa at the subspecies level generally took place during the last glaciation; that is, not earlier than 50,000 years ago.

The joint morphometric analysis of fossil and recent Apis species indicates two major steps in evolution: the first in the early or middle Caenozoic, when the Apis-type of wing venation appeared, very likely with biological characteristics of present tropical open-air nesting species (e.g. wax combs with hexagonal cells, swarm cluster formation, dance communication). The second step (multiple-comb cavity nesting, temperature homeostasis, wintering ability) occurred before or at the beginning of the Pleistocene and is represented by the cerana-mellifera-type of wing venation. The consequence is the existence of a conservative and a progressive phylogenetic line within the genus Apis. A preformation of this second line, as (rare) multi-comb dorsata nests and cavity nesting florea colonies has to be pointed out. The increasing speed of evolution within the progressive line can be demonstrated especially at the subspecies level (Fig. 8).

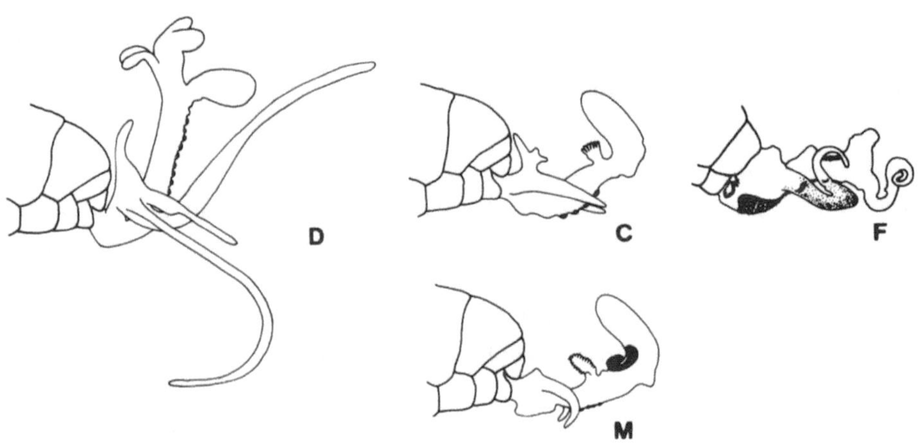

Fig. 4 - Endophallus of Apis species. C = cerana; D = dorsata; F = florea; M = mellifera.

MORPHOLOGY AND GENETICS

Endophallus

This unique, bizarre organ shows homologous structures in all four species: a membraneous tube with the ejaculatory duct inside, various hair plaques and several proturberances of the tube (Fig. 4). The most conspicious of these are two long, downwards bent "bursal cornua".

A.dorsata additionally has three pairs of thin dorsal cornua; they are clearly visible as a vestigial structure also in A. cerana, and even more reduced in A. mellifera. Thus a clear series of progressive reductions of the cornua can be seen, in the sequence dorsata-cerana-mellifera. A. florea takes a separate postion in the general structure of the whole organ.

Structure of melittin

The main component of bee venom, the protein melittin, is composed of 26 amino acids of known sequence (8). The sequence of cerana and mellifera melittin is identical (Fig. 5). Amino acids are substituted in three and five positions if compared with A.dorsata and with A.florea, respectively. Five amino acids are different in A.dorsate - A.florea.

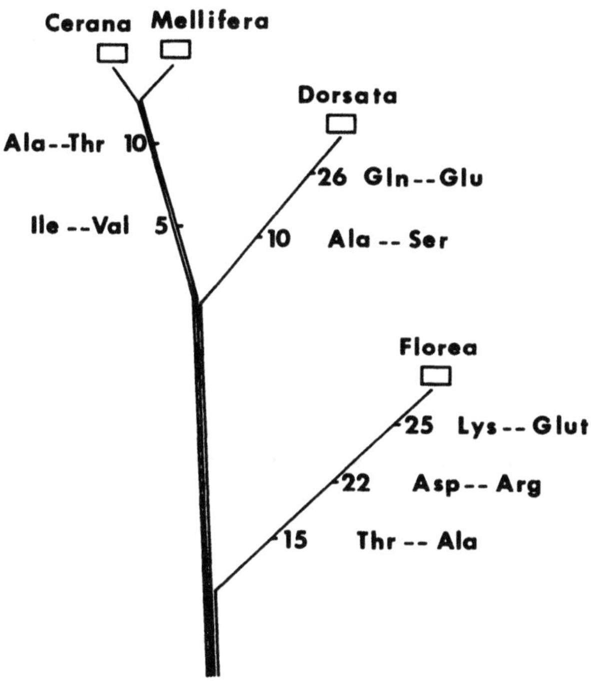

Fig. 5 - Changes of melittin structure. Numbers: position of amino acids (data from (8)).

BEHAVIOR

Communication

There is no need to describe the well-known differences in dance language among the Apis species. A. cerana-mellifera both hold the highest level with transposition of direction to the vertical plane and memorizing the position of the sun in the dark nesting cavity. A. dorsata shows directed dances only if an outlook to the sky is provided in the same situation, and A. florea varies in the communicative and geotactic behavior in several ways (6,8).

Nesting Behavior

Open-air nesting and cavity nesting are traditionally regarded as important differences between ancestral and derived species. Undoubtedly, cavity nesting is a prerogative for efficient temperature regulation and expansion of ecological adaptations. A. dorsata was described as "primitive" (3) on account of the differences between castes being smaller than in other species, irrespective of the differences in dance communication. A. florea, however, shows so many divergent features (19) that is seems appropriate to speak about a "spezialized" rather than a "primitive" species.

Recently (7, 18) a differing view of the phylogenetic relationships of Apis species was presented. Since all more primitive Apidae (Meliponinae and Bombinae) are cavity nesting, open-air nesting would more likely be a derived adaptation to tropical conditions. Two separate lines of descendence in honeybees are postulated, one ancestral (cavity nesting A. cerana-mellifera), the other derived (open-air nesting A. florea-dorsata). Analysis of wing venation indicates also two lines of evolution, but the venation type of open-air nesting species is surely very ancient (since the early Miocene, at least). Both cavity nesting species, however, are young, and only hypotheses can be presented about their common ancestors (see below).

As in the morphology of endophallus, a common nest architecture is found in the group dorsata-cerana-mellifera, A. florea being completely different.

Ecology

The two open-air nesting Apis species can be compared to Meliponinae in their ecological adaptation; that is, they are restricted to the tropics, or (to some degree) to warm subtropics. Both are excellently adapted in this zone, e.g., A. florea does better in an extremely hot and dry climate than a cavity nesting species. But evidently they have not been able to adapt to new ecological niches since the Caenozoic (leaving aside the very specialized A. laboriosa); they were expelled from Europe to SE Asia when the climate deteriorated. This is another argument for the relatively recent origin of cavity-nesting Apis species; if this type had existed in Europe in the late Caenozoic, with the same wing venation type as found in the fossil specimens from the Miocene, it should have been able to survive the Pleistocene in the southern Mediterranean or in the Caspian basin.

The most decisive step in honeybee evolution was multiple-comb cavity nesting, thermo-homeostasis and wintering ability. Cavity nesting and perfect temperature regulation are strictly correlated, but these two factors alone are not sufficient to secure the successful wintering of the whole colony. A number of additional physiological prerogatives are indispensable: restriction of swarming to a balance between reproductive need and colony strength; storage of ample food; special physiological condition of "winter bees", enabling brood rearing in flightless periods; capacity to retain feces over several months; "low-temperature blockade" of flight activity, irrespective of high light intensity. Several of these features are evidently new acquistions, existing only at the subspecies level.

The essential difference between tropical and temperate-zone mellifera races is demonstrated in South America, where temperate races are being rapidly replaced by tropical races: the mutual relation seems as if they were two different competitive species, and not races of one and the same species.

The significance of the unique change in fitness achieved by the cerana-mellifera group becomes evident if compared with Meliponinae, the most ancient family of Apidae. In spite of their abundant radiation and the evolution of big perennial colonies with sophisticated nest covers, they never succeeded in passing the limits of the tropics, although permanent contacts existed with temperate zones. In A. mellifera, the acquisition of wintering ability resulted in an extension of the distribution area across 30° lat. to the north. This bee is able to survive very cold winters with periods of no flight activity of up to six months. In Eurasia, the northern border of beekeeping with A. mellifera is marked by the line where rivers are covered by ice for less than 180 days. The major limiting factor for cavity nesting species, both in temperate as well as in tropical zones, is lack of suitable nesting sites rather than lack of food. The extraordinary adaptability of the species became evident when it was artificially transferred to other continents (such as to the Americas and Australia). It was immediately integrated into the new environment, even in feral conditions.

Honeybees are typical generalists as flower visiting insects; they collect sugar solutions where it is obtainable to them, provided a suitable kind of sugar (primarily monosaccharids and a few higher sugars like saccharose and melecitose) is present. Therefore, no co-evolution with flowers can be demonstrated in honeybees. They collect nectar from flowers and from extra-floral nectaries, honeydew excreted by insects and even the liquid from cut sugar cane. They immediately succeeded in exploiting a completely unfamiliar flora when introduced to the Americas and to Australia. But as generalists they are less efficient in pollinating a flower of a co-adapted partner of specialists such as Medicago sativa - Megachile rotundata. Attractivity to a food source is determined primarily by concentration and composition of the solution (5). Honeydew produced by the spruce coccide Lecanium is detected and exploited by honeybees in spite of the lack of signals (odor, color). Flower signals, of course, strongly influence the searching strategy of honeybees. To promote the deviation of field bees to the starting point of a highly rewarding honeydew flow, von Frisch (4) recommended the "Duftlenkung" by feeding colonies sugar syrup scented with emerging fir branches. Honeybees did not evolve the ability to discriminate food sources which are poisonous to them, as for example, nectar and pollen of some Ranunculus species, Tilia and Aesculus (1) or honeydews with a high amount of melecitose which cause winter mortality. The reason may be the limited local incidence of this source.

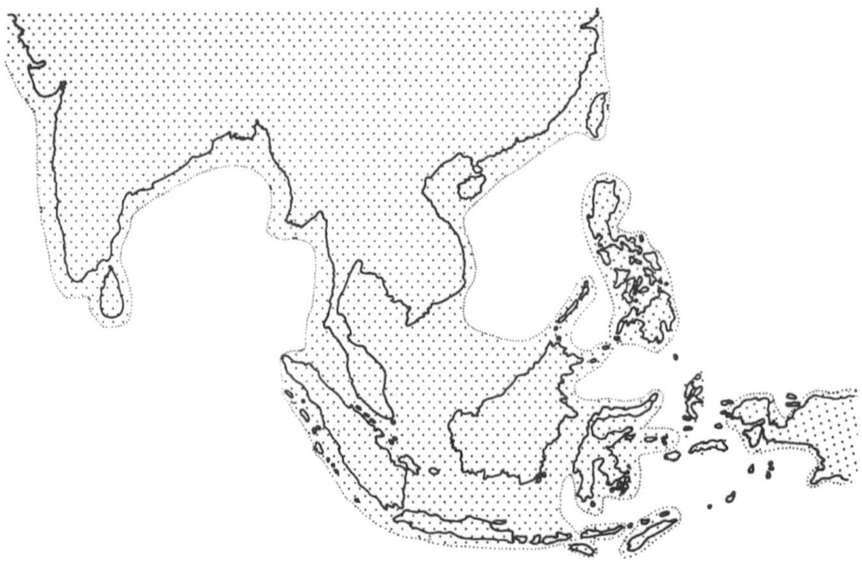

Fig. 6 - Map of SE Asia. Hatched: Asiatic continent during the Pleistocene.

EVOLUTION AND RADIATION OF APIS CERANA AND APIS MELLIFERA

Where and when did honeybees adapted to temperate climate evolve? The answer is found by consideration of the geographic situation. A. cerana is located east of the Iranian desert; A. mellifera west of it. Arabia and Africa were colonized by A. mellifera and not by A. cerana. A. mellifera is infested by parasites of A. cerana and A. dorsata, and vice versa, quite in contrast to the three sympatric Asiatic species which do not exchange parasites; this indicates a separate evolútion of A. mellifera, while A. cerana retained its partly tropical area. It is likely, therefore, that A. mellifera evolved in a temperate climate in the region where it is now closest to A. cerana. At present, both species are separated by 500 km of desert and dry steppe (at the closest point). The common ancestor of both species must have inhabited the southern slopes of the central Asiatic mountains, where adaptation to a cool climate is of selective advantage.

There is only one indication of the age of the first temperate-climate Apis species: its highly superior fitness and, in consequence of this, its rapid spread. It is very unlikely that no taxonomic radiation occurred immediately after establishing this crucial trait. Therefore, since only two temperate-climate speøies exist, the common ancestor cannot be much older than those.

It is not difficult to speculate about the process of isolation of the two present species. If, during a humid spell, the cerana-ancèstor succeeded in spreading farther west, to the mountains of Iran and to the depression of the Caspian Sea, the next drier period must have

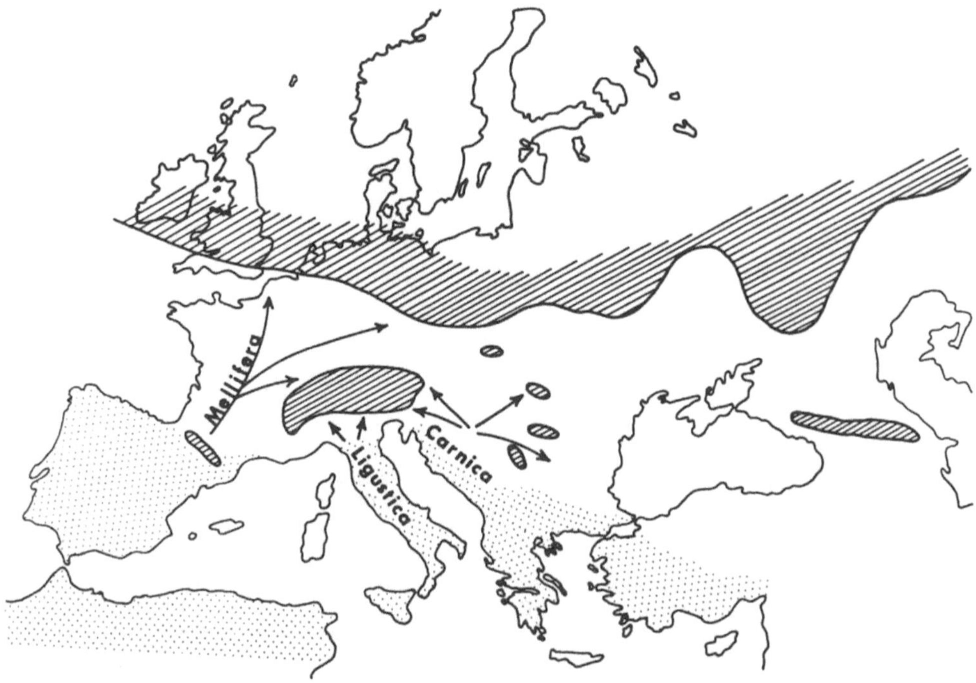

Fig. 7 - Refugial areas of European honeybee races and expansion in Holocene. Dark hatched: peak of glaciation. Light hatched: Deciduous forests in the Pleistocene.

separated this population from the main area. The central plateau of Iran was about as dry during most of the Pleistocene as it is today, and the so-called "pluvials" were mainly caused by lower temperature and evaporation (2). The Caspian region had a relatively warm and humid climate during main periods of glaciation where many Caenozoic plants were able to survive.

A fairly good estimate can be given about the approximate period when this speciation occurred. A. mellifera and A. cerana are true species - they are genetically isolated, but they are not "mature" species, since no pre-mating barriers and no sympatric areas exist (15). This indicates a geographic isolation during the Pleistocene, or at most, in the late Pliocene.

Apis cerana spread northeast as far as Ussuria, without morphological differentiation (as can be concluded from our data). In tropical South Asia, however, a distinctly different type is found; A. cerana indica is split into a number of island populations with only slight, overlapping inter-population variations. This gives another time table of evolution: the islands of southeastern Asia (including Sri Lanka) were connected with the continent by regression of the shore line during the last glaciation (Fig. 6) and were isolated only 8,000-10,000 years B.P. This is too short for the evolution of distinct subspecies. An exception is

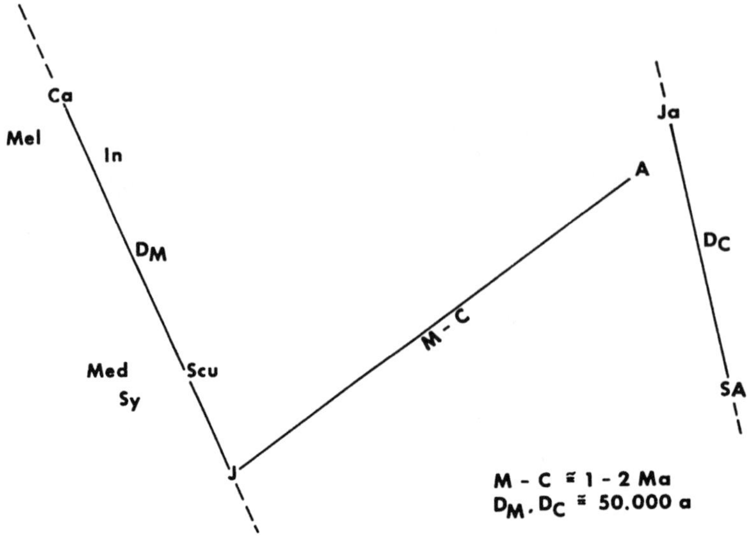

Fig. 8 - Statistical distance between centroids of races of A. mellifera, D_M and A. cerana, D_C (Discr. analysis of 16 venation angles. Dotted line: distance of extreme samples. M-C: nearest distance between centroids of A. mellifera. (J = A. m. yemenitica) and A. cerana.

the bee of Japan (A. c. japonica), which was partly separated from the continent in the early Pleistocene.

The diversification of A. mellifera was more complicated. Two lines of diversification are found: 1) to tropical Africa, via Arabia, where a further radiation into "eco-races" occurred (14). The highly disjunct area of A. m. monticola, found in mountain forests higher than 2400 meters in East Africa (Rwanda-Burundi, Tanzania, Kenya, Ethiopia), is a testimony of the last glaciation, when the snow line was 1000 meters lower. The area of monticola must have been much larger and more coherent than at present. 2) to the Mediterranean, most likely during the last interglacial (50,000 years ago). The climatic deterioration during the Würm glacial isolated various populations around the Mediterranean (9), which spread north in the postglacial (Fig. 7), remained stable or were diminished by desiccation (e.g., A. m. sahariensis). It has to be noted, therefore, that the mellifera populations were isolated substantially earlier than the cerana populations of the Sunda Islands. They show more distinct morphological differentiations, while only slight variations are observed within the territory colonized only during the Holocene.

The three major European races A. m. mellifera, ligustica and carnica were confined for climatic reasons to the three South-European islands during the last glaciation. In the postglacial warm period (Atlanticum, 6000 years B.P.), A. m. mellifera spread through West and Central Europe as far as Scandinavia and the Urals (Fig. 7); A. m. ligustica remained stuck on the Apenninian Peninsula by the Alps, while A. m. carnica expanded to the Danube valley, the Carpathians and to the Ukrainian plains (12).

The present taxonomic structure of the species A. mellifera, therefore, is mainly a result of the final period of the Pleistocene. Remarkable again is the increased speed of evolution, already mentioned for the step from A. armbrusteri (Sarmatian) to the recent species A. cerana-mellifera, as measured by changes in wing venation. Fig. 8 shows the intraspecies variations of A. cerana and A. mellifera: the maximal statistical distance between centroids of individual races is about the same as the nearest distance between the two species in spite of much shorter periods.

REFERENCES

(1) Böttcher, F.K., ed., 1984. Krankheiten der Biene. Stuttgart: Verlag E. Ulmer

(2) Brice, W.C., ed., 1978. The Environmental History of the Near and Middle East Since the Last Ice Age. London, New York: Academic Press.

(3) Buttel-Reepen, H.v. 1903. Die stammesgeschichtliche Entstehung des Bienenstaates. Leipzig: G. Thieme.

(4) Frisch, K.v. 1947. Duftgelenkte Bienen im Dienste der Landwirtschaft und Imkerei. Berlin, Heidelberg: Springer-Verlag.

(5) Frisch, K.v. 1967. The dance language and orientation of bees. Cambridge, Mass.: Harvard University Press.

(6) Gould, J.L.; Dyer, F.C.; Towne, W.F. 1985. Recent progress in the study of the dance language. In Experimental Behavioral Ecology: Fortschritte der Zoologie 31, eds. B. Hölldobler and M. Lindauer, pp. 141-161. Stuttgart, New York: G. Fischer.

(7) Koenige, K. 1976. Neue Aspekteder Phylogenie innerhalb der Gattung Apis. Apidologie 7: 357-366.

(8) Kreil, G. 1975. The structure of Apis dorsata melittin: Phylogenetic relationships between honeybees as deduced from sequence data. FEBS Letters 54: 100-102.

(9) Lindauer, M. 1956. Über die Verständigung bei indischen Bienen. Z. vergl. Physiol. 38: 521-577.

(10) Mayr. E. 1963. Animal Species and Evolution. Cambridge, Mass.: Harvard University Press.

(11) Michener, C.D. 1974. The Social Behavior of the Bees. Cambridge, Mass.: Harvard University Press.

(12) Ruttner, F. 1952. Alter und Herkunft der Bienenrassen Europas. Österr. Imker. 4: 8-10.

(13) Ruttner, F. 1985. Geographic variation and taxonomy of Apis cerana. Proc. 30th Int. Apicult. Congr. (in press).

(14) Ruttner, F., and Kauhausen, D. 1985. Honeybees of tropical Afirca: Ecological diversification and isolation. In Proc. 3rd Int. Conf. Apic. trop. Climates, Nairobi. 1984, pp. 45-51. Gerrards Cross, England: International Bee Research Association.

(15) Ruttner, F., and Maul, F. 1983. Experimental analysis of reproductive interspecies isolation of Apis mellifera L. and Apis cerana Fabr. Apidologie 14: 309-327.

(16) Ruttner, F.; Tassencourt L.; and Louveaux, J. 1978. Biometrical-statistical analysis of the geographic variability of Apis mellifera L. Apidologie 9: 363-381.

(17) Ruttner, F.; Wilson, E.C.; Snelling, R.; Vorwohl, G.; and Kauhausen, D. 1986. The evolution of honeybee wing venation. Apidologie 17: (in press).

(18) Sakagami, F.S.; Matsumura, T.; and Ita, K. 1980. Apis laboriosa in Himalaya, the litte known world largest honeybee (Hym., Apidae). Insecta Matsumurana, N.S. 19: 47-77.

(19) Whitcombe, R.P. 1984. The Biology of Apis Spp. in Oman with Special Reference to Apis florea Fab. Thesis, Zool. Dept., Univ. of Durham.

(20) Wille, A. 1979. Phylogeny and relationships among genera and subgenera of the stingless bees (Meliponinae) of the world. Rev. Biol. Trop. 27: 241-277.

(21) Williams, P.H. 1985. A preliminary cladistic investigation of relationships among the bumble bees (Hym. Apidae). Syst. Entomol. 10: 239-255.

(22) Winston, M., and Michener, C.D. 1977. Dual origin of highly social behavior among bees. Proc. Nat. Acad. Sci. USA, 74: 1135-1137.

(23) Zeuner, F.E.; Manning, F.J.; and Morris, S.F. 1976. A monograph on fossil bees (Hymenoptera: Apoidea). Bull. Brit. Museum (Nat. Hist.) 27: 149-268.

Behavior Genetics of Honeybees (Apis mellifera L.)

Robin F. A. Moritz[1] and Christian Brandes[1, 2]

[1]Institut für Bienenkunde (Polytechnische Gesellschaft), Johann Wolfgang Goethe Universität, Frankfurt/M., Karl-von-Frisch-Weg 2, D-6370 Oberursel/Ts., FRG

[2]Institut für Tierphysiologie, Neurobiologie der Freie Universität Berlin, Königin-Luise-Str. 28/30, D-1000 Berlin 33, FRG

Abstract. Behavioral genetic analysis in honeybees (Apis mellifera L.) allows for the documentation of gene expression in haploid and diploid individuals as well as in large groups. An example for the selection of learning behavior of individual workers illustrates the potential of the use of honeybees in behavioral genetics. Quantitative genetic models, originally designed for individual characters, have to be modified for all characters related to group behavior. The assembly of genotypes as well as interactions among the group members must be considered. The average intracolonial worker relationship, estimated in marker experiments, is a central issue for quantitative genetics of group characters.

HONEYBEES AS A BEHAVIORAL GENETIC TEST SYSTEM

The honeybee represents a unique organism for experiments in behavioral genetics. The knowledge concerning individual and social behavior of honeybees is detailed, and we can control matings with instrumental insemination, which allows for rapid selection of chosen characters. Maintenance of honeybee colonies is easy and breeding techniques are well developed. In addition, phenotypic mutants are available for experiments which require genetic markers (see appendix). The honeybee provides several characteristics which are of particular interest to behavioral geneticist. Honeybees are social insects and therefore individual as well as social behavior can be analyzed. Sociality, together with the male-haploid population structure, allows for genetic analysis of gene expression in haploid and diploid individuals, and in groups of individuals up to the size of colonies (50,000 individuals). In this light, honeybees are also of interest for other genetical disciplines and applications ranging from molecular genetic problems to complex sociogenetic topics.

INTRACOLONIAL WORKER RELATIONSHIP

For an accurate interpretation of results of genetic experiments with honeybees, the genetic structure of the colony must be understood. Fortunately, there is very detailed information on the reproduction of honeybees (29). Virgin queens mate with up to 17 drones during their nuptual flights. The semen is then vitally stored in the queen's spermatheca throughout sperm clumping in the spermatheca (28, 70), however, in most cases the sperm of the various drones which mated a queen is randomly mixed (33, 42, 44, 56, 67). Therefore, several patrilines of workers simultaneously coexist within a colony, which results in a large variation of relationships between workers in a colony (Fig. 1).

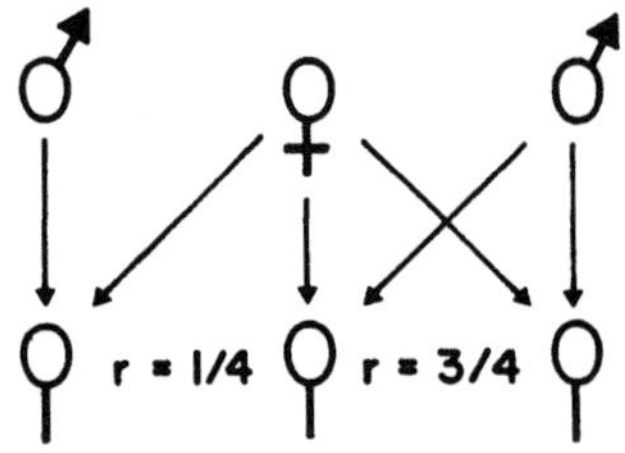

Fig. 1 - Possible worker relationships in a honeybee colony. Let us assume the queen has mated with z unrelated drones. Then we have to consider two possibilities. 1) Workers can have drone and queen in common (super sibs). This occurs in 1/z of all cases and r = 0.75. 2) Workers have only the mother in common (half sibs). This occurs in 1-1/z of all cases and r = 0.25.

Though there is mixing of sperm in the spermatheca, this does not mean that each drone which inseminates a queen contributes equal amounts of semen (33). Besides interindividual variation of sperm number per drone (41), phenomena indicating sperm competition have also been found (44). Observations on queens artificially inseminated in sequence with equal numbers of sperm from different mutant marker drones, revealed effects similar to a "last male advantage" (71). The last semen portion with which a queen was inseminated, appeared to be the most genetically effective (Fig. 2). As a result, the average intracolonial worker relationship, r_c, is lower than expected in the case of equal genetic effectiveness of drones. r_c has been estimated as 0.324 or 0.348 in the cases of queens inseminated with eight (44) or four drones (33) respectively, which is in contrast to the expected theoretical values, $r_{theoret} = 0.313$ or $r_{theoret} = 0.375$. These unequal contributions of drones remain constant over more than a two-year observation period (33), indicating a mixing of semen once it is in the spermatheca.

This phenomenon of mixed sperm at unequal ratios is not only of general evolutionary interest, but also has implications for estimating genetic variance components of behavioral characters of individual workers.

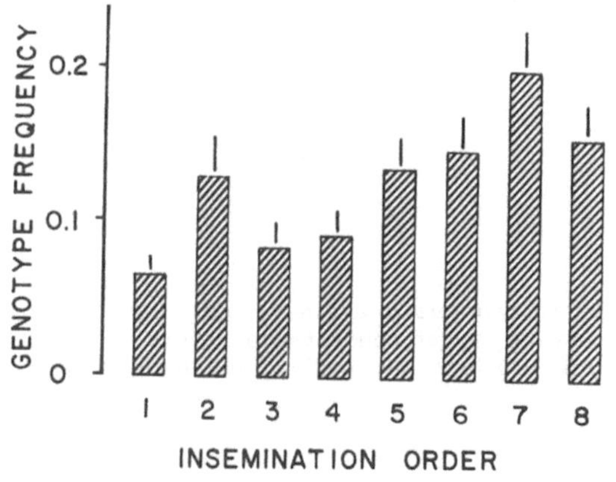

Fig. 2 - Genetic effeciency of semen. A queen was inseminated with equal numbers of sperm from eight drones. The insemination order is given on the x-axis (1 = first, 8 = last). Early injected semen proved to be genetically less effective than late injected semen. This effect was constant over time, indicating mixing of sperms in the spermatheca.

KIN SELECTION IN HONEYBEES

Intracolonial relationships of honeybee workers have implications for the inclusive fitness theory as established by Hamilton (23). The average relationship between workers is low with a high variance since workers within patrilines in a colony are closely related. Inclusive fitness will favor workers which have the ability to discriminate between super and half-sibs, and thereafter support related individuals.

Various experimental studies deal with the problem of kin recognition in honeybees. Concerning the recognition of queen larvae, there are conflicting reports. Some authors (52, 54) found that workers preferably rear related larvae whereas others (11) could not find any potential for kin discrimination in a similar experiment. In laboratory tests, workers attacked unrelated queens more often than related ones (8, 55). This behavior has been quantified in a metabolic bio-assay (48). Groups of 100 honeybee workers (test groups) respond with a typical increase in their metabolic activity when exposed to odors of queens, drones and other workers (Fig. 3). The oxygen concentration in the air which was passed over the test group in a flow-through system was used to measure the response.

Workers were able to discriminate between volatile odors of related and unrelated queens, drones and workers. The metabolic reaction of the workers was negatively correlated with the degree of relatedness (Fig. 4), thus an unrelated odor releases more "excitement" than related ones.

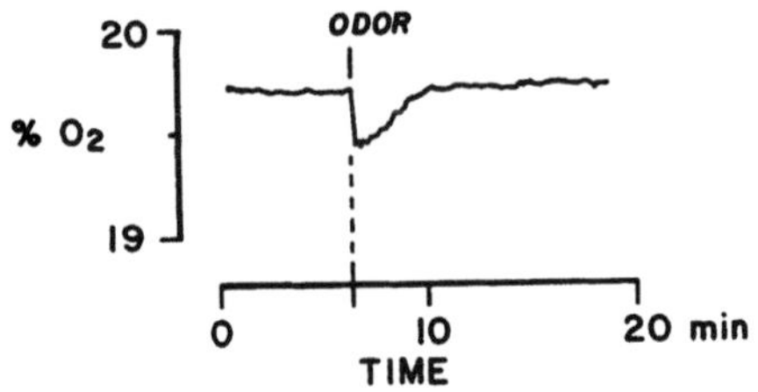

Fig. 3 - Typical metabolic response of a group of 100 workers to a 2 min exposure to volatile odors of an unrelated queen. The Y-axis represents the oxygen concentration in the air which has passed the workers. The difference between resting level and maximal metabolic activity is used for the quantification of the reaction.

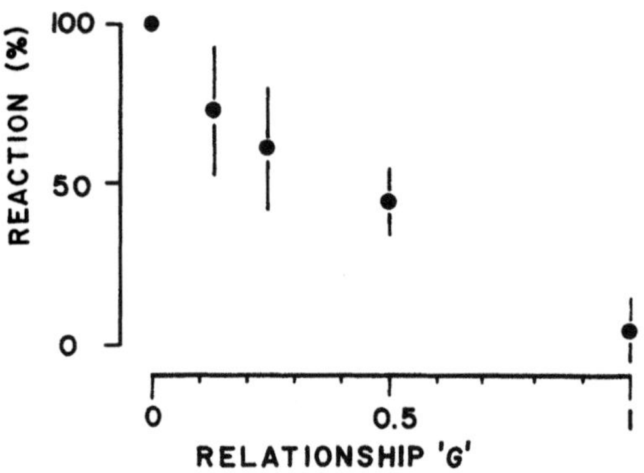

Fig. 4 - Regression of relative metabolic reaction of worker groups to queen odors (100 % = reaction to unrelated queens) on the pedigree coefficient of relationship G. Each dot represents mean ± SD of 7 independent test groups (48).

When swarming, honeybee workers are able to discriminate between related and unrelated queens (5). Getz et al. (18) claim that workers are also able to discriminate between super- and half-sisters during swarming. Their experimental approach, however, could not rigorously exclude other factors affecting the general behavior of swarming.

Though honeybee workers have the potential for discriminating related and unrelated queens, drones and workers, this does not give us an answer concerning its evolutionary significance. Under natural conditions genetic effects may be overridden by strong environmental components for the recognition of nest mates (27, 59). Furthermore, recognition abilities diminish in genetically mixed groups (12). The ability of workers to recognize kin, though predicted by inclusive fitness theory, does not mean that kin selection is the evolutionary force in social evolution. Within an already existing social system, inclusive fitness would favor the evolution of kin recognition systems. Though the kinship selection theory invokes the least preassumptions for explaining the evolution of social behavior, other models can also plausibly explain altruistic behavior (13).

ARTIFICIAL SELECTION IN HONEYBEES

In order to evaluate whether a given behavioral character is selectable, we have to discriminate between genetic and environmental effects on the expression of the phenotype. The phenotypic variance (S^2_P) of behavioral characters can be partitioned in various variance components which are either of environmental or genetic origin. In the classical quantitative genetic model (17), the total genetic variance (S^2_G) is composed of an additive (S^2_A) and a dominance (interaction) variance component (S^2_D). The ratio of total genetic variance to phenotypic variance is used as heritability in the broader sense ($S^2_G/S^2_P = h^2_{ibs}$). The heritability in the narrow sense ($h^2_{ins} = S^2_A/S^2_P$) is a more meaningful estimator for selection procedures since it expresses the selectability of a given character. If there are differences in the selectability of a character in disruptive selection projects, the estimation of the realized heritability (selection differential/parents mean) is useful, which accounts for asymmetries in genetic variances.

The estimation of h^2 is not only of interest for selection of particular behavioral traits, but also for insight into selection dynamics in natural populations. Characters under strong selective pressure and closely related to fitness have a small genetic variance and selectabilities in populations at equilibrium should be zero (26).

Genetic variance of individual characters

The general problem of selection of worker characters of honeybees is the caste system. The sexual reproductives often do not express behavior which is typical for workers. Several methods for the estimation of the heritability of characters of individual workers are known. Some techniques use data from breeding schemes involving artificial insemination (60), while others use data of workers from natural mated queens (40, 53). A different method for the estimation of heritabilities of individual worker characters involves using the laying workers of Apis mellifera capensis which produce parthenogenetically diploid female offspring (thelytoky). In this system, selection can be performed on the level of workers. Single selected worker bees are introduced in queenless colonies of Apis mellifera . The introduced bees lay eggs since the Cape bees develop faster than those of the Carnolian bees. Parthenogenetically produced offspring of these bees can be used for queen rearing, because caste difference in bees is dependent on the food of the larvae. The queens are then inseminated with drones produced by unfertilized queens which were also reared from selected worker bees. This method has also been used to select bees with high and low learning scores (Brandes unpubl.). Learning was characterized by proboscis extension reflex (PER) conditioning. In this paradigm excitatory classical conditioning of PER relies on temporal pairing of an initial neutral and later conditional stimulus (CS) and a sugar water stimulus (US), which unconditionally evokes the PER by touching the bees antennae or its proboscis. For disruptive selection bees were trained in discriminative procedures where several conditioned stimuli (CS+) were paired with the US, whereas other stimuli (CS-) were unpaired with the US. Tests of worker offspring of queens, reared as described above, show

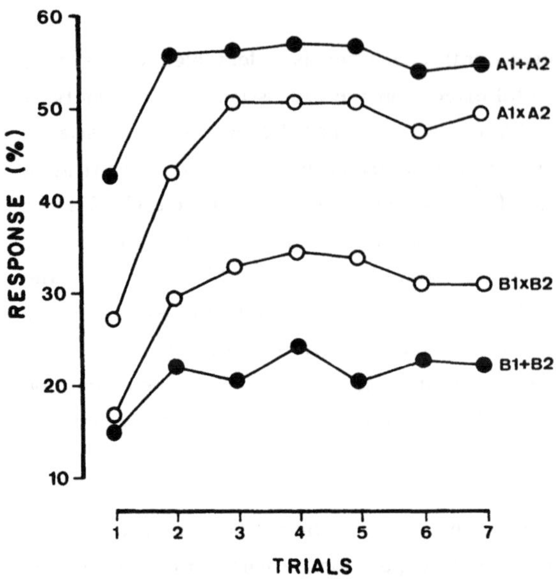

Fig. 5 - Response of disruptive selection of conditioning of proboscis extension reflex (PER). During the tests different conditioned stimuli were given paired (CS+) or unpaired (CS-) with an unconditioned sugar water stimulus. Each of the CS+ and CS- were tested and trained in 7 trials, and between 39 and 80 individuals were trained per group. With h^2 estimations (6) it can be shown that environmental effects are lowest if trials of different tests are combined. y-axis: percentage of the combined PER response; x-axis: consecutive trials; (•) = parthenogenetic groups; (o) = sexual offspring groups produced by the queens.

that in one generation significant differences between high and low lines appear. In addition the PER response was selected exclusively with laying Capensis workers and non-sexual produced offspring were tested (Brandes unpubl.). This selection prcedure enables selections in a much shorter time because it is not necessary to rear queens and drones. In Fig. 5 selection of PER response is compared for the two methods. A1 + A2 and B1 + B2 represents the PER response of a high (A) and a low (B) parthenogenetic line. Each curve illustrates the mean data of two parthenogenetic groups, one of them (index 2) was used for rearing unfertilized queens which produced drones. These drones were then used to inseminate queens reared from the second parthenogenetic group (index 1). A1 x A2 and B1 x B2 show response of the offspring produced by these queens. Except for crossover there are no genetic differences between queens and corresponding parthenogenetic groups, the drones representing the gametes of the parthenogenetic groups. Thus, differences between the sexual and asexual groups occur because of recombination of the genes in the sexual groups of the original A1 + A2 or B1 + B2 groups. In case PER response is exclusively determined by additive gene effects we would not expect any differences between A1 + A2 and A1 x A2 or between B1 + B2 and B1 x B2. The difference between the parthenogenetic groups, however, is larger than the difference between the sexual groups. This shows that the response levels are also affected by non-additive effects. Furthermore Fig. 5 illustrates that in selections which are done only with parthenogenetic groups, non-additive as well as additive effects can be maintained. However, because there is a very low recombination by the non-sexual production of offspring, the selected differences of the first generation only slightly increase in further generations. In selection of the PER-response it was not possible to increase the difference between the lines of the first generation by selection of a second generation (7). Increase of learning differences in four consecutive selected generations were only obtained if queens and drones were produced from selected worker bees in each generation and sexual gene recombination was possible.

An overview over various heritability estimates of individual worker characters is given in Table 1. Particularly interesting are the high estimates for characters closely related to individual worker fitness.

TABLE 1 - Estimates of heritabilites of individual characters of honeybee workers. Values with * indicate estimates including h^2_{ins} and h^2_{ibs}. Values with ** represent estimates of realized heritabilities including h^2_{ins} and h^2_{ibs}.

character	heritability	reference
morphological	0.1-0.95*	(20, 39, 46, 53)
cold resistance	0.15-0.37	(25)
metabolic activity	0.13-0.41	(25)
pupal development	0.87	(43)
learning	0.38-0.44**	(6)
longevity	0.2-0.32*	(38, 61)
trophallactic behavior	0.32	(47)
production of queen substance	0.89	(47)
reproduction	0.27-0.57	(47)

In an intact colony, the direct individual fitness of a worker should be 0 since only the sexual reproductives are able to produce offspring. In queenless colonies, however, workers are able to develop ovaries and begin with oviposition. Since the loss of a queen during mating can be a frequent event in honeybee populations (30% on the average, (67)), there is a considerable potential for worker reproduction, and worker fitness will be substantially larger than 0. Though the selectability of fitness characters is expected to be small, the estimates for h^2_{ibs} can be as high as 0.89 in the case of laying A.m. capensis workers. One reason for these high estimates could be strong dominance effects on the tested characters since fitness is known to be highly affected by heterotic mechanisms. Another explanation for the large genetic variance of worker fitness is a balanced system between group and individual selection (47).

Genetic variance of group characters

Since honeybees are eusocial insects, many behavioral traits are closely linked to a social context. Temperature regulation in the colony, ventilation and regulation of humidity in the nest are typical group characters where the colony as a whole is necessary for the expression

TABLE 2 - Estimates of heritabilities of group characters of honeybees. Values with * indicate estimates of h^2_{ins}.

character	h^2	reference
honey production	0.07-0.75	(1,16,21,30,36,58,69)
brood production	0.10-0.90	(1,16,21,58,69)
defensive behavior	0.01-0.93*	(14,51)
hoarding behavior	0.44-0.71*	(14)
alarm reaction	0.03-1.28*	(14,45,61)

of the behavior. Genetic variance components of typical group characters have been repeatedly estimated (Table 2). The alarm reaction, hoarding and hygenic behavior of groups of worker bees are particularly well documented, since these behavioral properties can easily be studied in laboratory experiments under controlled conditions. Rothenbuhler (63) suggested that hygenic behavior, which causes resistance to American foul brood disease, might be controlled by two loci. Workers which display hygenic behavior have the ability to detect dead larvae, uncap the cell and remove the dead brood. A quantitative genetic model, however, assuming nest cleaning to ba a pleiotropic character might give a better fit to some of Rothenbuhler's data.

When dealing with groups instead of individuals, the underlying genetic model is complex. One has to consider the group phenotype and the genetic composition of the group, for the accurate estimation of genetic variance components. Griffing (22) showed in a series of papers how complex a consequent extension of a genetic model for individuals to a genetic model for groups may become. Various interactions between additive and dominance effects have to be considered, most of which cannot be estimated with the classical mating schemes discussed above. A simple model in which the more complex interactions are ignored and the group is treated as a "superorganism" with intraindividual genetic variation may be more helpful for the analysis of experimental data (45). In this model, only additive gene effects and interaction effects between genes within the group are considered. Classical dominance effects between genes and interactions between genotypes are lumped together for the estimation of one overall interaction component. Using this simplified model, it is possible to obtain estimates of the additive genetic variance component and the interaction component with classical diallel or hierarchical mating schemes and parent-offspring regression.

An experimental approach to quantify the effect of interactions among group members on the group phenotype is given by Moritz and Southwick (49). Workers of a high and low line for defensive behavior were combined at various ratios, and the resulting group phenotype was analysed. For the tested alarm reaction, only linear interactions were found and there was no deviation from a plain additive model.

Another problem in the analysis of group characters in honeybees arises when composed characters of queen and workers are to be analysed (eg., brood production). In this case, an analysis as suggested by Wilham (75) regarding direct maternal effects, direct worker effects and the covariance between both on the expression of the group phenotype might be appropriate to estimate genetic variance components (2). Gene or genotype interactions, however, cannot be regarded in this model.

TOWARDS A SOCIOGENETIC ANALYSIS?

As we have shown, we have some knowledge concerning the mode of inheritance of a few basic behavioral characters of individual worker. Some of these characters are directly related to the polyethism in honeybee colonies. Indeed, these are the first reports of a genetically determined polyethism in honeybees which, to date, was believed to be mainly environmentally determined (34, 62, 68). The presence of strong environmental effects on polyethism does not mean that there is no genetic variation for these characters per se. Of course, we do not know presently whether these phenomena, mainly found for A.m. capensis, are general feature of the honeybee. A first step, however, is complete and we feel that further investigation in this direction will increase our knowledge of the mode of polyethism in general.

The other wide-open field concerning the behavioral genetics of honeybees is the genetic analysis of group behavior. The theoretical basis is small and empirical data, especially relating to the effects of genotype interactions within groups, are rare. The synthesis of genetic analyses of both individual and group behavior, a sociogenetic analysis, might increase and change our understanding of social behavior and sociality as a whole. Honeybees can, and hopefully will, provide us with the keys to the experimental answer of some of these questions.

Acknowledgement. This work was partially funded by the Alexander von Humbolt-Stiftung (RFAM) and the Deutsche Forschungsgemeinschaft (CB, RFAM).

REFERENCES

(1) Bar Cohen, R.; Alpern, G.; and Bar Anan, R. 1978. Progeny testing and selecting Italian queens for brood area and honey production. Apidologie 9: 95-100.

(2) Bienefeld, K. 1986. Heritabilitätsschätzungen von Leistungseigenschaften bei der Honigbiene. Apidologie 17(4): in press.

(3) Boch, R., and Morse, R.A. 1979. Individual recognition of queens by honey bee swarms. Ann. Entomol. Soc. Am. 72: 51-53.

(4) Boch, R., and Morse, R.A. 1981. Effects of artificial odors and pheromones on queen discrimination by honey bees (Apis mellifera L.). Ann. Entomol. Soc. Am. 74: 66-67.

(5) Boch, R., and Morse, R.A. 1982. Genetic factor in queen recognition odors of honey bees. Ann. Entomol. Soc. Am. 75: 654-656.

(6) Brandes, Ch. Estimation of heritability of learning behaviour in honeybees (Apis mellifera capensis), submitted.

(7) Brandes, Ch. Genetic differences of learning behavior in bees (Apis mellifera capensis), submitted.

(8) Breed, M.D. 1981. Individual recognition and learning of queen odors by worker honey bees. Proc. Natl. Acad. Sci. USA 78: 2635-2637.

(9) Breed, M.D. 1983. Nestmate recognition in honey bees. Anim. Behav. 31: 86-91.

(10) Breed, M.D. 1985. How honeybees recognize their nestmates: a re-evaluation from new evidence. Bee World 66: 113-119.

(11) Breed, M.D.; Velthuis, H.H.W.; and Robinson, G.E. 1984. Do worker honey bees discriminate among unrelated and related larval phenotypes? Ann. Entomol. Soc. Am. 77: 737-739.

(12) Breed, M.D.; Butler, L.; and Stiller, T.M. 1985. Kin discrimination by worker honey bees in genetically mixed groups. Proc. Natl. Acad. Sci. USA 82: 3058-3061.

(13) Brockmann, H.J. 1984. The evolution of social behavior in insects. In Behavioral Ecology: An Evolutionary Approach, eds. J.R. Krebs and N.B. Davies. Oxford: Blackwell.

(14) Collins, A.M.; Rinderer, T.E.; Harbo, J.R.; and Brown, M. 1984. Heritabilities and correlations for several characters in the honey bee (Apis mellifera L.). J. Hered. 75: 135-140.

(15) Drescher, W. 1971. Selektionsversuch an einem Merkmal mit polygener Basis bei Apis mellifica L. 23rd Internat. Apic. Cong. Moscow., pp. 390-391. Bucharest, Rumania: Apimondia Publishing House.

(16) El-Banby, M. 1967. Heritability estimates and genetic correlation for brood-rearing and honey production in the honeybee. XXIst Int. Apic. Cong., p. 498. Bucharest, Rumania: Apimondia Publishing House.

(17) Falconer, D.S. 1981. Introduction to Quantitative Genetics. London, New York: Longman.

(18) Getz, W.M.; Brückner, D.; and Parisian, Th.R. 1982. Kin structure and the swarming behavior of the honey bee Apis mellifera. Behav. Ecol. Sociobiol. 10: 265-270.

(19) Getz, W.M., and Smith, K.B. 1983. Genetic kin recognition: honey bees discriminate between full and half sisters. Nature, 302: 147-148.

(20) Goncalves, L.S. 1972. Investigations of the morphological characteristic "number of hamuli" in Apis mellifica. In Controlled Mating and Selection of the Honey Bee. International Symposium, Lunz am See, pp. 70-73. Bucharest, Rumania: Apimondia Publishing House.

(21) Grankin, N.N. 1978. Analytische Auslese zentralrussischer Bienen in der Region Orlow. In Genetik, Selektion und Reproduktion bei der Honigbiene, eds. V. Harnaj and G.D. Bilash, pp. 249-251. Bucharest, Rumania: Apimondia Publishing House.

(22) Griffing, B. 1982. A theory of natural selection incorporating interaction among individuals. X. Use of groups consisting of a mating pair together with haploid and diploid caste members. J. Theor. Biol 95: 199-223.

(23) Hamilton, W.D. 1964. The genetical evolution of social behavior I and II. J. Theor. Biol. 7: 1-52.

(24) Hemmling, C.; Koeniger, N.; and Ruttner, F. 1979. Quantitative Bestimmung der 9-Oxodecensäure im Lebenszyklus der Kapbiene (Apis mellifera capensis Escholtz). Apidologie 10: 227-240.

(25) Hillesheim, E., and Moritz, R.F.A. 1986. Genetic variance of physiological characters of workers in the Cape honeybee (Apis mellifera capensis Esch.) J. Apic. Res., submitted.

(26) Istock, C.A. 1983. The extent and consequences of heritable variation for fitness characters. In Population Biology. Retrospect and Prospect., eds. Ch.E. King and P.S. Dawson, Proc. Annu. Biol. Colloq., Vol. 41, pp. 61-96. New York: New York Columbia University Press.

(27) Kalmus, H., and Ribbands, C.R. 1952. The origin of the odors by which honeybees distinguish their companions. Proc. Roy. Soc. B 140: 50-59.

(28) Kerr, W.E.; Martinho, M.R.; and Concalves, L. 1980. Kinship selection in bees. Rev. Bras. Genet. 3: 339-344.

(29) Koeniger, G. 1986. Reproduction and mating behavior. In Bee Breeding and Genetics, ed. T.E. Rinderer, pp. 255-280. New York: Academic Press.

(30) Kriwzow, N.I. 1978. Erblichkeit und Reproduzierbarkeit ökonomisch wertvoller Merkmale bei der zentralrussischen Biene. In Genetik, Selektion und Reproduktion bei der Honigbiene, eds. V. Harnaj and G.D. Bilash, pp. 96-98. Bucharest, Rumania: Apimondia Publishing House.

(31) Kulincevic, J.M., and Rothenbuhler, W.C. 1975. Selection for resistance and susceptibility to hairless-black syndrome in the honey bee. J. Invert. Path. 25: 289-295.

(32) Kulincevic, J.M., and Rothenbuhler, W.C. 1982. Selection for length of life in the honeybee (Apis mellifera). Apidologie 13: 347-352.

(33) Laidlaw, H.H., and Page, R.E. 1984. Polyandry in honeybees (Apis mellifera L.). Sperm utilization and intracolony relationships. Genetics 108: 985-997.

(34) Lindauer, M. 1952. Ein Beitrag zur Frage der Arbeitsteilung im Bienenstaat. Z. Vergl. Physiol. 34: 299-345.

(35) Mackensen, O., and Nye, W.P. 1966. Selecting and breeding honeybees for collecting alfalfa pollen. J. Apic. Res. 5: 79-86.

(36) Malkow, W.W.; Timoschonowa, A.E.; and Tschjapligin, W.P. 1978. Variabilität und Vererbung der ökonomisch wertvollsten Charakteristika bei den Bienen des Oka-Ökotypus. In Genetik, Selektion und Reproduktion bei der Honigbiene, eds. V. Harnaj and G.D. Bilash, pp. 196-198. Bucharest, Rumania: Apimondia Publishing House.

(37) Maynard Smith, J. 1964. Group selection and kin selection: A rejoinder. Nature 201: 1145-1147.

(38) Milne, C.P. 1985a. An estimate of the heritability of worker longevity or length of life in the honeybee. J. Apic. Res. 24: 137-139.

(39) Milne, C.P. 1985b. An estimate of the heritability of the corbicular area of the honeybe. J. Apic. Res. 24: 137-139.

(40) Milne, C.P., and Friars, G.W. 1984. An estimate of the heritability of honeybee pupal weight. J. Heredity 75: 509-510.

(41) Moritz, R.F.A. 1981. Der Einfluß der Inzucht auf die Fitness der Drohnen von Apis mellifera carnica. Apidologie 12: 41-55.

(42) Moritz, R.F.A. 1983. Homogeneous mixing of honeybee semen. J. Apic. Res. 22: 249-255.

(43) Moritz, R.F.A. 1985. Heritability of the postcapping stage in Apis mellifera L. and its relation to varroatosis resistance. J. Hered. 76: 267-270.

(44) Moritz, R.F.A. 1986a. Intracolonial worker relationship and sperm competition in the honey bee (Apis mellifera L.). Experientia 42: 455-458.

(45) Moritz, R.F.A. 1986b. Estimating the genetic variance of group characters: social behaviour of honeybees (Apis mellifera L.) Theor. Appl. Genet., in press.

(46) Moritz, R.F.A., and Klepsch, A. 1985. Estimation heritabilities of worker characters: a new approach using laying workers of the Cape honeybee (Apis mellifera capensis Esch.). Apidologie 16: 47-56.

(47) Moritz, R.F.A., and Hillesheim, E. 1985. Inheritance of dominance in honeybees (Apis mellifera capensis Esch.). Behav. Ecol. Sociobiol. 17: 87-89.

(48) Moritz, R.F.A., and Southwick, E.E. 1986a. Analysis of queen recognition by honey bee workers (Apis mellifera L.) in a metabolic bio-assay. Exp. Biol., in press.

(49) Moritz, R.F.A., and Southwick, E.E. 1986b. Phenotype interaction in groups of honey bees (Apis mellifera L.). Behav. Genet., submitted.

(50) Moritz, R.F.A.; Southwick, E.E.; and Breh, M. 1985. A metabolic test for the quantitative analysis of alarm behavior of honey bees. J. Exp. Zool. 235: 1-5.

(51) Moritz, R.F.A.; Southwick, E.E.; and Harbo, J.B. 1986. Genetic analysis of defensive behaviour of honeybees (Apis mellifera L.) in a field test. Apidologie, in press.

(52) Noonan, K.C. 1985. Studies of worker recognition of brood in the honey bee (Apis mellifera). Ph.D. thesis. University of Wisconsin, Madison.

(53) Oldroyd, B., and Moran, C. 1983. Heritability of worker characteristics in the honeybee (Apid mellifera). Aust. J. Biol. Sci. 362: 323-332.

(54) Page, R.E., and Erickson, E.H. 1984. Selective rearing of queens by worker honey bees: kin or nestmate recognition. Ann. Entomol. Soc. Am. 77: 578-580.

(55) Page, R.E., and Erickson, E.H. 1986. Kin recognition and virgin queen acceptance by worker honey bees (Apis mellifera L.). Anim. Behav., in press.

(56) Page, R.E.; Kimsey, R.B.; and Laidlaw, H.H. 1984. Migration and dispersal of spermatozoa in spermathecae of queen honeybees (Apis mellifera L.). Experientia 40: 182-184.

(57) Page, R.E., and Metcalf, B. 1982. Multiple mating, sperm utilization, and social evolution. Am. Nat. 119: 263-281.

(58) Pirchner, F.; Ruttner, F.; and Ruttner, H. 1960. Erbliche Unterschiede zwischen Ertragseigenschaften von Bienen. XI. Internat. Congr. Entomol., Vienna, 2: 510-516.

(59) Renner, M. 1960. Das Duftorgan der Honigbiene und die physiologische Bedeutung ihres Lockstoffes. Z. vergl. Physiol. 43: 411-468.

(60) Rinderer, T.E. 1977. Measuring the heritability of characters of honeybees. J. Apic. Res. 16: 95-98.

(61) Rinderer, T.E.; Collins, A.M.; and Brown, M.A. 1983. Heritabilities and correlations of the honey bee: response to Nosema Apis, longetivity, and alarm response to isopentyl acetate. Apidologie 14: 79-85.

(62) Rösch, G.A. 1925. Untersuchungen über die Arbeitsteilung im Bienenstaat. I. Die Tätigkeiten im normalen Bienenstaate und ihre Beziehungen zum Alter der Arbeitsbienen. Z. Vergl. Physiol. 12: 571-631.

(63) Rothenbuhler, W.C. 1964. Behavior genetics of nestcleaning in honeybees IV. Responses of Fl and backcross generations to disease-killed brood. Am. Zool. 4: 111-123.

(64) Rothenbuhler, W.C.; Kulincevic, J.M.; and Thompson, V.C. 1979. Successful selection of honeybees for fast and slow hoarding of sugar syrup in the laboratory. J. Apic. Res. 18: 272-278.

(65) Ruttner, F. 1976. Die Bienenrassen Afrikas. XXVth Internat. Apic. Congr., pp. 344-364. Bucharest, Rumania: Apimondia Publishing House.

(66) Ruttner, F., and Hesse, B. 1981. Rassenspezifische Unterschiede in der Ovarentwicklung un Eiablage von weisellosen Arbeiterinnen der Honigbiene Apis mellifera L. Apidologie 12: 159-183.

(67) Ruttner, H. 1980. Haltung der Königinnen während der Paarungszeit. In Königinnenzucht, ed. F. Ruttner, pp. 225-268. Bucharest, Rumania: Apimondia Publishing House.

(68) Seeley, T.D. 1982. Adaptive significance of the age polyethism schedule in honeybee colonies. Behav. Ecol. Sociobiol. 11: 287-293.

(69) Soller, M., and Bar Cohen, R. 1967. Some observations on the heritability and genetic correlation between honey production and brood area in the honeybee. J. Apic. Res. 6: 37-43.

(70) Taber, S. 1955. Sperm distribution in the spermatheca of multiple-mated queen honey bees. J. Econ. Entomol. 48: 522-525.

(71) Thronhill, R., and Alcock, J. 1983. The Evolution of Insect Mating Systems. Cambridge, Mass.: Harvard University Press.

(72) Tucker, K.W. 1980. Tolerance to carbaryl in honeybees increased by selection. American Bee Journal 120: 36-46.

(73) Velthuis, H.H.W. 1970. Ovarian development in Apis mellifera worker bees. Ent. Exp. Appl. 13: 377.394.

(74) Verma, S., and Ruttner, F. 1983. Cytological analysis of the thelytokous parthenogenesis in the Cape honeybee (Apis mellifera capensis ESCHOLTZ). Apidologie 14: 41-57.

(75) Willham, R.L. 1956. The covariance between relatives for characters composed of components contributed by related individuals. Biometrics 19: 18-27.

Appendix

List of phenotypical mutants in A. mellifera. Names of alleles in parentheses.

locus	symbol	phenotype freshly emerged	phenotype old imagines
albino	a	non pigmented integument, normal eye pigment	
bayer	by	white eye color	reddish-orange

Appendix (Continued)

List of phenotypical mutants in A. mellifera. Names of alleles in parentheses.

locus	symbol	phenotype: freshly emerged	phenotype: old imagines
black	bl	dark body color	
	bl^{y}	partly yellow body (yellow)	
	bl^{ac}	only workers partly yellow (abdome castarito)	
brick	bk	red eye color	red brown
chartreuse	ch	yellow green eye color	reddish-brown
	ch(1)	yellow green	brown
	ch(2)	green	reddish-brown
	ch(B)	green (Benson green)	olive to reddish
	ch(c)	oo dark red (cherry), oo yellow to red brown	
	ch(r)	purple red (red)	red brown
	ch(li)	yellow (limao)	reddish-brown
cordovan	cd	light brown body color	
cream	cr	white eye color	white
cyclops	-	compound eyes merged over verrex	
diminuitive	di	short wings	
droopy	D	flat separated wings, lethal in homozygote	
einäugig	-	one compound eye missing	
eyeless	e	no facets	
facetless	f	eye facets vestigal	
garnet	g	garnet red eye color	wild type
hairless	h	no body hairs	
haarlos	H	only hairs on tomentum, lethal in homozygote	
ivory	i	white eye color	white
	i(ro)	rose pink (rose)	pink
	i(u)	peach pink (umber)	orange-brown
lethal	l	lethal	
laranja	la	orange eye color	reddish-brown
ocelos claros	oc	compound eyes: rose	brown
		ocelli: rose	glassy white
pink	p	pink eye color	pink
pearl	pe	white eye color	white
reduced facet	rf	small number of facets in atrophied eyes	

Appendix (Continued)

List of phenotypical mutants in A. mellifera. Names of alleles in parentheses.

locus	symbol	phenotype freshly emerged	phenotype old imagines
rudimental wing	rw	atrophied wings	
schwarz-süchtig	s	hairs missing	
short	sh	small wings, abnormal venation	
snow	s s(t) s(la)	white eye color white (tan) orange (laranja)	white yellow-brownish reddish-brown
split-sting	sps	lancets separated from stylet	
spade	sp	rose pink eyes	red
truncate	tr	wings truncated in middle, abnormal venation	
white	-	white eyes	
wrinkled	wr	wrinkled wings	

The Foraging Honeybee

Social Foraging by Honeybees: How a Colony Tracks Rich Sources of Nectar

Thomas D. Seeley and Royce A. Levien
Department of Biology, Yale University, New Haven, Connecticut 06511, USA*

Abstract. This paper examines how the behavioral acts of the thousands of foragers in a honeybee colony are combined to produce the coordinated foraging behavior of a whole colony. We focus on a colony's ability to quickly adjust the distribution of its foraging efforts following changes in the spatial distribution of rich nectar sources. The analysis begins by examining the factors that influence an individual nectar forager's response to a patch of flowers (Fig. 1). These include variables, such as distance from the nest, nectar sweetness, and nectar abundance (Fig. 4), that are associated with the patch itself, as well as variables, such as weather conditions and the colony's rate of nectar intake (Fig. 2), that are not associated with a particular patch of flowers. These non-patch variables affect a forager's response to her patch of flowers by changing her thresholds in patch quality for abandoning or recruiting nestmates to a patch (Fig. 3). Foragers evidently assess their colony's rate of nectar intake while unloading nectar to receiver bees. The ease of unloading varies inversely with the rate of nectar flow into the colony. The responsiveness of nectar foragers to this indicator of their colony's foraging status enables a colony to swiftly redirect its nectar collection efforts following changes in the spatial distribution of rich nectar sources. Whenever the quality of a major nectar source declines, its foragers reduce their rate of visits to the patch, which depresses the colony's total rate of nectar intake, which in turn stimulates recruitment to whichever patches remain high in quality (Figs. 6 and 7). The paper concludes by presenting some generalizations about colony integration in social insects that emerge from this research.

INTRODUCTION: OVERVIEW AND QUESTIONS

Foraging by honeybees is a social enterprise, one in which the thousands of foragers in a colony cooperate to find and exploit rich patches of flowers. The heart of this system of social foraging is the waggle dance, a communication behavior through which colony members share information about the locations of profitable food sources. By pooling the reconnaissance of its thousands of foragers, a colony monitors a vast area, often more than 100 square kilometers, for patches of flowers rich in nectar and pollen. By then focusing its foragers on the richest patches that have been found across this expanse a colony achieves high efficiency in food collection (6, 8, 12, 15, 28, 29, 30, 31, 33).

*Current address: Section of Neurobiology and Behavior, Cornell University, Ithaca, New York 14853 USA

A critical component of the honeybee's system of social foraging is the set of processes that focus a colony's foragers on high quality forage patches despite constant shifts in the spatial distribution of these patches. In previous works (29, 30) one of us (T.D.S.) has argued that a colony's ability to track prime food sources emerges directly from a colony's thousands of foragers each following two basic behavioral programs: (1) the grading of behavior in relation to patch quality such that at one extreme (poor patch) a bee abandons her patch, while at the opposite extreme (rich patch) she recruits nestmates to her patch; and (2) the following of recruitment dances when a new patch of flowers needs to be found. The consequence of these two programs being executed en masse is a steady migration of foragers away from poor patches, back to their nest where they follow recruitment dances, and finally out onto rich patches of flowers.

This report summarizes recent progress in studies of the first behavioral program, i.e., how a honeybee forager grades her behavior in accordance with the quality of her flower patch. To date, this question has been probed only in the context of bees foraging for nectar, so this discussion will be limited to the particular, though not peculiar (3, 20), situation of honeybees specializing in nectar collection. We start by briefly describing the spectrum of responses by foragers to patches of flowers. Next we review an experiment which shows that a bee's response to a patch of flowers depends on her colony's overall foraging status. Then we consider a model of how a bee integrates information about her patch with information about her colony's foraging status. After this we examine how a forager evaluates a patch of flowers, and how she senses one key aspect of her colony's foraging status--its rate of nectar intake. Presentation of a model of the information-processing performed by foragers rounds off the discussion from the perspective of individual forager. Next we turn to the question of how colony- and individual-level behaviors are related. A systems model of colony integration in foraging, based on the results of "two-feeder experiments", is presented to explain how the foraging behavior of the colony as a whole emerges from the behavior of its individual foragers. We end by relating these studies to general observations about the integration of colonies of social insects.

INDIVIDUAL-LEVEL VIEW: HOW A BEE RESPONDS TO A PATCH OF FLOWERS

The Spectrum of Responses

A worker bee shows a wide range of responses to a patch of flowers. These are portrayed in Fig. 1. At one extreme, a forager simply abandons the patch; at the other, she performs repeated, high-tempo trips to the patch combined with vigorous recruitment dances while back at the nest. Between these two extremes of response there is a regular series of intermediate behavior patterns created by foragers grading such behavioral variables as the rate of visits to the patch, the size of their nectar load, and the intensity of their recruitment activity (5, 6, 7, 12, 17, 18, 19, 24, 25, 26).

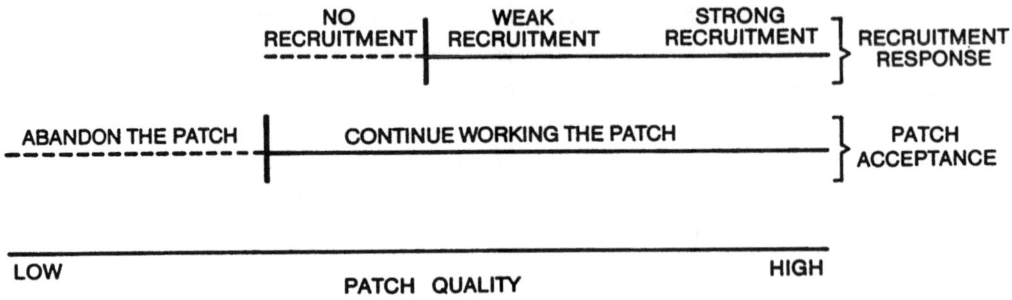

Fig. 1 - A graphical representation of the response spectrum of a bee to a patch of flowers. Responses range from abandoning a poor patch to vigorously working and recruiting nestmates to a rich patch.

Foragers Integrate Information about Patch and Non-patch Variables

How does a bee decide what point along this response spectrum she should adopt for her particular patch of flowers? It is clear that this decision-making must reflect certain properties of the flower patch itself, including its distance from the nest and its nectar sweetness (discussed in detail in the following section). Furthermore, it is clear that certain variables independent of any particular patch of flowers also influence a bee's response to her patch of flowers. These non-patch variables include the weather conditions (1, 27), the general availability of nectar (12), and probably also the amount of honey stored in the forager's colony (12, 22).

We have recently demonstrated experimentally that the rate of nectar intake by a colony is a major factor influencing the decisions of its nectar foragers (31). The design of our experiment was quite simple. A colony was taken to a densely wooded location with little or no natural forage, and there provided with two widely spaced feeders. One feeder was used to manipulate the colony's rate of nectar intake by regulating between 0 and 90 the number of bees bringing back nectar from this feeder. At the second feeder a record was kept of the rate at which 30 labelled foragers recruited unmarked nestmates. This was used to measure changes in the labelled bees' response to the second feeder (whose properties did not change) following changes in the colony's nectar intake rate (manipulated at the first feeder). All recruits to either feeder were captured to prevent any buildup of foragers at the two feeders. Fig. 2 shows clearly how the recruitment rate for the second (south) feeder rose or fell dramatically in synchrony with a decrease or increase, respectively, of the colony's nectar intake from the first (north) feeder. The conclusion from this experiment, briefly stated, is that the higher the colony's rate of nectar intake, the higher a forager's standards of patch quality for recruitment to a patch.

One way to visualize how a forager integrates information about patch quality and non-patch variables, such as the colony's rate of nectar intake, is shown in Fig. 3, which illustrates our

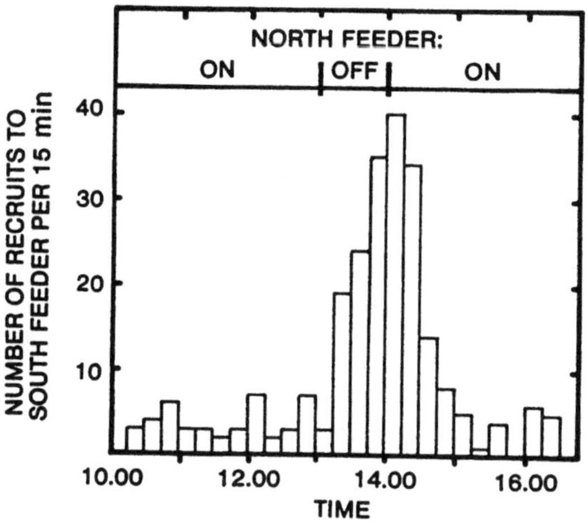

Fig. 2 - Results of an experiment testing the effects of change in a colony's rate of nectar intake (altered by turning the north feeder on or off) on its recruitment to a food source of fixed quality (the south feeder). The experiment was conducted in a vast, heavily forested area which was essentially devoid of flowers. When the north feeder was "on", a total of 60 bees (30 from the north feeder and 30 from the south feeder) brought nectar into the colony. When the north feeder was off, only the 30 bees from the south feeder could continue foraging. Thus shutting off the north feeder cut in half the colony's rate of nectar intake. This reduction in the flow of nectar into the colony triggered a rapid intensification of recruitment to the unchanged feeder in the south.

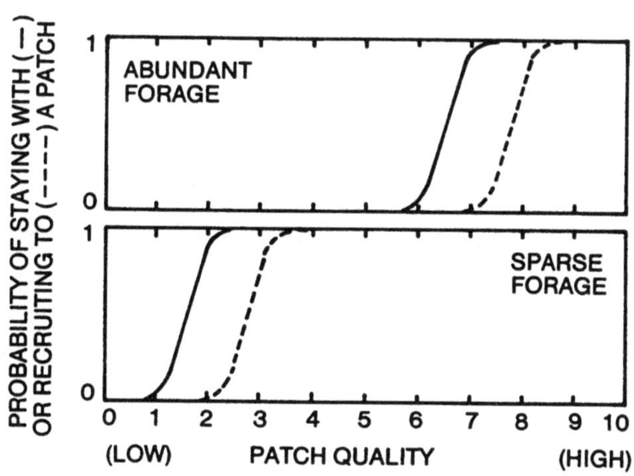

Fig. 3 - A graphical representation of how foragers may integrate information about patch quality and forage abundance in deciding how to respond to a patch of flowers. In this model, a forager makes an assessment of her patch's overall quality and adjusts the thresholds of patch quality for accepting and recruiting to a patch in relation to the abundance of forage. By raising these thresholds when forage is abundant, a forager focuses her efforts on only extremely high quality patches, and by lowering them when forage is sparse, a forager broadens her range of acceptable patches. As is explained in the text, the abundance of forage is evidently perceived by foragers by sensing, through interactions with receiver bees, the rate of nectar intake by the colony as a whole.

"threshold-adjustment" model. According to this model, a forager forms an assessment of her patch's overall quality, and ranks the patch on a scale of quality, represented by the x-axis in Fig. 3. This information-processing skill is closely analogous to the assessment ability (Einschätzungsvermögen) that Lindauer (14, 15) demonstrated scout bees use in selecting a nest site. A forager's responsiveness to various non-patch variables is incorporated in the Fig. 3 model by changes in the thresholds of patch quality for various responses, such as acceptance of and recruitment to a patch.

Thus, for example, when forage is sparse and little nectar flows into a colony, a forager's thresholds for acceptance and recruitment are low and a patch of intermediate quality will elicit acceptance and even vigorous dancing (Fig. 3, bottom). Conversely, during times of abundant forage, a forager's thresholds are high and a patch of intermediate quality will be rejected (Fig. 3, top)

The ability of foragers (and thus of the colonies they form) to change patch selectively in relation to forage abundance and other factors seems highly adaptive. For example, when forage is abundant, a colony probably enjoys a wide choice among forage patches and so high standards of patch quality are appropriate. But when forage is sparse, a colony may struggle to find work sites for all of its foragers and then lower standards of patch quality are appropriate. Beggars cannot be choosers.

The model of information processing expressed in Fig. 3 emphasizes the importance of understanding how nectar foragers assess patch quality and non-patch variables, such as nectar availability. These are the two puzzles we will consider next.

Assessing the Quality of a Patch of Flowers

Here we face several interrelated questions. What properties of a flower patch enter into a bee's evaluation of the patch's quality? What is the fundamental currency of patch quality? How steeply do bees grade their behavior in relation to patch quality? Numerous investigators have probed the first question and have consistently identified the following three properties of nectar source as important to bees: (1) sweetness of the nectar (5, 12, 17, 26, 31, 34, 35), (2) availability of the nectar (4, 17, 18, 19, 25, 26, 34, 35), and (3) distance from the nest (1, 19, 26, 31). A bee's sensitivity to these patch properties is what enables her to forage effectively. Other traits of nectar sources, such as purity of the sweet taste, presence of a floral fragrance, and form of the food container, also influence the decisions of foragers in experimental settings (10, 12), but probably are irrelevant to bees foraging from flowers in nature.

The second question - how information about the properties of a nectar source is integrated in forming an overall assessment of patch quality--is knottier than the first and still lacks a totally conclusive answer. Nevertheless, some important pieces of information are at hand. Many models of optimal foraging are concerned with the rate at which a forager gains energy (11, 21, 36) so a starting hypothesis for the currency of patch quality is the rate of energy intake achieved by a bee in foraging from a patch. If bees do seek to maximize their rate of energy delivery to their colony, it seems that it is the net rate of energy delivery (gain - cost /time), not simply the gross rate (gain/time) that is important, since several studies indicate that bees are sensitive to the costs of foraging (2, 9, 34, 35). An alternative hypothesis for the currency of patch quality, one which also incorporates cost, is the net energy efficiency of foraging from a patch (gain - cost/cost). Three studies have explicitly compared these two currencies--net rate of energy delivery and net energetic efficiency--in predicting the foraging behavior of bees (25, 26, 31). All three report that the behaviors of bees (the degree of crop filling and the intensity of recruitment) were much more consistent with predictions based on maximization of rate of energy delivery to the hive. However, none of these three studies eliminates the possibility that some more complex currency is involved, so the issue is not yet completely settled.

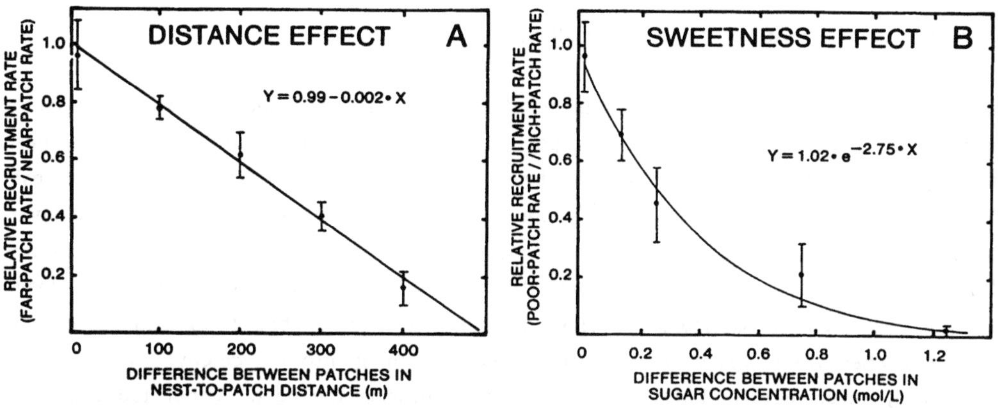

Fig. 4 - Relative recruitment to two food sources as a function of the difference between the two sources in distance from the nest or in concentration of sugar solution. These plots illustrate the steepness with which workers grade their recruitment behavior in relation to two major variables which influence the quality of a patch of nectar-bearing flowers.

Even without a firm understanding of the currency of overall patch quality, we can measure how strongly foragers respond to differences in quality between patches. This was done by training two groups of 30 bees out to two widely spaced feeders which differed either in distance from the hive or in concentrations of the sucrose solution they provided and then tediously measuring the rates of recruitment to the two feeders (31). More than 2000 counts were made of the number of recruits arriving at a feeder per 15 min period. What emerges from these investigations is a picture of the steepness with which workers grade their recruitment behavior in relation to two major variables of patch quality. This is shown in Fig. 4, where we see that a patch at 700m from the nest receives recruits 40 percent less rapidly than one at 500m, even though the 200m difference is but a few percent of the more than 10,000 m radius of a typical colony's foraging activities (33). Likewise, a patch providing a 2.00 mol/L sucrose solution receives recruits 50 percent less rapidly than one with a 2.25 mol/L solution, and again the 0.25 mol/L difference represents only a small fraction of the range of sugar concentrations for nectars collected by honeybees, roughly 0.5 to 2.5 mol/L (31). From these patterns we can conclude that bees are keenly sensitive to differences in quality between nectar sources, and respond strongly to the differences they detect. Although these are properties of individual bees, they nevertheless relate to the foraging behavior of colonies since these skills of individuals underlie the ability of whole colonies to choose wisely among patches of flowers.

Assessing the Availability of Nectar to the Colony

As discussed earlier, a nectar forager bases her response to a patch of flowers on both the patch's quality and on the state of several non-patch variables. A recent study (31) sheds light on how a bee is able to assess one of these variables: the rate of nectar intake by the colony. The subject is an intriguing one since it requires that individual foragers acquire information about conditions within their colony as a whole. This is generally considered a difficult achievement for a social insect worker, especially for ones like honeybee workers which live in colonies containing many thousands of members (37, p. 224). How then does a worker honeybee sense her colony's overall rate of nectar intake?

In 1948 Lindauer suggested that this piece of information is encoded in a nectar forager's experiences upon return to her nest, especially her reception by receiver bees (the bees, slightly younger than foragers, that unload nectar from foragers and store it in the combs). This hypothesis is supported by observations of interactions between foragers and receiver bees made during the experiments involving manipulations of a colony's rate of nectar intake (Fig. 2). As is indicated in Table 1, when there was a heavy flow of nectar into the colony, foragers experienced considerable delay in finding a receiver bee to unload them. In contrast, when there was only a trickle of nectar coming into the colony, foragers were mobbed by eager receiver bees immediately upon entering the nest. Other features of a forager's reception by receiver bees--including the maximum number of receiver bees simultaneously unloading a forager, the number of aborted food transfers, and the intensity of antennation during nectar transfer--were also affected dramatically by a colony's rate of nectar intake. Of course, these correlations between elements of the unloading process and colonial intake rate do not prove that foragers actually use some feature of the former as a sign of the latter. Conclusive proof of this awaits an experimental demonstration that the patch selectivity of foragers changes in response to changes in the unloading experience alone, that is, in the absence of any actual changes in the colony's rate of nectar intake.

It is worth digressing here for the sake of perspective, especially since our conclusions about the type of information transferred from receiver bees to nectar foragers run counter to prevailing views (see 1, p. 106; 6, p. 250; 13, p. 421; 23, p. 90; 30, p. 97). In 1954 Lindauer suggested that the information encoded in a nectar forager's experiences with receiver bees is not the colony's rate of nectar intake, as he had proposed six years earlier, but is instead the sweetness of each forager's nectar relative to that of her nestmate's nectars. This switch in Lindauer's interpretation probably stemmed from his then recent discovery about the regulation of water collection in honeybee colonies. Lindauer (13) observed that when a colony needs water desperately to prevent nest overheating, its receiver bees exert preferences among foragers. They speedily unload those with water or dilute nectar but tend to ignore foragers with concentrated nectar. This stimulates the water collectors to continue gathering water and to recruit others to their task (in other words, it lowers their thresholds for acceptance of and recruitment to water sources). Lindauer evidently surmised that when a colony needs food (sugar) rather than water, its receiver bees will continue discriminating among foragers, though preferentially unloading ones with concentrated nectar rather than water or dilute nectar.

Variable	Colonial intake rate	
	High (N feeder:90 bees)	Low (N feeder:30 bees)
Time to start of unloading (sec)	27.6 ± 20.5	13.8 ± 7.8
Time to end of unloading (sec)	82.1 ± 30.0	49.7 ± 22.3
Maximum number of simultaneous receivers	1.2 ± 0.4	2.1 ± 0.5
Aborted food transfers	1.4 ± 1.9	0.3 ± 0.5
% Intense antennations	25	93

TABLE 1. Comparisons of the experiences of foragers unloading nectar to receiver bees during times of high and low rates of nectar intake by the colony. The foragers which were observed came from a feeder to the south of the observation hive. The colony's rate of nectar intake was manipulated by varying the number of bees working a feeder to the north of the hive. All differences are significant at the level of P 0.01.

It is worth digressing here for the sake of perspective, especially since our conclusions about the type of information transferred from receiver bees to nectar foragers run counter to prevailing views (see 1, p. 106; 6, p. 250; 13, p. 421; 23, p. 90; 30, p. 97). In 1954 Lindauer suggested that the information encoded in a nectar forager's experiences with receiver bees is not the colony's rate of nectar intake, as he had proposed six years earlier, but is instead the sweetness of each forager's nectar relative to that of her nestmate's nectars. This switch in Lindauer's interpretation probably stemmed from his then recent discovery about the regulation of water collection in honeybee colonies. Lindauer (13) observed that when a colony needs water desperately to prevent nest overheating, its receiver bees exert preferences among foragers. They speedily unload those with water or dilute nectar but tend to ignore foragers with concentrated nectar. This stimulates the water collectors to continue gathering water and to recruit others to their task (in other words, it lowers their thresholds for acceptance of and recruitment to water sources). Lindauer evidently surmised that when a colony needs food (sugar) rather than water, its receiver bees will continue discriminating among foragers, though preferentially unloading ones with concentrated nectar rather than water or dilute nectar.

It now seems clear that this hypothesis, though reasonable, is incorrect. The critical test of the hypothesis was a comparison of the receptions by receiver bees of foragers from two groups, working simultaneously but gathering sucrose solutions of two different concentrations (1.50 and 2.00 mol/L). No significant differences were observed (31, Table 3). Evidently there exists an important difference between the social regulation mechanisms for water and nectar collection. The former involves receiver bees discriminating among foragers on the basis of sugar concentration whereas the latter does not. The adaptive significance of this switch in receiver bee behavior seems evident. On the other hand, when a colony collects water to prevent disastrous overheating of the nest, it is essential to get water as swiftly as possible and so receiver bees preferentially unload foragers bearing water. On the other hand, when a colony collects nectar to fill a long-term need for energy, it is most important to gather the energy as efficiently as possible. Receiver bees, confined to the nest, cannot know which foragers are working the most profitable patches (determined by numerous variables, including patch distance, nectar sweetness, and nectar abundance; see section 2.c), thus they should not show preferences among foragers, but should instead unload all foragers as rapidly as possible. By behaving in this manner, the receiver bees provide the foragers with a clear indication of the colony's rate of nectar intake.

Summary and Speculations

The most striking feature of decision-making by foragers described so far is its integration of a multiplicity of perceptions: patch properties, receiver bee behavior, weather conditions, and possibly still others, as is illustrated in Fig. 5. How this information processing occurs in the bee's nervous system remains a riddle, though generally speaking we know that the inputs about non-patch variables affect the thresholds of responses to patch quality (section 2.b), and we have already some insights into the integrated currency of patch quality (section 2.c).

Fig. 5 also emphasizes that a bee's response to her particular patch of flowers is tuned to her colony's foraging status, and that a bee can sense her colony's foraging situation through interactions with receiver bees. On this point we have included the speculation that the amount of empty storage space for nectar, like the colony's rate of nectar intake, affects the behavior of receiver bees and so influences a forager's thresholds in patch quality. Actually, this is not pure speculation. Both Lindauer (12) and Rinderer (22) report that reducing the amount of empty comb in a colony results in reduced recruitment to a feeder, but the precise connection between these two phenomena is not known. If the link is a change in the ease of unloading by receivers, then we should view the interactions between foragers and receiver bees as providing nectar foragers with a message richer in meaning than simply the colony's rate of nectar intake, i.e., a message of the colony's need for a higher rate of nectar intake. This need will be high only if both the colony's intake rate is low and the colony contains abundant storage space for additional nectar.

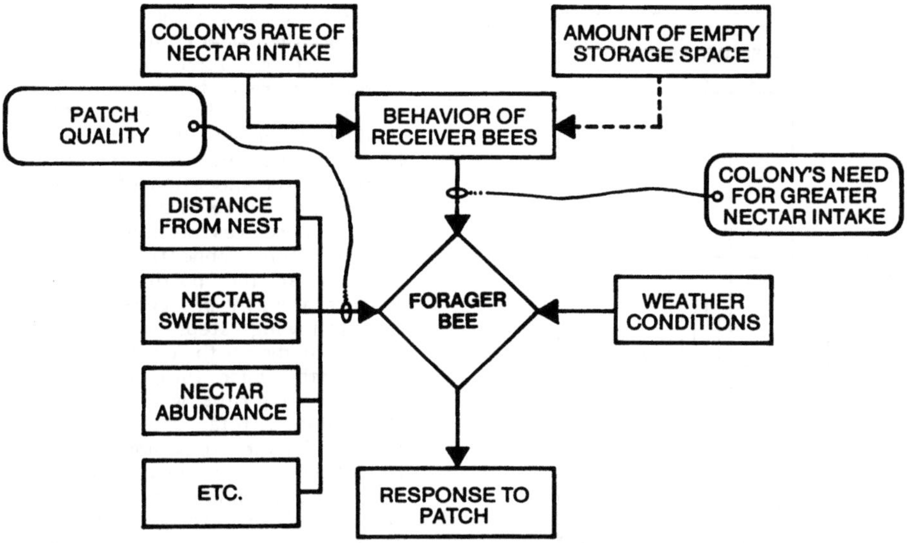

Fig. 5 - Flow diagram showing the multiplicity of perceptions which a forager integrates in deciding how to respond to a patch of flowers. These can be summarized as (1) patch quality (section 2.c), (2) colony's need for a greater rate of nectar intake (sections 2.b and 2.d), and (3) weather. A forager's response to a patch can range from abandoning the patch to vigorously recruiting nestmates to the patch (section 2.a). The dashed line indicates a link which is not yet proven by experiment.

It should be added that the ideas expressed in Figs. 3 and 5 are our current best bets about the information processing underlying a nectar forager's carefully graded response to a patch of flowers. They are not firm facts. Further research over the next few years will refine and perhaps strongly alter these models. Nevertheless, they provide powerful insights into the way the actions of whole colonies emerge from the behaviors of their component workers. This is the topic to be discussed next.

COLONY-LEVEL VIEW: HOW A COLONY RESPONDS TO CHANGE IN THE LANDSCAPE

The Two-Feeder Experiment

The outstanding characteristic of the foraging behavior of whole colonies of honeybees is the constant, day-by-day, if not hour-by-hour, change in the foci of a colony's recruitment and foraging efforts (33). These spatial dynamics in foraging activity almost certainly mirror changes in the foraging opportunities. To study this colony-level process in greater detail, a simplified foraging array was established in which a colony collected nectar from just two sources. Creating this situation involved transporting a colony to a virtually flowerless study area deep in the northern woods of New York State and providing the colony with two widely separated sources of sucrose solution. We then followed in detail how the colony as a whole, and how its workers as component parts, responded to changes in the relative qualities of these food sources. These changes were induced by keeping constant the concentration of the sucrose solution at one feeder (2.0 mol/L) while varying it at the other feeder (0.5 to 2.0 mol/L) (for details, see ref. 31).

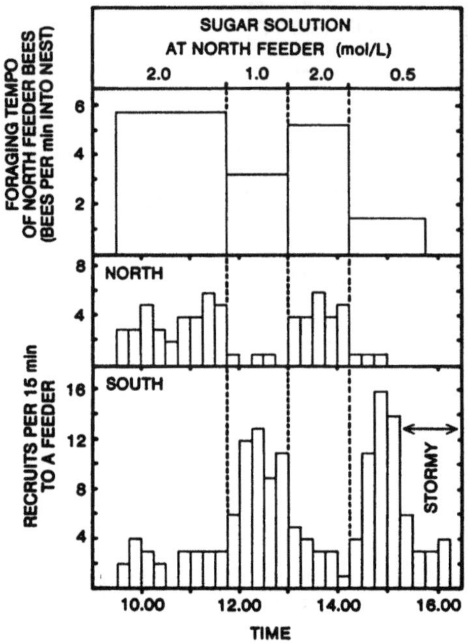

Fig. 6 - Results of an experiment showing the effect of change in quality of one food source (north feeder) on recruitment to a food source of fixed quality (south feeder). Whenever the food source in the north deteriorated, the colony increased its allocation of foragers to the food source in the south even though there was no change in its quality. The connection between changes at the north and south feeders probably proceeded through the following steps. When the quality of the north feeder declined, the north-feeder foragers lowered their foraging rate, which depressed the colony's total rate of nectar intake. This led to a more vigorous reception of foragers by the receivers, signalling an increase in the colony's need for greater nectar flow, which stimulated recruitment by the south-feeder foragers.

The colony's responses to these manipulations were quick and tightly coordinated. Within 15 min of the decline in quality of one food source, the colony had begun to restrict the nectar flow from the inferior source (north), by slowing its foraging there, and simultaneously had begun to expand it from the superior source (south), by intensifying recruitment to this source. This is expressed graphically in Fig. 6. What is the mechanism that produces these coordinated shifts in a colony's foraging efforts? In particular, how can we explain the rises in recruitment to the south feeder whenever the quality of the north feeder declined, even though conditions were held constant at the south feeder? No doubt it partly reflects the disappearance of competition for recruits between the north and south feeder forager groups. However, this can account for at most a doubling of the recruitment rate to the south feeder, whereas this actually multiplied by a factor of 5 to 10. Clearly, loss of competition for recruits plays a minor role in redirecting a colony's foraging operations. The major influence is probably the drop in a colony's rate of nectar intake whenever an important nectar source deteriorates. When the quality of the north feeder declined in the two-feeder experiment, the north-feeder foragers lowered their foraging rate, which depressed the colony's total rate of nectar intake, and so stimulated recruitment to the south feeder. Let us now consider how these numerous lines of interaction are interwoven to form a colony's total system for control of foraging effort.

A Systems View of Colony Integration in Foraging

Fig. 7 expresses in a schematic diagram our current understanding of the relationships among elements of honeybee colony and its nectar sources which enable a colony to track rich sources of nectar.

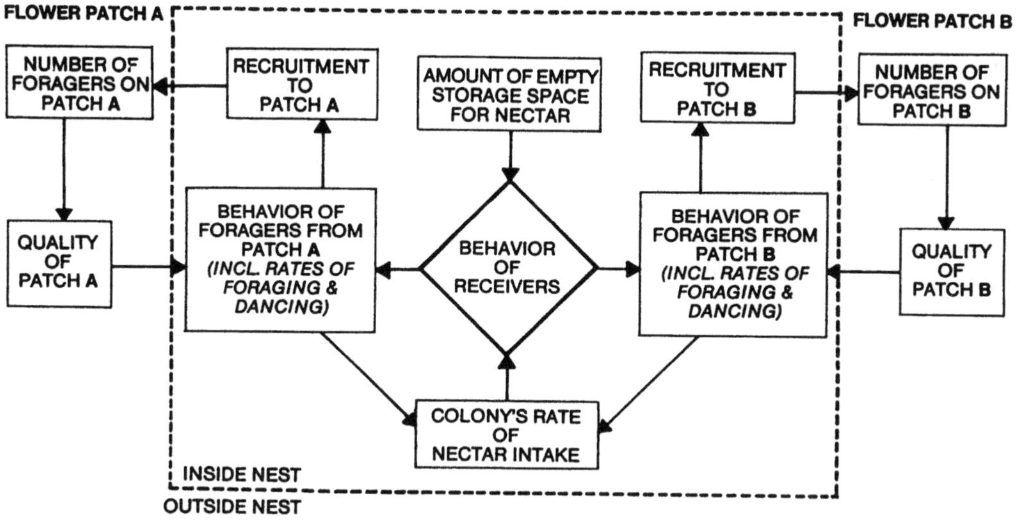

Fig. 7 - Schematic diagram showing the relationships among elements of a honeybee colony and its food sources that regulate the colony's allocation of foragers to these food sources. The diagram shows that both the amount of empty storage space for nectar in a colony's nest and the nectar intake rate of a colony influence the behavior of receiver bees. It also shows that a forager combines information about her colony's foraging status (coded in the behavior of receiver bees) with information about her forage patch (A or B) in deciding how strongly to recruit to her patch of flowers. Furthermore, the diagram shows how the foraging activities of the bees working one patch can influence the behavior of receiver bees and so affect the recruitment behavior of bees working another patch. Thus this figure illustrates the central role of receiver bees in regulating a colony's allocation of foragers among patches of flowers.

Let us highlight some of the main features of this system:

1) The colony's rate of nectar intake and probably also the amount of empty storage space for nectar influence the behavior of receiver bees.

2) A forager combines information about her colony's foraging status (coded in the behavior of receiver bees) and weather conditions (not shown) with information about the quality of her forage patch in deciding how strongly to forage from and recruit to her patch.

3) Recruitment to a patch will tend to reduce patch quality by reducing the nectar abundance at the patch.

4) The foraging activities of bees working one patch can strongly influence the behaviors of bees working a second patch without any direct contact or communication between the two forager groups. This occurs as bees of the first group influence the colony's rate of nectar intake, which affects the behavior of receiver bees, which ultimately sways the foraging decision of the bees in the second group.

5) Receiver bees play a central role in regulating a colony's allocation of foragers among different sources of nectar.

In summary, Fig. 7 illustrates how the behavior of each individual nectar forager is tuned to the quality of her flowers and to the foraging status of her colony, and in turn has effects which spread throughout a colony's entire foraging operation. The net effect of this tight linking of a bee's behavior to conditions both inside and outside her colony, multiplied over the thousands of foragers in a colony, is the foraging "wisdom" of a whole colony of honeybees. This colony "wisdom" includes the ability to raise and lower patch selectivity in response to colony need and forage abundance, and the ability to rapidly redirect the forager force as different flower patches wither and bloom. Thus a colony's forager force, although composed of thousands of physically independent individuals, functions as an integrated whole.

DISCUSSION: THE BRIDGING OF LEVELS OF DESCRIPTION

In 1971, Edward O. Wilson wrote that "the reconstruction of mass behavior from a knowledge of the behavior of single colony members is the central problem of insect sociology." This bold statement reflects two basic truths about the social insects. One is that their most remarkable achievements are mass phenomena: cooperative construction of properly proportioned nests, precise regulation of elevated temperatures inside nests, efficient performance of group foraging raids, and numerous other forms of coordinated mass action. The second fundamental fact is that at present we can only dimly visualize how the group phenomena of social insects emerge from the collective behaviors of a colony's members. In short, the social insects present us with two distinct levels of description--individual and colony--but we have difficulty in bridging the two levels. The studies summarized here have addressed this challenge in the context of honeybee colonies tracking rich sources of nectar, and have yielded the specific findings presented above. Let us now consider what generalizations about the integration of insect societies are suggested by the research.

One general conclusion is that sophisticated achievements of a colony as a whole can reflect a small set of underlying rules of individual behavior. For example, it seems that the two behavioral programs stated in the introduction--(1) grading of behavior in relation to patch quality, and (2) following recruitment dances--are sufficient to account for the ability of colonies to track rich sources of nectar. Thus there is a certain simplicity hidden beneath the complexity of a honeybee colony's foraging activities. But this simplicity should not destroy our wonder about the achievements of colonies. These two behavioral programs, although easily summarized, are highly complex. The first one requires that a worker bee can integrate information about patch quality, her colony's foraging status, meterological conditions, and possibly still other factors in deciding how to respond to a patch of flowers. Furthermore, this behavioral program requires that she can send recruitment signals to other foragers and can receive from receiver bees signals indicating the colony's foraging status. Given this behavioral complexity, it should be clear that identifying a small set of rules that explain the amazing abilities of a whole colony need not destroy our wonder about a mass behavior, such as colonial tracking of rich nectar sources. New fascination must arise about the intricacy of the behavioral programs that create this mass behavior (Fig. 5) and about the way they are assembled to create a coordinated colonial behavior (Fig. 7).

A second general message about the interrelations of the behaviors of individuals and the actions of colonies concerns the awareness of individuals about conditions within their colony as a whole. As a rule, this awareness is extremely low (37). Nevertheless, a high level of awareness by individuals of certain colony-level variables is possible, and when it does exist, it provides a special opportunity for integrating the actions of individuals into a colony-level behavior. This is illustrated in the present research by foragers being able to sense their colony's overall rate of nectar intake, jointly adjusting their thresholds of patch quality in relation to the colony's intake rate, and so producing a coordinated shift in a colony's patch selectivity.

The phenomenon of nectar foragers responding to their colony's rate of nectar intake suggests two further generalizations about the design of insect societies. One is that feedback loops between individuals and their colony can be crucial to regulating a colony's activities. In other words, it is important to recognize that not only do the behaviors of individuals shape the actions of their colony, but also that conditions within their colony shape the behaviors of these individuals. For example, the foraging behaviors of individuals determine their colony's rate of nectar intake, and reciprocally, this colonial intake rate of nectar influences the foraging behavior of individuals. The second, and related, point is that both external stimuli and a colony's internal configuration determine the behaviors of a colony's members. Thus the nectar foragers of a honeybee colony respond not only to the properties of their flowers and to the weather, but also to the needs of their colony. Because of this intricate intertwining of the responses of individuals to conditions outside and inside the nest, a colony as a whole is capable of both perception and self-perception. This remarkable fact explains much of the behavioral delicacy, self-involvedness, and capacity for cognition (16) that is so fascinating about colonies of social insects.

We are still a long way from understanding how colonies of insects translate the numerous behavioral acts of their members into higher order effects. This challenge is not a trivial one because, as the generalizations just stated emphasize, colonies of social insects are composed of complex parts integrated through complex rules of interaction--they are truly "complex systems" (32). Nevertheless, we believe that the results of our studies of colonial foraging in honeybees should leave the reader with a sense of optimism, with the feeling that it is possible to make solid progress toward solving the "central problem of insect sociology."

Acknowledgements. The research reported in this review has been supported by National Science Foundation grant BNS-8105391.

References

(1) Boch, R. 1956. Die Tänze der Bienen bei nahen und fernen Trachtquellen. Z. vergl. Physiol. 38: 136-167.

(2) Cheverton, J.; Kacelnik, A.; and Krebs, J.R. 1985. Optimal foraging: constraints and currencies. Fort. Zool. 31: 109-126.

(3) Free, J.B. 1960. The behaviour of honeybees visiting the flowers of fruit trees. J. Anim. Ecol. 29: 385-395.

(4) Frisch, K. von. 1923. Über die "Sprache" der Bienen, ein tierpsychologische Untersuchung. Zool. Jb. (Physiol). 40: 1-186.

(5) Frisch, K. von. 1934. Über den Geschmackssinn der Bienen. Z. vergl. Physiol. 21: 1-156.

(6) Frisch, K. von. 1967. The Dance Language and Orientation of Bees. Cambridge: Harvard University Press.

(7) Frisch, K. von, and Lindauer, M. 1955. Über die Fluggeschwindigkeit der Bienen und ihre Richtungsweisung bei Seitenwind. Naturwissenscnaften 42: 377-385.

(8) Heinrich, B. 1978. The economics of insect sociality. In Behavioural Ecology: An Evolutionary Approach, eds. J.R. Krebs and N.B. Davies, pp 97-129. Sunderland, Mass.: Sinauer Associated Press.

(9) Kacelnik, A., and Houston, A.I. 1984. Some effects of energy costs on foraging strategies. Anim. Behav. 32: 609-614.

(10) Kappel, I. 1953. Die Form des Safthalters als Anreiz für die Sammeltätigkeit der Bienen. Z. vergl. Physiol. 34: 539-546.

(11) Krebs, J.R.; Stephens, D.W.; and Sutherland, W.J. 1983. Perspectives in optimal foraging. In Perspectives in Ornithology, eds. A.H. Brush and G.A. Clark, pp 165-216. New York: Cambridge University Press.

(12) Lindauer, M. 1948. Über die Einwirkung von Duft- und Geschmacksstoffen sowie anderer Faktoren auf die Tänze der Bienen. Z. vergl. Physiol. 31: 348-412.

(13) Lindauer, M. 1954. Temperaturregulierung und Wasserhaushalt im Bienenstaat. Z. vergl. Physiol. 36: 391-342.

(14) Lindauer, M. 1955. Schwarmbienen auf Wohnungssuche Z. vergl. Physiol. 37: 263-324.

(15) Lindauer, M. 1961. Communication among Social Bees. Cambridge: Harvard University Press.

(16) Markl, H. 1985. Manipulation, modulation, information, cognition: some of the riddles of communication. Fort. Zool. 31: 163-194.

(17) Núnez, J.A. 1966. Quantitative Beziehungen zwischen den Eigenschaften von Futterquellen und dem Verhalten von Sammelbienen. Z. vergl. Physiol. 53: 142-146.

(18) Núnez, J.A. 1970. The relationship between sugar flow and foraging and recruiting behavior of honey bees (Apis mellifera L.). Anim. Behav. 18: 527-538.

(19) Núnez, J.A. 1982. Honeybee foraging strategies at a food source in relation to its distance from the hive and the rate of sugar flow. J. Apic. Res. 21: 139-150.

(20) Parker, R.L. 1926. The collection and utilization of pollen by the honeybee. Cornell Univ. Agric. Expt. Sta. Mem. 98: 1-55.

(21) Pyke, G.H.; Pulliam, H.R.; and Charnov, E.L. 1977. Optimal foraging: a selective review of theory and tests. Q. Rev. Biol. 52: 137-154.

(22) Rinderer, T.E. 1982. Regulated nectar harvesting by the honeybee. J. Apic. Res. 21: 74-87.

(23) Rinderer, T.E. 1983. Regulation of honey bee hoarding efficiency. Apidologie 14: 87-92.

(24) Schmid, J. 1964. Zur Frage der Störung des Bienengedächtnisses durch Narkosemittel, zugleich ein Beitrag zur Störung der Sozialen Bindung durch Narkose. Z. vergl. Physiol. 47: 559-595.

(25) Schmid-Hempel, P.; Kacelnik, A.; and Houston, A.I. 1985. Honeybees maximize efficiency by not filling their crop. Behav. Ecol. Sociobiol. 17: 61-66.

(26) Schmid-Hempel, P. 1986. Efficient nectar-collecting by honeybees. I. Economic models. J. Anim. Ecol. In press.

(27) Schuà, L. 1952. Untersuchungen über die Einfluss meteorologische Elemente auf das Verhalten der Bienen. Z. vergl. Physiol. 34: 258-277.

(28) Seeley, T.D. 1983. Division of labor between scouts and recruits in honeybee foraging. Behav. Ecol. Sociobiol. 12: 253-259.

(29) Seeley, T.D. 1985a. The information-center strategy of honeybee foraging. Fort. Zool. 31: 75-90.

(30) Seeley, T.D. 1985b. Honeybee Ecology. A Study of Adaptation in Social Life. Princeton: Princeton University Press.

(31) Seeley, T.D. 1986. Social foraging by honeybees: how colonies allocate foragers among patches of flowers. Behav. Ecol. Sociobiol. In press.

(32) Simon, H.A. 1962. The architecture of complexity. Proc. Amer. Phil. Soc. 106: 467-482.

(33) Visscher, P.K. and Seeley, T.D. 1982. Foraging strategy of honeybee colonies in a temperate deciduous forest. Ecology 63: 1790-1801.

(34) Waddington, K.D. 1982. Honeybee foraging profitability and round dance correlates. J. Comp. Physiol. 148: 297-301.

(35) Waddington, K.D. 1985. Cost-intake information used in foraging. J. Insect Physiol.31: 891-897.

(36) Waddington, K.D. and L.R. Holden. 1979. Optimal foraging: on flower selection by bees. Amer. Nat. 114: 179-196.

(37) Wilson, E.O. 1971. The Insect Societies. Cambridge: Harvard University Press.

New Perspectives on the Dance Orientation of the Asian Honeybees

Fred C. Dyer
Department of Zoology, Michigan State University, East Lansing, Michigan 48824, USA

Abstract. Several recent studies of the Asian honeybees, Apis florea, A. dorsata, and A. cerana, have greatly extended our understanding of dance orientation in honeybees. From early studies, the dances of A. florea and A. dorsata were thought to be somewhat primitive in comparison with those of the other species of Apis. Now it is clear that each exhibits capabilities of information processing that are no less sophisticated than any seen in A. cerana and in the European species, A. mellifera. Apis dorsata forages on moonlit nights, even by the light of a half moon, and performs waggle dances that are oriented not to the moon but instead apparently to the hidden sun. Apis florea, once thought to be capable of orienting dances only in the horizontal plane and in the presence of celestial cues, can actually orient without a view of the sun and blue sky by referring to landmarks visible from the exposed dance area. Furthermore, A. florea will dance on steep, even vertical, slopes. In such dances a bee continues to orient to the horizontal projections of celestial cues, instead of to their projections onto the plane on which she is dancing (as the other species do if presented with celestial cues during a vertical dance). In addition to raising a host of new questions about the mechanisms underlying the dances of A. florea and A. dorsata, these results challenge previous assumptions about the evolution of the dance language in Apis.

INTRODUCTION

Martin Lindauer's insightful early studies of dance orientation in the honeybees of Asia (13) revealed striking differences among these three species and the European bee, Apis mellifera (reviewed in 8, 14). The differences in the dances parallelled differences in nesting behavior, and on the basis of these two lines of comparison, Lindauer proposed that the extant species of Apis exhibit modern evidence of a phylogenetic progression in the honeybee dance language. Specifically, the little bee, A. florea, was thought to be primitive in both nesting behavior and dance orientation. This species builds exposed nests consisting of a single sheet of comb suspended from a small branch in a tree or shrub. Its recruitment dances are usually performed only in an approximately horizontal plane--on a rounded extension of the comb above the branch--and only in the presence of celestial orientation cues (the sun and polarized skylight). Von Frisch (8) established that A. mellifera can orient horizontal dances to celestial cues; however it normally dances on vertical surfaces, indicating the location of food through a transposition of light and gravity such that the angle of a waggle run relative to the upward direction encodes the angle of the forager's flight relative to the sun. This form of dance orientation was assumed to be evolutionarily advanced, as was the nesting behavior of A. mellifera: colonies inhabit dark cavities, building several parallel, vertical honey combs, where the dances are performed. Lindauer found that the Asian hive bee, A. cerana, closely resembles A. mellifera in both its nesting behavior and its dances. However, he placed the giant honeybee, A. dorsata, at an intermediate phylogenetic position. Although dances of this species are performed in a vertical plane and have the same relationship with gravity as A. mellifera's and A. cerana's, its nests consist of single exposed combs similar to A. florea's (albeit much larger and lacking a flattened upper surface). Furthermore, Lindauer observed bees to dance only on the parts of the nest that were exposed to a view of the sky, and he could stop their dancing by blocking the sky from view. Hence A. dorsata dancers seemed to resemble A. florea in being dependent upon a view of the sky. Figure 1 illustrates some of the differences among the Apis species in nesting and dancing behavior.

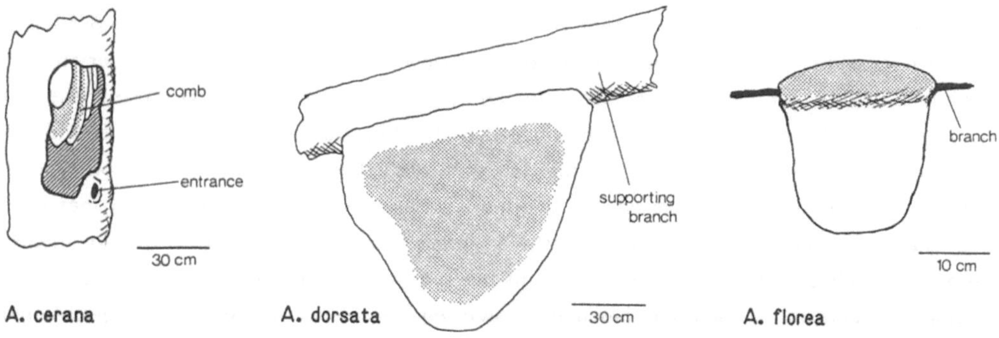

FIG. 1 - Nests of each of the Asian honeybee species. Stippled area indicates the region on the comb where dances are performed. The nest of the European bee, A. mellifera, is very similar to that of A. cerana.

Recent studies inspired by Lindauer's original work have revealed hidden complexities in the dances of A. florea and A. dorsata, and as a consequence, have sharpened our assumptions regarding the origin and subsequent evolution of the dance language. As envisaged by Lindauer, the dance first arose in a bee which, like A. florea, nested on an exposed comb, and originally consisted of excited movements on a horizontal platform which were crudely oriented with respect to celestial cues used on the flight. Subsequently, the dance was modified to incorporate, in all species but A. florea, the ability to transpose light and gravity and to dance on a vertical surface. Apis dorsata was thought to represent a transitional form still somewhat dependent upon celestial cues. The most advanced form of the dance presumably would have provided bees the flexibility to dance when no celestial cues were visible from the nest, and ultimately permitted the progenitors of A. mellifera and A. cerana to move into cavities. Despite some objections (10), Lindauer's hypothesis concerning the origin of dance communication seems highly credible. The results in this paper, which are based largely upon my studies in India (1-3; see also 9), bear upon his suggestions concerning subsequent evolutionary changes in the dance. I will show that the dances of A. dorsata and, in particular, A. florea cannot be viewed merely as contemporary representatives of simpler forms of dance communication on a linear scale of complexity culminating in the dance of A. mellifera. Instead, each is capable of complicated, but previously undetected, feats of orientation. Hence, these findings both open new questions about the mechanisms of information processing underlying the dances of the Asian honeybees and clarify the interspecific differences that any evolutionary speculations must address.

DANCE ORIENTATION ON CLOUDY DAYS

The supposed primitiveness of A. florea was inferred from its apparent dependence upon a view of celestial cues during the dance. Such a dependence would suggest that dance communication should be impaired when the sky is overcast, and so an important implication of Lindauer's observations (13) was that a need for flexibility in the dance may have led to the incorporation of gravity as a more reliable reference for dance orientation. But a bee that dances under a cloudy sky may well have just flown under one. An ability to orient her dances to gravity--or to any other non-celestial reference--would be of little use if she had no way of locating the sun on the flight since it is the direction of flight relative to the sun that is the information conveyed by the dance. Thus, these two steps in the process of orienting a dance have to be considered together. I have shown with A. mellifera that bees are unable to see celestial cues directly on most overcast days, but can nevertheless determine their direction of flight relative to the sun by referring to a memory of the sun's course in relation to familiar landmarks seen en route to the food (4). Directional information obtained in this way on the flight is expressed in dances oriented to gravity. Subsequently, I found A. cerana to exhibit identical orientation behavior on overcast days, underlining the similiarity between this species and A. mellifera (1).

Broad features of the landscape are probably widely used by insects as a frame of reference for learning about solar movement (5). Hence both A. florea and A. dorsata presumably share with A. mellifera and A. cerana the ability to obtain information about the sun's position relative to their line of flight when they have flown under a cloud cover. However, according to Lindauer's observations (13), A. florea should be unable to communicate this information in dances under overcast skies, and A. dorsata's communication may also be partially or wholly disrupted. Lindauer's studies were essentially preliminary in their scope, and the more recent work discussed here focuses on new discoveries concerning A. florea's and A. dorsata's orientation under conditions in which celestial cues are obscured or otherwise changed.

NOCTURNAL ORIENTATION OF APIS DORSATA

Koeniger and Koeniger (11) were the first to show that A. dorsata dancers are undisturbed when deprived of a view of the sky. I have also observed well oriented dances on colonies hanging from an arched ceiling from which no sky could be seen, but I obtained even more dramatic evidence of the sophistication of A. dorsata's information processing abilities when I discovered this species to fly and dance at night. At one low-nesting colony that I watched in South India, foragers flew from the nest in large numbers on moonlit nights, and upon returning they performed consistently oriented dances to natural sources of nectar and pollen (2). In the distances and directions indicated, these dances sorted into a few obvious, discrete groups, and since dancers indicating the same information carried the same species of pollen, I concluded that the groups referred to different floral patches in the landscape, each probably a single flowering tree.

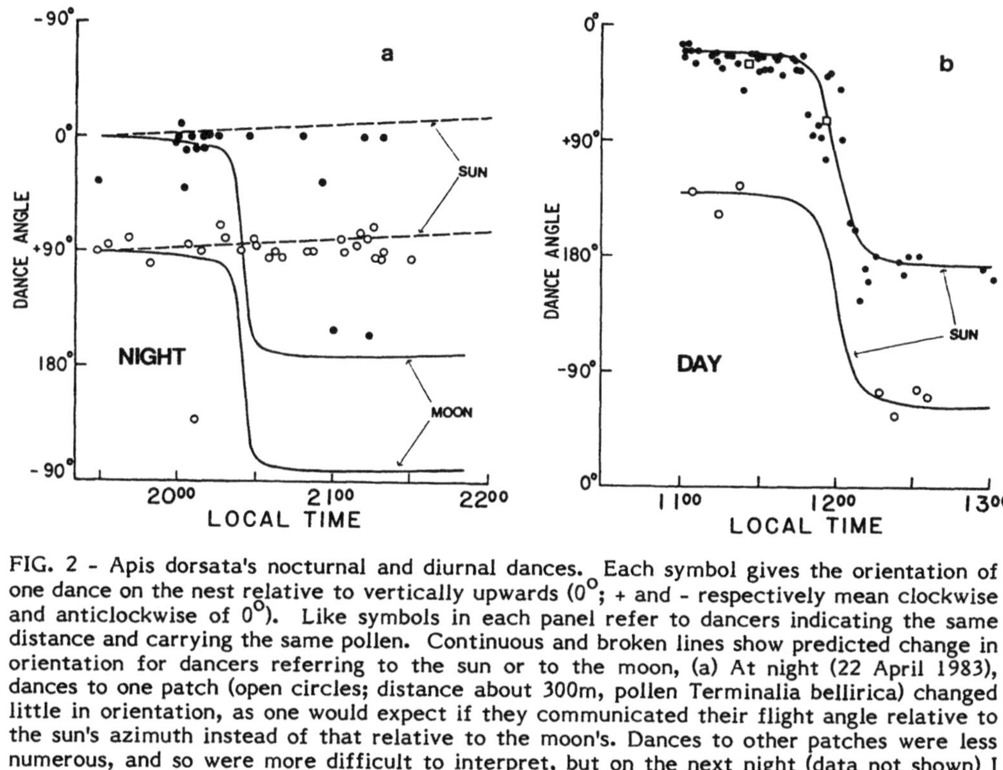

FIG. 2 - Apis dorsata's nocturnal and diurnal dances. Each symbol gives the orientation of one dance on the nest relative to vertically upwards (0°; + and - respectively mean clockwise and anticlockwise of 0°). Like symbols in each panel refer to dancers indicating the same distance and carrying the same pollen. Continuous and broken lines show predicted change in orientation for dancers referring to the sun or to the moon, (a) At night (22 April 1983), dances to one patch (open circles; distance about 300m, pollen Terminalia bellirica) changed little in orientation, as one would expect if they communicated their flight angle relative to the sun's azimuth instead of that relative to the moon's. Dances to other patches were less numerous, and so were more difficult to interpret, but on the next night (data not shown) I observed the same tendency of dances not to shift with lunar movement. (b) During the day (3 May 1983), dances to two sites did change rapidly as the sun's azimuth shifted rapidly along the horizon at noon. For further details see Ref. 2.

With this assumption I could examine what celestial reference provides the basis for communication in nocturnal dances. Since the light of the moon is apparently necessary for bees to forage at night (2), one obvious possibility was that foragers monitor their direction of flight relative to the moon's azimuth, and then express this angle in their dance angle relative to gravity. Alternatively, by analogy with the behavior of A. mellifera and A. cerana on cloudy days, nocturnal foragers might rely upon the sun to obtain information for use in the dance, even though it is not visible. For example, during the flight, bees could measure their bearing relative to familiar features of the landscape, and then by reference to the point of sunset, they could extend their memory of the sun's movement into the night. Over periods at night when the moon's azimuth shifted rapidly, but the sun's azimuth (actual or extrapolated from solar movement before sunset) changed little, I observed that dances indicating a specific floral patch did not shift, and therefore must have referred to the sun and not the moon (Fig. 2). Many questions remain concerning the mechanism underlying A. dorsata's nocturnal orientation (2). However, it is clear at least that the ability of this species to obtain information on the flight about the sun's position and then to orient its dances is no less sophisticated than what is observed in A. mellifera and A. cerana on cloudy days, and may even be more complicated in some ways.

ORIENTATION OF A. FLOREA'S DANCES TO LANDMARKS

Although Lindauer found that A. florea dancers were disoriented when he denied them a view of the sun and blue sky, Koeniger et al. (12), using slightly different techniques, successfully induced bees to continue dancing with consistent orientation when no celestial references were visible. I confirmed this finding in a series of experiments, which also were designed to determine what environmental references, if not celestial ones, were responsible for the orientation of the dancers (3). When I blocked the sky from the view of the dancers on the top of the nest, they continued to align their waggle runs according to their previous orientation relative to landmarks visible from the nest. When I shifted the position of a conspicuous striped pattern that I had placed next to the nest, the orientation of the dancers shifted by a corresponding degree (Fig. 3). Although in some experiments bees oriented ambiguously to the pattern, they oriented exclusively to it and not to other possible references. For example, their dance orientation over the series of experiments was independent of the actual compass bearing of the feeding station that they were indicating, and was independent of the topography of the surface on which they danced, ruling out slope as a reference by itself. Moreover, when I provided neither landmarks nor celestial cues, dancers were completely disoriented.

I frequently observed A. florea to dance with good orientation on overcast days. In this species, as in the other, the dancer indicates the angle she has flown relative to the sun, and hence she can presumably locate the sun's azimuth in relation to landmarks seen en route if celestial cues are not available. However, whereas the other species communicate this information in a waggle dance relative to gravity, an A. florea dancer, as my results show, orients her dances to landmarks near the nest. Such landmarks are likely to be completely different from those used on the flight, since nests are generally built in dense vegetation (16). For the dances to be meaningful, as they apparently are since A. florea can recruit effectively on overcast days, dancers and dance followers both must be able to locate the sun's position relative to the panorama of landmarks visible from the nest. Then, once they fly from the nest and these landmarks are no longer visible, bees must locate the sun by reference to a different panorama of landmarks on their way to the food.

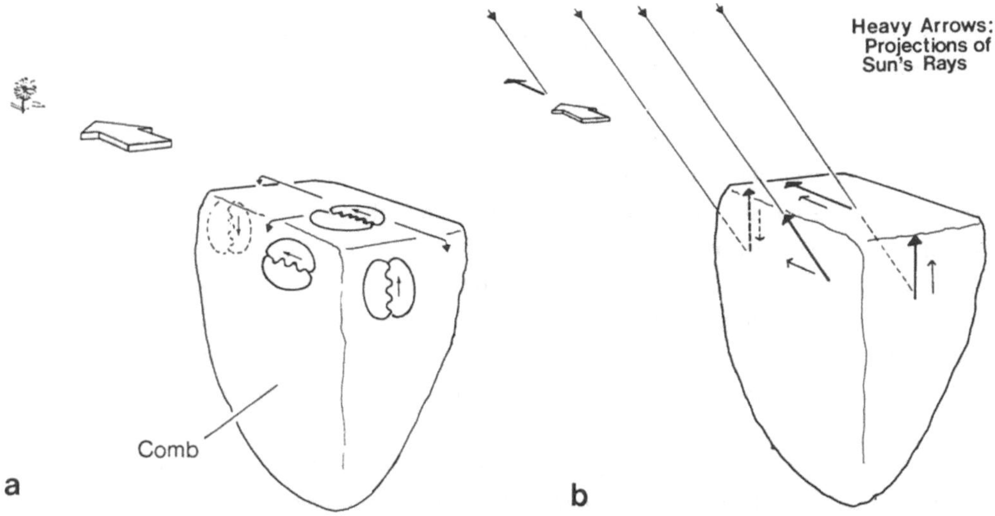

FIG. 3 - Dances on top of A. florea nest (viewed from above) relative to the direction of the food (vector F), comb orientation, and a striped pattern positioned near the nest (horizontal angle, 135°; height, 30cm. Open vector gives mean angle of distribution, in which smallest bar is 1 waggle run. (a) Dancers have view of blue sky during dance. (b) Sky blocked from view. (c) Sky still not visible, and pattern rotated 90° anticlockwise. Dance angles changed relative to original compass direction and original slope on comb, but were not different from the orientation relative to the pattern in a and b. From Ref. 3.

These new findings raise the quesion of whether the other species of Apis are capable of such behavior under unusual circumstances (the others would certainly never need to orient their dances to terrestrial references since gravity is normally always available). Whatever the answer to this question, at least we can be certain that A. florea's dance incorporates specializations which endow it with some of the flexibility that the other species of Apis enjoy by virtue of their ability to transpose light and gravity and, therefore, to dance without direct reference to celestial cues. However, it seems likely that A. florea's system of orientation still constrains its nesting behavior. Since dances in relation to landmarks are only meaningful insofar as they can be related to the sun's position, nests would have to be constructed in sites from which dancers could occasionally see at least part of the sky. I have observed this invariably to be true in India, even for colonies that have nested inside rotted tree trunks or under the eaves of houses. In Oman, A. florea frequently nests in shallow rock caves although the original reports of these nesting sites (reviewed in Ref. 7) provide no detailed evidence as to whether they are exposed to the sky, the colonies are easily photographed from the outside, and so the sites presumably are usually sufficiently open to provide dancers with celestial references. Still, a systematic study of dance orientation in such colonies would be of considerable interest (7).

APIS FLOREA'S DANCES ON SLOPES

When Lindauer (13) prevented A. florea dancers from reaching the near-horizontal upper surface of the nest, so that they had to dance on the vertical sides of the colony, he observed that they either were disoriented or were oriented in a way that was not easy to account for. In my own preliminary observations, I often saw consistently oriented dances on steep, even vertical, slopes. Because these dancers had flown to a feeder in a known location, I could easily confirm Lindauer's conclusion that A. florea does not transpose light and gravity to orient in a way that the other species of Apis do (3). An alternative possibility, since the dancers could see the sky, was that they orient on an inclined surface so as to match their view of celestial cues with that which they remember from the flight or from a dance on the upper surface of the nest. This is how A. mellifera orients its dances on a vertical plane if presented with a view of the sky; the sun/gravity transposition rule is ignored and the dancer simply aligns herself relative to the projection of the sun onto that plane in the way she would be aligned relative to the solar azimuth in the horizontal plane (6, 8).

Apparently A. florea orients according to yet a different set of rules. I performed a series of experiments (3) in which bees were allowed to dance only on one vertical flank of the nest, which was then rotated so that the dancers on it were exposed to different views of the same patch of sky. The bees exhibited a striking pattern of orientation which did not change as the sun moved, as would be expected of both of the mechanisms by which the other species can orient on slopes (sun/gravity transposition and matching). Instead, the orientation depended only upon the position of the vertical plane in relation to the direction of flight. Fig. 4a summarizes the pattern of dance orientation that I observed in these experiments.

Significantly, the same pattern of orientation can commonly be seen in dances on most natural colonies. Because of the tendency of dancers to advance slightly with each waggle run in the direction being indicated (12), they move over slopes of various inclinations on the vaulted nest (see Fig. 1) during the same dance. Let us follow a fairly typical dance from start to finish. A returning forager may land on any part of the nest; we will consider a bee that lands on the side opposite the source of food she has just visited. If her dance begins immediately, each waggle run is aligned directly up the slope, no matter what the position of the sun. As mentioned, the dancer moves forward with each waggle run, and so her dance soon brings her to the top of the nest. At this point she is on a more or less horizontal plane, and her waggle runs are aligned exactly with the direction of the food, in the orientation one would also expect of any of the other species on a horizontal surface. After she moves over the crest of the comb, her waggle runs are oriented down the incline, and when she finally reaches the side of the nest closest to the food, she may be dancing on a nearly vertical plane again, but now with each waggle run oriented exactly downwards. Sometimes a forager lands and begins dancing on a surface that is aligned approximately in the same direction as her flight to the food (see Fig. 4a). In this case, or in the case of a dancer that marches over the upper surface of the nest to one side of its highest point, each waggle run is always aligned approximately towards the direction of the food source, and hence is inclined relative to the direction of the slope.

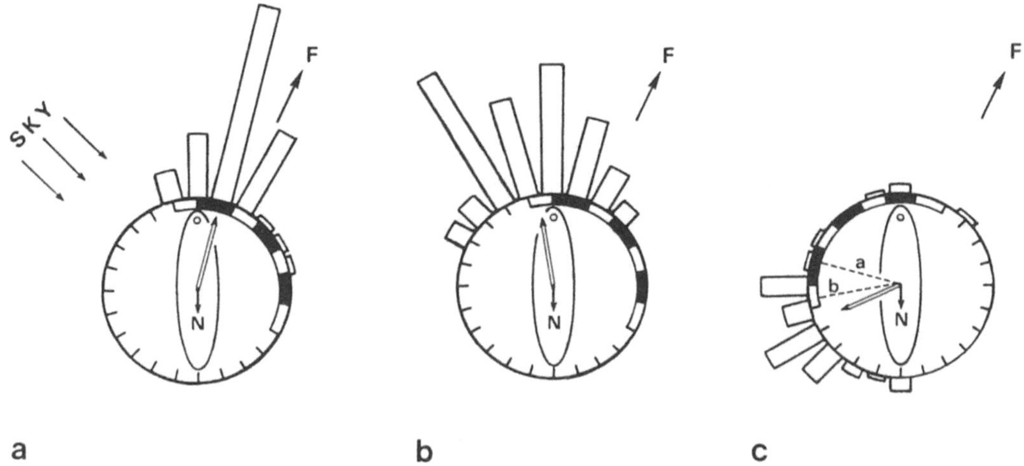

FIG. 4 - (a) Schematic summary of experiments (in September 1983) which revealed A. florea's pattern of dance orientation on different vertical planes relative to the direction of flight (large open arrow), and in relation to the orientation of a dance in the horizontal plane. This pattern is essentially identical no matter what the position of the sun. (b) The same pattern of dance orientation (light arrows on comb), shown with sun's azimuth in direction of flight, to contrast A. florea's dances with A. mellifera's expected orientation on the same planes. The latter tends to orient waggle runs to the sun's projection, on whatever plane, so as to match the view of the sun with that seen during the flight (6). In this case, A. mellifera would orient in the direction of the heavy arrows, and on all planes would see the sun "straight ahead;" in some cases A. florea's view of the sun seems to be exactly opposite, although in other cases it is similar. Adapted from Ref. 3.

The contrast between this pattern of orientation and that exhibited by the other honeybee species during orientation to celestial cues (as inferred from studies on A. mellifera: 6, 8) is shown in Fig. 4b. First, as mentioned, the pattern of orientation on vertical planes by A. florea does not change with the movement of the sun, even though the sun is used for orientation, while the other species do shift their dance orientation so as to maintain a current match with the solar angle seen during the flight. Hence, A. mellifera's pattern of orientation with the sun in a different position from that in Fig. 4b would be different, while A. florea's would be the same. Moreover, A. florea's system will in some cases expose the dancer to a veiw of celestial references that is very different from what she had during the flight, and different from what A. mellifera dancers would experience by their system of sensory matching on a vertical plane. In Fig. 4b the difference is most apparent on the side of the comb nearest the food. As a final point, note that A. mellifera's system of orientation to celestial cues on a vertical plane results in orientation that is very close (always less than 90°) to the orientation that is expected when gravity is substituted as a reference for the sun (upward dances expected on all vertical planes in Fig. 4b). Apis florea's orientation may differ by 180° from this expected direction.

How then does A. florea set a dance angle on a slope? One clue is evident in the close relationship between the pattern of dance orientation on inclined surfaces and the orientation in a horizontal plane. Consider the example in Fig. 4a. Imagine rotating the horizontal plane to each of the three vertical planes while maintaining the angle of the dance relative to the axis of rotation. In each case the resulting dance orientation would be identical to that observed. Or, consider the bee described earlier that moved over various non-vertical slopes during her dance. If one projects the vector described by any waggle run to the horizontal plane, its orientation is the same as that of a waggle run actually performed on a perfectly horizontal surface. This relationship suggests that A. florea dancers reference their waggling angle to the horizontal world even when on a slope, instead of simply orienting to obtain the best sensory match of celestial information projected to whatever plane they find themselves on, as A. mellifera does (6). To accomplish this, a bee must compensate for the different views her eyes have of celestial references during dances on different inclines. Perhaps she integrates gravitational information with visual information to make this compensation. Alternatively, perhaps she simply rotates her head during the dance to keep it fixed as well as possible with respect to the horizontal plane as she orients to celestial cues, and thereby determines her body orientation on a particular slope. In any event, A. florea obviously responds to celestial cues very differently on non-horizontal planes from the way A. mellifera and the other species do.

DIVERGENT SYSTEMS OF DANCE ORIENTATION

These results modify our understanding of the differences among the dances of the four species of Apis in two important ways. First, A. dorsata's system of dance orientation is very similar to that of A. mellifera and A. cerana, and is certainly not hindered by the absence of celestial orientation cues. In fact, its ability to perform dances that refer to the sun at night implies considerable sophistication in the underlying information processing, though this may simply involve an extension of the ability, already documented in A. mellifera and A. cerana (1, 4), to compensate by memory for the sun's movement during long overcast periods. The specializations that permit A. dorsata's nocturnal activities may actually be visual ones; the other Asian species (unpublished observations) as well as the Italian race of A. mellifera (2) all have difficulty flying by the light of the moon. Second, A. florea's system of dance orientation is obviously not simply a restricted, primitive version of that seen in the three other species (3). Instead, it has diverged from the others, and this divergence seems to involve fundamental differences in the way celestial and gravitational information is processed. Both modern systems of dance orientation, of course, refer to flight orientation in relation to the azimuthal projections of celestial cues. Apis florea's dances continue to be oriented to the same horizontal frame of reference, even if the dancer is on a different slope or cannot see the sky and must use celestial cues via reference to the landmarks near the nest. Dancers of the three other species, on the other hand, all shift their frame of reference to the plane on which they are dancing, whether orienting to projections of celestial cues or to the projection of the gravity vector (6). Furthermore, the orientation of A. florea's waggle dances on overcast days seems to depend upon dancers and recruits memorizing the course of the sun in relation to two arrays of landmarks, those seen on the flight and those near the nest. Apis mellifera and A. cerana are only known to use the former.

CONCLUSION

I conclude by summarizing how these findings affect our thinking about the origin and evolution of the honeybee dance. First, as mentioned, it still seems reasonable to assume that the original Apis dance was, like A. florea's, performed on a horizontal portion of an exposed nest (13). Koeniger (10) has disputed this assumption, arguing that since there are no extant social bees that nest in the open, this nesting behavior must be a derived condition unique to A. florea and A. dorsata. Koeniger presents various other arguments in support of the hypothesis that the original dance actually occurred in dark cavities, and was oriented to gravity. However, much about the social behavior of Apis is unique (15), and indeed eusociality itself may have arisen independently on the phylogenetic line that led to honeybees (17), so it is not hard to imagine that the precursor to today's Apis was unique among bees in nesting in the open. More important, the orientation of horizontal dances shows very clear links to the mechanisms of orientation used in flight by bees and other insects (5). Since all four species can use these mechanisms on a horizontal plane (including A. dorsata (1), which normally never dances on a horizontal), while only A. florea lacks the ability to translate the flight angle into a dance relative to gravity, it seems most reasonable to interpret the gravity-based system as derived. It is less easy to imagine A. florea having this elaborate set of behavioral mechanisms and then losing it than it is to conclude that for some reason an evolutionary divergence led to A. florea's acquistion of a different set of additions to the basic system of dance orientation in the horizontal plane.

Ever since Lindauer's pioneering work (13), most speculations about the evolution of the honeybee dance have focused upon how and why the ability to substitute gravity as a reference for the sun evolved from dances that were primitively horizontal. Traditionally, it has been assumed that this ability provided the flexibility needed so that communication could occur on cloudy days, or so that the dance language could work in a nest built in a dark cavity (8, 14). The directional frame of reference in the gravity-based dance--in which a waggle run vertically upwards signifies a flight towards the sun's azimuth--has been explained as a derivative of the behavioral equivalence between positive phototaxis and negative geotaxis that many insects exhibit (8). However, it is difficult to reconcile these ideas with our new understanding of the Asian bees--particularly A. florea. For example, A. florea's system of orientation to landmarks seems inherently no less well suited to communication on overcast days than the gravity-based system exhibited by the other species. Furthermore, in A. florea's dances on inclined planes when celestial cues are available, waggle runs often deviate markedly from the orientation expected if there were an intrinsic equivalence of positive phototaxis and negative geotaxis. Hence these new findings support the notion that the orientation system seen in A. florea must be very different from the original dance language whose evolutionary modification led also to the system exhibited by the other species of Apis. Now the question of how and why the original dance language was modified must address two different general results.

My intention here is not to solve these various evolutionary riddles, but instead to highlight what appear to be two incompatible systems of information processing in the extant dance languages of honeybees. The two systems clearly share a common heritage. In Thailand, recently, I induced A. cerana foragers to join an A. florea colony, collect sugar syrup from a nearby feeder, then perform dances that were followed by their heterospecific nest-mates. These two species must, therefore, share a constellation of behavioral signals and motor patterns involved in recognizing nest-mates, soliciting food from a returning forager, inducing the forager to commence dancing, and circling in tandem with the dancer. The A. florea followers were even recruited to the feeder a few meters away; although they could have used olfactory cues to find the food, at least they were successfully alerted to its presence and induced to search. Superimposed upon these similarities, however, are the profound differences that I have already discussed. It seems almost certain that in dances to a distant feeding site during cloudy weather or on certain vertical planes, such interspecific communication could result in considerable confusion.

More experiments are necessary to dissect further the mechanisms of information processing underlying the dance orientation of each of the Apis species. Already an experimental analysis combined with interspecific comparisons has both exposed more clearly the design of the orientation systems of the bees, and sharpened certain evolutionary questions. Further studies could reveal additional differences among the four species, but they could also reveal latent similarities. Either outcome would futher clarifly our understanding of the behavioral system that is among the most remarkable that evolution has produced.

Acknowledgements. I thank T.D. Seeley and R.A. Levien for valuable comments on the manuscript. The Smithsonian Institution and the Fulbright Foundation supported my studies in India. The National Science Foundation and a Seesel-Anonymous Grant (Yale University) supported the preparation of the manuscript.

REFERENCES

(1) Dyer, F.C. 1984. Comparative Studies of the Dance Language and Orientation of Four Species of Honey Bees. Ph.D. Thesis, Princeton University.

(2) Dyer, F.C. 1985. Nocturnal orientation of the Asian honey bee, Apis dorsata. Anim. Behav. 33: 769-774.

(3) Dyer, F.C. 1985. Mechanisms of dance orientation in the Asian honey bee, Apis florea. J. Comp. Physiol. A 157: 183-198.

(4) Dyer, F.C., and Gould, J.L. 1981. Honey bee orientation: a backup system for cloudy days. Science 214: 1041-1042.

(5) Dyer, F.C., and Seeley, T.D. 1987. Orientation and foraging in honey bees. In Insect Flight, eds. G.C. Goldsworthy and C.H. Wheeler. Cleveland, Ohio: CRC Press, in press.

(6) Edrich, W. 1977. Interaction of light and gravity in the orientation of the waggle dance of honey bees. Anim. Behav. 25: 342-363.

(7) Free, J.B. 1982. The biology and behaviour of the honeybee Apis florea. In Social Insects in the Tropics, ed. P. Jaisson, pp. 181-187. Université Paris-Nord.

(8) Frisch, K.v. 1967. The Dance Language and Orientation of Bees. Cambridge, Mass.: Belknap/Harvard.

(9) Gould, J.L.; Dyer, F.C.; and Towne, W.F. 1985. Recent progress in the study of the dance language. Fortschr. Zool. 31: 141-161.

(10) Koeniger, N. 1976. Neue Aspekte der Phylogenie innerhalb der Gattung Apis. Apidologie 7: 357-366.

(11) Koeniger, N., and Koeniger, G. 1980. Observations and experiments on migration and dance communication of Apis dorsata in Sri Lanka. J. Apic. Res. 19: 21-34.

(12) Koeniger, N.; Koeniger, G.; Punchihewa, R.K.W.; Fabritius, Mo.; and Fabritius, Mi. 1982. Observations and experiments on dance communication of Apis florea in Sri Lanka. J. Apic. Res. 21: 45-52.

(13) Lindauer, M. 1956. Über die Verständigung bei indischen Bienen. Z. vergl. Physiol. 38: 521-557.

(14) Lindauer, M. 1961. Communication Among Social Bees. Cambridge, Mass.: Belknap/Harvard.

(15) Sakagami, S.F. 1971. Ethosoziologischer Vergleich zwischen Honigbienen und stachellosen Bienen. Z. Tierpsychol. 28: 337-350.

(16) Seeley, T.D.; Seeley, R.H.; and Akratanakul, P. 1982. Colony defense strategies of the honey bees in Thailand. Ecol. Monogr. 52: 43-63.

(17) Winston, M.L., and Michener, C.D. 1977. Dual origin of highly social behavior among bees. Proc. Nat. Acad. Sci. USA 74: 1135-1137.

Perception of Foraging Costs and Intakes, and Foraging Decisions

Keith D. Waddington

Department of Biology, University of Miami, Coral Gables, FL 33124, USA

Abstract. Honeybees use information acquired in the field and in the hive to make foraging decisions. I review recent work designed to understand bees' perceptions of foraging costs and intakes and the use of this information for making foraging decisions. Findings include: 1) costs are weighted in relation to intakes, 2) perceptions of costs are more variable than those of intakes, and 3) individuals vary in their perceptions. Information on costs and intakes is used by bees to choose among flowers and to plot a path through a single-species patch of flowers.

INTRODUCTION

Foraging is a complex behavior for which many of an animal's facilities come to bear. Information is received and processed, and decisions and responses are made. The studies of honeybees by Karl von Frisch and his colleagues on sensory physiology, learning, memory, orientation and navigation were aimed at understanding general principles of animal physiology and behavior, but their work is the solid foundation on which we now extend work on foraging behavior.

Scout bees leave the hive to search for food and return loaded with nectar and pollen and a nervous system full of new information. Landmarks are learned and a locale "map" constructed so that the bee can navigate between hive and field. The bee learns associations between colors, shapes and, scents of flowers and quantity and quality of food inside the flowers. Flowers have different morphologies that require different motor patterns to be learned through trial and error for acquiring food. All of this information and more is used to choose between flowers of different species, plot a path between flowers in a patch, choose when to leave a patch for another or for the hive, and to make other decisions.

The purpose of this paper is to focus on a line of inquiry that attempts to understand and predict some aspects of foraging behavior based on the energetics of foraging. During the past quarter century, the "energetics" approach has been a major focus of behavioral ecologists for studying foraging behavior of numerous species (9). I will summarize the recent history of this approach. Then, three questions are addressed: 1) what is a foraging bee's schedule of actual costs and intakes? 2) what is the nature of perceptions of these costs and intakes? 3) how is information on costs and intakes used to make some foraging decisions?

PROXIMATE AND ULTIMATE CAUSATION

Much work in behavioral ecology is aimed at assessing how and to what extent animals articulate beneficial and detrimental aspects of their environment in order to make decisions. Often the researcher's quest is to determine the payoffs and costs associated with performing alternative behavioral patterns. This is a view of behavior from an ecological perspective that helps us understand the evolution of behavior by natural selection. Niko Tinbergen was the early champion of the "natural selection" approach to studying behavior. That removal of egg shells from the nest by adult herring gulls lowers risk of predation on chicks is a classic example of this approach. Tinbergen's experimental approach to studying ultimate causation of complex behavior has continued, but it has been supplemented by attempts to formalize evolutionary arguments using mathematical models. These models are based on the notion that complex behavior is molded by natural selection, given certain constraints (both real and imagined!), and they are used to predict the behavior that maximizes fitness.

Evolutionary models of foraging behavior begin with very general biological considerations and are usually used to make very general qualitative but sometimes quantitative predictions about performance (e.g. choice of food; 4). Predictions of foraging models have been tested using many taxa, but with mixed results in predicting behavior. The advantage of the modelling approach is that sometimes a considerable amount of variation in behavior is explained by using a relatively simple formulation. The main disadvantage is that when predictions and observations are discordant, little can be learned about the deviations. Several explanations of discrepancies are possible: 1) a simple assumption of the model is incorrect (e.g., the way food is encountered or assessed as to "value" is different from assumed; 2) an assumption has been omitted; 3) behavior is a compromise between maximizing food intake and other considerations such as predator avoidance; and 4) other, including historical considerations and drift.

Recently mathematical models have been used as frameworks for experimental work aimed at deciphering behavioral and physiological mechanisms which underlie foraging behavior. In some cases, the work is motivated by a hope to patch up an evolutionary model. Also, the resurgence of interest in mechanisms and experimental work is part of a general trend in behavior and ecology to pay more attention to what animals are actually doing and less attention to evolutionary models which are sometimes too vague and of limited long-term value. Gould and Marler (7) expressed it this way - "As biologists we are interested in the underlying mechanisms rather than in superficial "laws" which beg both physiological and evolutionary questions." This is an extreme view; a rewarding protocol might be to draw the best from both approaches. I have found mathematical models useful for orienting some questions on mechanisms.

ACTUAL COSTS AND INTAKES

Honeybees obtain nectar and pollen from many species of flowering plants. Nectar is the bees' primary source of energy. It consists primarily of sugars and water, but it may also contain trace quantities of amino acids, proteins, lipids, and other organic and inorganic compounds. The concentration of sugars (sucrose, glucose and fructose) in nectar and the volume of nectar per flower varies greatly within and between species of plants. Millions of returns are made to the colony, each bee carrying some 40 mg of nectar, in order to fuel the colony through the growing season and winter. Pollen serves as the major source of lipids, proteins, vitamins and minerals. Worker honeybees use pollen to produce rich glandular secretions which are fed to larvae.

Acquistion of nectar and pollen comes only with costs. Time and energy are spent during all foraging activities. Activities can be broadly divided into flight and non-flight. Flight costs of a bee weighing 0.1 g about 0.67 calories per minute and expenditure is independent of air temperature over a wide range of flight temperatures (metabolic rate is 80-85 ml O_2/g body weight/h and 1 ml of O_2 consumed is equivalent to about 5.0 calories expended; (8)). Energy expended to handle flowers (which is usually assumed equivalent to "resting" expenditures) varies with air temperature. Handling expenditures of thermoregulating bees at low air temperatures approximate light-expenditures. However, at 30°C a 0.1 g bee expends just 0.1 calorie per min (3).

Flight time and energy spent in flight during foraging are a function of distance to the floral patch, velocity of the wind, and distribution of plants and of flowers on plants. Handling costs are affected by floral morphology and the quantity and concentration of nectar. Scouts also use time and energy to perform the recruitment dance inside the hive.

In addition to the above "direct" costs of foraging which can be measured in time and energy, there are more difficult to measure, intangible costs. Foraging is a strenuous, physically demanding activity (compared with tending brood or cleaning cells) that results in wear and tear on the bee's structural and perhaps biochemical machinery. Neukirch (12) demonstrated that once a bee begins foraging it has a fixed total flight performance of about 800 km before it quite suddenly dies. Foragers may also be subject to considerable risk of predation and accidental death.

PERCEPTION OF COSTS AND INTAKES

No animal is better suited than the honeybee for studying perception of costs and intakes because honeybees communicate information on these parameters in their recruitment dance (6, 18). The dance, which can be quantified by a human observer, reflects the dancer's perception of its experience in the field. Frisch (6) and his colleagues studied perception of "profitability" using the waggle dance. Several aspects of the waggle dance vary with changes in costs and intakes: probability of dancing, duration of the dance, and frequency of acoustic bursts. These studies indicate that bees perceive information on intakes and costs such as sweetness, viscosity, quantity of nectar, and energy required to fly between hive and resource. Boch's (2) work on the waggle dance indicates that bees integrate information on costs and intakes. The greater the distance between a feeder containing sugar solution and the hive, the more concentrated must be the solution in order to release dancing.

Waddington (18) trained a bee to fly between two artifical flowers; handling and flight costs were manipulated as were intakes per floral visit. An aspect of the round dance, the rate that sharp turns were performed (called RATE), varied inversely with the costs to fly to a flower to suck sugar solution and directly with the caloric intake per visit. These results corroborate Boch's finding that bees integrate information on costs and intakes and encode the composite information in the dance. The question remains, what is a bee's formulation of this integration on costs and intakes?

Foraging models, in fact most models in behavioral ecology used to predict complex behavior, assume that costs and intakes are additive along the same scale. For instance, a bee foraging at a floral patch will perceive the patch as having profitability X. If the costs to forage are increased, the profitability will be reduced to say X-c. The assumption is generally that the original profitability can be restored by increasing the intake by g, where $c = g$. Waddington (19, 21) tested this assumption.

Costs and intakes were varied for a bee to forage between two flowers. Rate of the round dance was "read" inside the hive. A stepwise multiple regression analysis was used to create a "surface" of the perception of costs and intakes (RATE was the dependent variable). Fifteen bees were tested singly at the floral patch. The assumption that assessments of costs and intakes are additive on the same scale is met if the regression coefficients for the two energy variables have the same absolute magnitude. Three significant findings of this study are presented below.

First, costs and intakes were assessed differently. Costs were weighted in relation to intakes; apparently costs loom larger than intakes (Fig. 1). The mean of the absolute values of the regression coefficients for cost (14 of 15 coefficients were negative) was about five times greater than the coefficients for intake. This is a potentially important finding especially if other animals assess costs and intakes this way; weighting may apply to other complex behaviors where costs and gains are important for making decisions (e.g., reproductive strategies). Human beings also weight losses in relation to gains to make decisions (1, 16). This analogy is clear and potentially interesting, but presently the

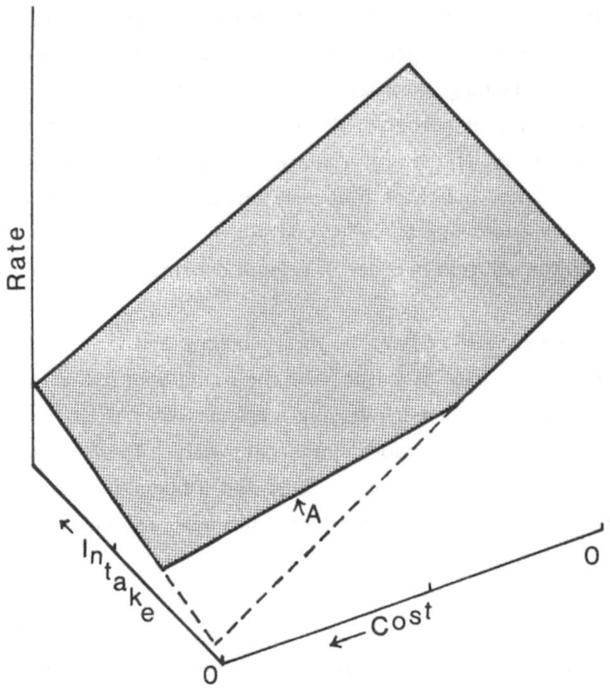

FIG. 1 - Surface portraying a bee's perception of costs and intakes per floral visit. The rate of sharp turns in the path of the round dance is used as a measure of perception. Shaded area indicates the combinations of costs and intakes which elicit dancing; line A is the dance threshold. This surface is hypothetical, but it shows that bees weight costs in relation to intakes (Waddington, 1985). A linear formulation is presented for simplicity, scaling would result in a reduced rate of change in RATE when costs are low and intakes are high.

significance of the analogy is dubious. The ultimate and proximate causations may very well be different.

Why weight costs? The only gains of foraging are food, but costs in addition to expended energy are associated with foraging. These include risk of predation, loss of time that could be put toward other activities, and wear and tear on the bee's body. Neurkirch's (12) discovery that bees have a fixed allotment of flight energy before they die places a premium on cost that may be reflected in a bee's assessments and dance. A simple example shows how intuitively obvious this phenomenon is. If intakes were offset exactly by costs, the gain would be the same whether or not the bee decided to forage, but only a foolish bee would make the trip.

Schmid-Hempel et al.(14) also found that bees weight costs in deciding when to stop foraging and return home. They developed equations to predict the number of floral visits before departure. Two currencies were used in their equations: net caloric intake per time, (G-C)/T,

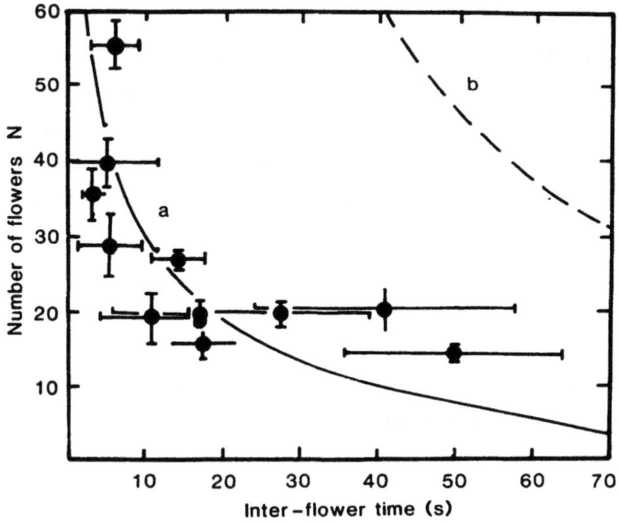

FIG. 2 - The number of flowers visited as a function of inter-flower time. The numbers predicted by the two models (curves) correspond to the behavior that maximizes net energetic gain/energy expenditure (curve a) or maximizes net energetic gain/energy expenditure (curve a) or maximizes net energetic gain/time (curve b). The observations of twelve different bees are shown (•: mean standard deviation). Bees appear to maximize net energetic gain/energy expenditure (From 13).

(where G = caloric gain, C = caloric cost, T = duration of foraging) and energetic efficiency (G-C)/C; the equations predicted the number of visits that maximized each of the currencies per foraging trip. In the field three artificial flowers were set out 30 m from the hive and each provided the bee with 2.4 calories per visit. The time to fly between flowers was varied by controlling with a sliding cover the interval between leaving one flower and landing on another flower. Each model predicted an inverse relationship between inter-floral flight time and the optimal number of floral visits. However, the efficiency model more clearly predicted the bees' behavior (Fig. 2). Schmid-Hempel et al. (14) conclude that the bees' departure behavior can be predicted by assuming that the workers maximize energetic efficiency per foraging trip. This effect is to weight costs.

A second finding of Waddington's (21) study was that dance behavior differed among individuals. The regression coefficients for costs ranged between 3 and -127 for the 15 bees and the coefficients for intakes ranged between -5 and 15. Their perception of the energy variables may have differed because of age or social context. For example, since allotment of cost is fixed (12), and the amount of a bee's energy remaining would usually be an inverse function of age, older bees may weight costs more than younger bees. Also, conditions of the colony, such as amount of stored food, may have changed during the experiment and affected the bees' perception of the energy variables at the patch (food stores affect the release of dancing;(6, p. 243)).

Third, the bees' assessments of cost were more variable than their assessments of intakes. The standard errors of the regression coefficients for costs ranged between 4 and 53 for the 15 bees and between just 1 and 7 for coefficients of intakes. Costs may be physiologically more difficult to assess than intakes involving quality and quantity of nectar, or cost could be more variable than intakes. The latter could result from different schedules of thermoregulation (in this study costs were estimated by measuring time and multiplying time by a constant rate of energy expenditure). Human beings, for whatever reason, also show greater variation in decisions based on losses than in those based on gains (15).

FORAGING DECISIONS

The question remains - how is information used to make decisions during foraging? Two kinds of decisions by foraging honeybees have been examine most closely in relation to costs and intakes: 1) floral choice and 2) flight path. Here I summarize this work.

Floral Choice

The cost-benefit approach has proven useful for studying choice of food by many animals. Enlightening results have come from studies of nectivores, including bumblebees (Bombus), honeybees and hummingbirds. Studies of floral choice by honeybees focused until recently on the notion that individuals are "flower-constant" (reviewed by 5, 20); that is, bees tend to visit a single plant species during a foraging bout. The earlier research was not designed to explain deviations from species fidelity (deviations which are observed) nor was it useful for understanding how individuals decided among flowers. Recently, there have been attempts to examine how choice in mixed-species arrays is related to costs and intakes.

Honeybees can assess and base decisions on concentration of sugars. Bees collected sucrose solutions in the 30-50% range in preference to higher or lower concentrations (23). Given a choice between two types (colors) of artificial flowers, bees generally chose flowers providing the higher expected reward per floral visit (21, 22). Wells and Wells (24) found high fidelity to one of two colors of artificial flower generally without regard to the concentration or volume of sucrose solution inside the flowers. This may have occurred because the caloric intakes from their flowers were always "large". Waddington (21) found that bees chose flowers with 2ul of 20% sucrose solution over flowers with 1ul of the same solution when handling costs were high, but they did not select on the basis of volume when the handling costs were low. Psychophysical scaling may explain this; physical measurements and subjective measurements along a scale do not coincide. Similar to the perception of other stimuli, two stimuli which are "intense" must be more different to discriminate than two stimuli of "low" intensity because the stimulus-response function of the receptors saturate for strong stimuli.

Costs also play a role in the bees' choice. Bees given a series of binary choices between artificial flowers with the same sucrose solution but different color and length of the tubular corollas (which influenced handling costs directly) chose the shorter corolla (21). Likewise, bees appear to minimize their flight costs. Marden and Waddington (11) also gave bees a series of binary choices between blue and yellow artificial flowers. Bees specialized on one color when the two flowers were equidistant from a star point, but when the flowers were spaced unequally, they flew to the closer flower and minimized flight costs.

Few data are available to examine whether bees weight costs when choosing between flowers. One bit of evidence indicates that they do not (21). Bees were given a binary choice between two different color flowers. Choosing either flower would give the bee about the same net rate of intake but the costs and intakes differed. One flower had high handling costs and intakes while both the costs and intakes were lower at the other flower. Bees weighting costs would visit the latter, lower cost flower. Eleven bees were given this problem. Some bees preferred each type, and some preferred neither, indicating that they had difficulty discerning the more profitable type. Additional work is needed on this problem.

Flight Distance and Direction

Plants often grow in single-species patches. After visiting a flower, a bee must decide where to fly next for food. Visual and olfactory cues may not be available to facilitate a choice between more and less profitable flowers. Research conducted primarily on bumblebees indicates that cost-intake information is used to plot a course and this behavior seems to enhance foraging returns. A few studies have been of honeybees.

Honeybees tend to leave a flower and alight on a neighboring flower which minimizes flight costs (10). They also tend to maintain a straight path through the patch (17) which minimizes unrewarding repeat visits. This general pattern of behavior is modified as the bees experience particular costs and intakes. Waddington (17) arrayed artificial flowers horizontally; some contained sucrose solution and some were empty. When a filled flower was encountered, a bee flew to a close neighboring flower, but when an empty flower was encountered, the next floral visit was more distant. Information from previous visits also influenced flight distance; flight distance increased with the number of preceding, uninterrupted, nonrewarding floral visits increased. This behavior likely enhances foraging returns because nectar abundance is probably patchy in plant populations. Flight directionality (i.e., tendency to keep a straight course) did not vary with presence or absence of nectar in Waddington's study.

However, Schmid-Hempel (13) found that costs to handle artificial flowers do affect flight directionality. Increased handling costs resulted in decreased directionality. Reduced directionality may have resulted from decay in memory of the arrival direction during the visit. This is a case where information on cost is not used to make decisions, rather it is a constraint on the bee's decision behavior.

SUMMARY

Optimal foraging theory has recently become a primary organizing concept for understanding and predicting foraging behavior, yet no model has been soundly built on empirically-derived behavioral and physiological assumptions. The honeybee is ideal for study to fill this gap. The puzzle of honeybee foraging behavior, using pieces of information on mechanisms, development, and evolution, is partially complete. The picture will take form quickly over the near future as more is learned about the bees' use of information on costs, risks, and intakes, decision processes, and as all of this is viewed in context of the bees' ecology.

Acknowledgements. I thank Randy Breitwisch for comments on a draft of the manuscript. My work reported here is a product of NSF grant BNS 8004537.

REFERENCES

(1) Anderson, N.H., and Norman, A. 1964. Order effects in impression formation in four classes of stimuli. J. Abnormal Soc. Psych. 69: 467-471.

(2) Boch, R. 1956. Die Tänze der Bienen bei Nahen und fernen Trachtquellen. Z. Vergl. Physiol. 38: 136-167.

(3) Cahill, K., and Lustick, S. 1976. Oxygen consumption and thermoregulation in Apis mellifera workers and drones. Comp. Biochem. Physiol. 55A: 335-357.

(4) Charnov, E.L. 1976. Optimal foraging: attack strategy of a mantid. Am. Nat. 110: 145-151.

(5) Free, J.B. 1963. The constancy of honeybees. J. Anim. Ecol. 32: 119-131.

(6) Frisch, K.v. 1967. Dance Language and Orientation of Bees. Cambridge, Mass.: Harvard University Press.

(7) Gould, J.L., and Marler, P. 1984. Ethology and natural history of learning. In The Biology of Learning, eds. P. Marler and H.S. Terrace, pp. 47-74. Berlin: Springer-Verlag.

(8) Heinrich, B. 1980. Mechanisms of body-temperature regulation in honeybees, Apis mellifera. II. Regulation of thoracic temperature at high air temperatures. J. Exp. Biol. 85: 73-87.

(9) Krebs, J.R., and McCleery, R.H. 1983. Optimization in behavioural ecology. In Behavioural Ecology: An Evolutionary Approach, eds. J.R. Krebs and N.B. Davies, pp. 91-121. Oxford: Blackwell Scientific Publications.

(10) Levin, D.A., and Kerster, H.W. 1969. The dependence of bee-mediated pollen and gene dispersal upon plant density. Evolution 23: 560-571.

(11) Marden, J.H., and Waddington, K.D. 1981. Floral choices by honeybees in relation to the relative distances to flowers. Physiol. Ent. 6: 431-435.

(12) Neukirch, A. 1982. Dependence of the life span of the honeybee (Apis mellifica) upon flight performance and energy consumption. J. Comp. Physiol. 146: 35-40.

(13) Schmid-Hempel, P. 1984. The importance of handling time for flight directionality in bees. Behav. Ecol. Sociobiol. 15: 303-309.

(14) Schmid-Hempel, P.; Kacelnik, A.; and Houston, A.I. 1985. Honeybees maximize efficiency by not filling their crop. Behav. Ecol. Sociobiol. 17: 61-66.

(15) Swalm, R.O. 1966. Utility theory - insights into risk taking. Harvard Bus. Rev. 44: 123-136.

(16) Tversky, A., and Kahneman, D. 1981. The framing of decision and choice. Science 211: 453-458.

(17) Waddington, K.D. 1980. Flight patterns of foraging bees relative to density of artificial flowers and distribution of nectar. Oecologia 44: 199-204.

(18) Waddington, K.D. 1982a. Honey bee foraging profitability and round dance correlates. J. Comp. Physiol. 148: 297-301.

(19) Waddington, K.D. 1982b. Information used in foraging. In The Biology of Social Insects, eds. M.D. Breed, C.D. Michener and H.E. Evans, pp. 24-27. Boulder: Westview Press.

(20) Waddington, K.D. 1983. Floral visitation sequences by bees: models and experiments. In Handbook of Experimental Pollination Biology, eds. C.E. Jones and R.J. Little, pp. 461-473. New York: Van Nostrand-Reinhold.

(21) Waddington, K.D. 1985. Cost-intake information used in foraging. J. Insect Physiol. 31: 891-897.

(22) Waddington, K.D., and Holden, L.R. 1979. Optimal foraging: on flower selection by bees. Am. Nat. 114: 179-196.

(23) Waller, G.D. 1972. Evaluating responses of sugar solutions using an artificial-flower feeder. Ann. Entomol. Soc. Am. 65: 857-862.

(24) Wells, H., and Wells, P.H. 1983. Honey bee foraging ecology: optimal diet, minimal uncertainty or individual constancy? J. Anim. Ecol. 52: 829-836.

The Bee's E-Vector Compass

Samuel Rossel and Rüdiger Wehner
Department of Zoology, University of Zürich, Winterthurerstrasse 190,
CH-8057 Zürich, Switzerland

INTRODUCTION

In the late forties, the discovery by Karl von Frisch that bees detect the e-vectors of polarized skylight (Fig. 1), and that they can use these e-vectors as a compass came as a real surprise (von Frisch, 1949). It was greeted as the discovery of a qualitatively new sensory capacity of animals. By presenting an answer to the question of how bees use the celestial patterns for navigation we show that polarization vision is not as exotic a capacity as hitherto surmised.

A number of important properties of the bee's e-vector detecting system had already been discovered by von Frisch (1965) - namely that e-vector detection was done exclusively in the short wavelength range of the spectrum, that the degree of polarization was not used as a compass cue (it had only to exceed 10 percent before the bees were able to detect the e-vector), and that a single small patch of blue sky was sufficient for compass orientation. The principal question, however, had not been answered: How does the bee's e-vector compass work?

On closer scrutiny, there are three major problems to be solved. First: What are the e-vector sensitive structures (analyzers) in the bee's eye? Second: How does a bee detect a particular e-vector in the sky? Third : What "knowledge" of the whole celestial e-vector pattern does the bee use for steering a compass course?

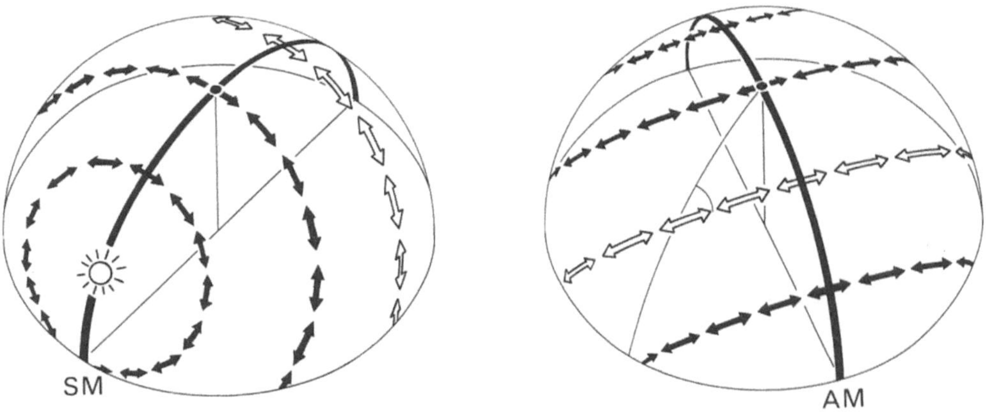

Fig. 1 - The pattern of polarized light in the sky. The two celestial spheres are rotated relative to each other. SM and AM denote the solar and antisolar meridian respectively. The arrows indicate the directions of polarization (e-vector directions). In general the e-vectors form concentric circles around the sun. Direct sunlight is unpolarized; the degree of polarization increases gradually to a maximum along a circle 90° from the sun (open arrows). The solar and antisolar meridian constitute a prominent axis of symmetry; the e-vector pattern on both sides of these meridians are mirror images to each other.

The answer to the first question is clear: The analyzers in the compound eyes of arthropods are the photoreceptors themselves. Due to the preferential alignment of the visual pigments within the photoreceptor membrane (6) each microvillus of the receptor is highly dichroic, and due to the alignment of all microvilli within one receptor, the receptors exhibit high polarization sensitivities. Furthermore, they employ a number of tricks to increase their polarization sensitivity beyond what the photoreceptor membrane already achieves, or - on the other hand - to decrease or even destroy polarization sensitivity (18). In fact, it is known for bees that only a small part at the dorsal rim of the eye (POL region) participates in polarization vision (14, 17, 20), and that within this specialized region only the UV photoreceptors are sensitive to polarized light (7, 10).

The second problem has been a subject of much debate and speculation. In principle, the direction of an e-vector could be determined by either a successive or a simultaneous method (8). The successive method implies that an analyzer is rotated about its direction of view, and that the e-vector direction of the stimulus is inferred from the angular position of the analyzer at which the maximum response occurs. The insect might find it difficult to employ such a strategy in the sense just described, because it cannot rotate its photoreceptors within the eyes. The simultaneous method avoids this difficulty in assuming a stationary relationship between the photoreceptors and the e-vector to be detected (Fig. 2). In this case, however, at least three analyzers, each with its own analyzer direction, must simultaneously look at the e-vector and properly compare their outputs, when the e-vector direction is to be determined unambigously. This is for the simple theoretical reason that light emanating from a particular

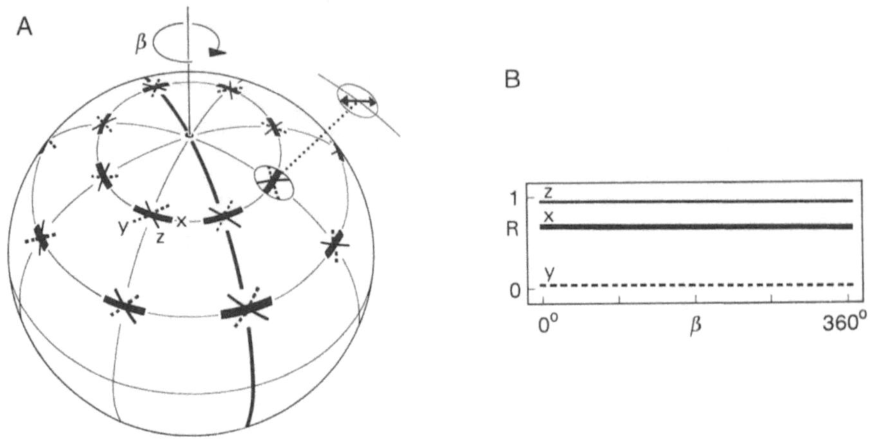

Fig. 2 - Determination of an e-vector by the simultaneous method. A. A set of at least three analyzers (x, y, z) with different analyzer directions is necessary. Several such sets are shown within the visual sphere of the animal (the meridian marked by the heavy line defines the animal's medial plane). The x-, y- and z-type analyzers of all sets must be orientated consistently within the retinal system of coordinates. A and B. When the array of sets of analyzers sweeps through a particular e-vector (rotation β), the response (R) of all analyzers belonging to the same type do not change. Different e-vectors vary in the relative effect that they have on the three analyzers. Thus a particular ratio of analyzer outputs provides the basis for an unambigous discrimination of e-vector directions.

celestial point varies in three dimensions: e-vector direction, degree of polarization, and intensity. As only one spectral type of receptor is involved in e-vector detection, the ultraviolet receptor, a fourth dimension (the spectral dimension) is not needed.

Even more has been speculated about how the bee could solve the third problem. Endowed with the capacity to determine individual e-vector directions in the sky, the bee could apply a number of strategies like performing spherical geometry in the sky to calculate the position of the sun, or relying on memory information about e-vector patterns. A number of such possibilities have been discussed (1, 4, 5, 9, 17), but the experimental data at hand were not complete enough to vindicate any of these hypotheses.

Recently we have proposed a new model for e-vector detection and orientation in bees which combines the second and third problem discussed above and solves them in a single step. In the following we first outline this model and explain how it has been derived from behavioral and neurobiological observations.

MODEL FOR POLARIZED LIGHT DETECTION AND ORIENTATION

Imagine that the bee's eye were equipped with an array of analyzers in which each analyzer direction occupied a specific azimuthal direction (Fig. 3a). For example, the analyzers which are maximally sensitive to horizontal e-vectors point in the back and forward direction of the eye i.e. lie in the bee's medial plane; the vertical analyzers point laterally i.e. lie at right

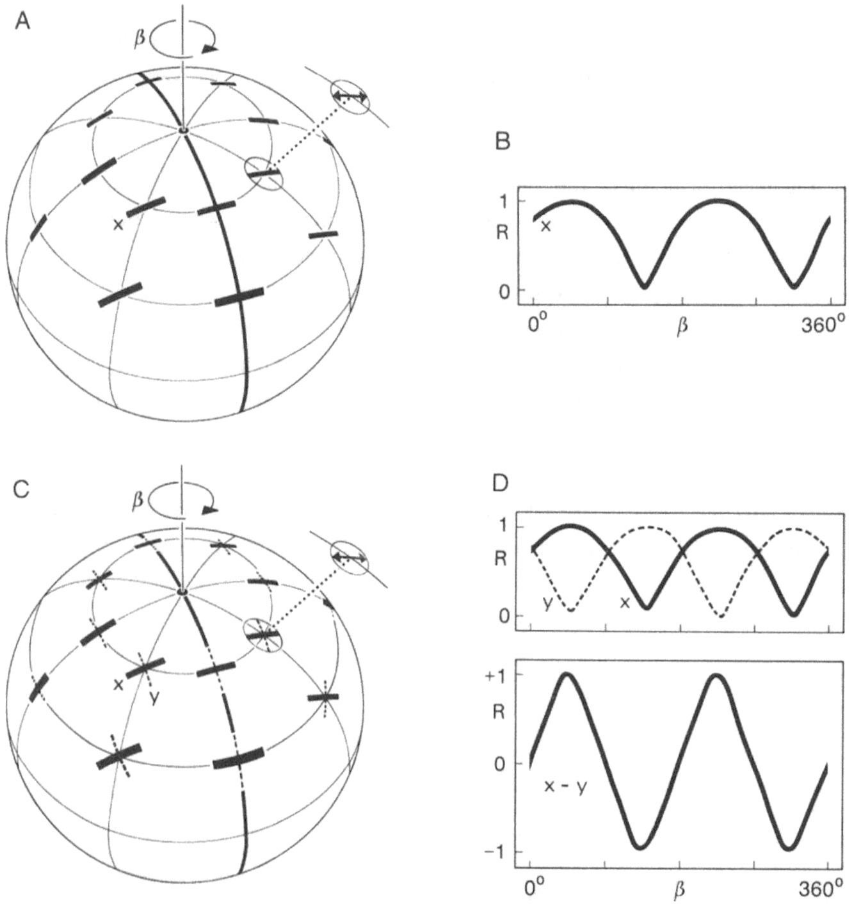

Fig. 3 - Scanning model of e-vector detection. A. One-analyzer array. The sphere marks the visual field of the animal (the meridian marked by the heavy line defines the medial plane). The black bars indicate the analyzer directions. B. Responses (R) of the analyzers (x) when the analyzer array scans an external e-vector (rotation ß). The particular shape of the curve reflects the logarithmic intensity coding characteristics of the photoreceptors. Note that a maximum output is produced by the array, when the e-vector direction is matched by a suitably orientated analyzer direction. C. Two-analyzer array. Each eye position is occupied by a pair of orthogonally arranged analyzers (x and y) which interact to give a differential output. D. Responses (R) of the x- and y-type analyzers (upper graph) and the difference between the two (lower graph).

angles to the horizontal ones; and all other analyzer directions are spread out between. Consider now what happens to the output of each analyzer when a bee, which views a single e-vector in the sky, rotates about a vertical axis. The e-vector is positioned at 60° above the horizon and stimulates successively a ring of analyzers as the bee rotates. Once every revolution, the output of each analyzer rises to a peak or falls to a trough as the e-vector comes within its receptive field of view, with the amplitude of the peak varying according to the angle between the direction of the analyzer and the direction of the e-vector (Fig. 3B).

A maximum output will occur in that analyzer whose direction is parallel to the celestial e-vector. Since in each eye the analyzer directions vary through 180°, the bee, while scanning the sky, can discriminate any given e-vector, simply by recording which analyzers within the array generate the largest output.

Without altering the basic principles, the scanning model can be improved by substituting each analyzer by a set of two mutually perpendicular analyzers whose outputs are differentially compared. In Fig. 3C, one of these analyzers is denoted by X (and coincides with the directions shown in Fig. 3A), the other by Y. We assume that X and Y interact so that the output will reach a maximum when X is parallel to the e-vector and will reach a minimum when the e-vector is parallel to Y. When again swept through a particular e-vector in the sky, an array of such antagonistic pairs of analyzers "sees" much larger and sharper response modulations than is the case with the single analyzer array (compare Fig. 3B and D).

Let us now consider how the bee can use its analyzer array to obtain compass bearings from the polarization patterns in the sky. As an example we shall take the polarization pattern

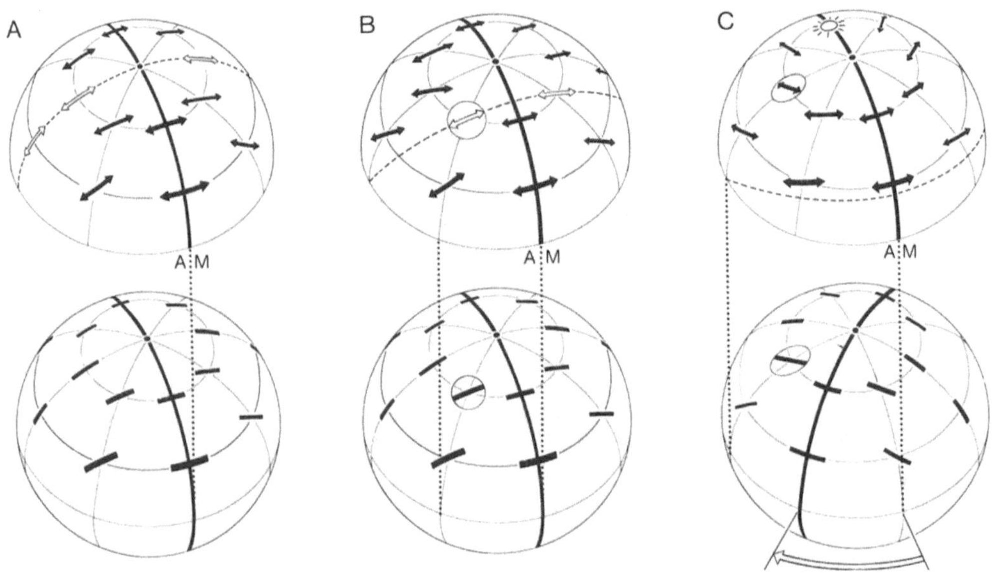

Fig. 4 - Use of the scanning model in deriving compass information from the polarization patterns in the sky. A. Upper hemisphere: e-vector pattern when the sun is at the horizon. AM denotes the antisolar meridian. The dashed circle and the open arrows mark the band of maximum polarization. Lower sphere: model eyes with analyzer array (only x-type analyzers are shown). Note that the distribution of e-vectors is closely matched by the array of analyzers when the median plane of the eyes (heavy line) is aligned with the solar and antisolar meridian. B and C. Polarization patterns for sun elavations of 25° (B) and 65° (C). The eyes are orientated so that suitably arranged analyzers match the encircled e-vectors in the sky. The medial plane of the eyes coincides with the symmetry plane of the celestial patterns when the matched e-vectors lie along the band of maximum polarization (B), but substantial deviations may occur for other celestial e-vectors (C).

that is present at dawn and dusk. When the bee is aligned with the solar and antisolar meridian of such a pattern an important feature of the analyzer array becomes evident, namely that the distribution of analyzers closely matches the distribution of the e-vectors in the sky (Fig. 4A). Thus our scanning model proposes that the bee turns until the analyzers match the e-vectors visible in the sky. When this is achieved, the analyzers produce a maximum signal, telling the bee that she is aligned with the solar and antisolar meridian. Once the bee has aligned herself with these reference meridians, she must turn until she faces in her desired orientation.

The simple strategy of determining compass bearings is bound to result in mistakes when the bee navigates underneath a daytime polarization pattern (Fig. 4B and C). This is due to the fact that the e-vector directions do not lie on fixed bearings relative to the solar and antisolar meridian but change their position with the elavation of the sun (see Fig. 1). As a consequence the spatial layout of analyzers deviates from the e-vector pattern in the sky. These deviations are generally small along the most polarized band in the antisolar half of the sky but increase substantially towards the sun. The scanning mechanism therefore provides the bee with a rather accurate estimate of the solar and antisolar meridian when the e-vectors visible in the sky are highly polarized, but errors must occur for all other e-vectors. This in turn should lead to errors of orientation expressing the discrepancy between the e-vector pattern and the array of analyzers. Our previous experiments have shown that such orientation errors do in fact occur, and this has led us to formulate the scanning model proposed (11, 12, 13, 19).

Our experimental paradigm was essentially the same as the one used by von Frisch (1965). Bees trained to an artificial feeder performed their waggle dances on a horizontal comb. The comb was surrounded by an opaque Plexiglass hemisphere which depolarized the natural e-vector pattern completely and closely matched the radiance field of a fully overcast sky.

Under these conditions the waggle dances were orientated randomly unless the bees could view a small patch of naturally or artificially polarized light through one of the apertures which could be opened in the hemisphere. When artificial stimuli were used, the light entering the aperture was provided by a Xenon arc and polarized by a polarizing filter (for further details see 12 and 19). The results obtained from recording more than 10, 000 waggle runs showed that the bees made consistent orientation errors depending on the elavation of the sun and the e-vector direction. Thus the position assumed by the bee for a particular e-vector direction does not necessarily correspond to its actual position in the sky but deviates from the latter by an angle which equals the orientation error. This finding allowed us to reconstruct the bee's map of the polarization patterns in the sky. According to this map bees invariably treat a given e-vector as though it were at a fixed azimuthal angle relative to the antisolar meridian irrespective of the elevation in the sky or the time of day. For instance, bees treat a horizontal e-vector as if it lay along the antisolar meridian and a vertical e-vector as if it were positioned at right angles to the antisolar meridian, with the azimuthal angles inferred for all other e-vectors spread out in between (Fig. 5). Finally, we assumed that this simplified e-vector map was embodied in the array of polarization analyzers, such that the azimuth which is associated by the bee with a particular e-vector direction in the sky corresponded with a suitably arranged analyzer direction within the eyes (compare Figs. 5 and 3).

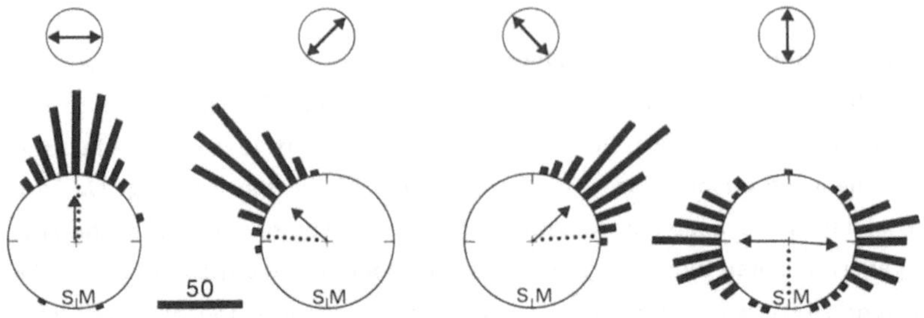

Fig. 5 - Dance orientation to polarized light. Four different e-vector directions (horizontal e-vector, +45° e-vector, -45° e-vector and vertical e-vector; see diagrams from left to right), were presented by means of a beam of artificially polarized UV light. The light source was at 60° above the horizon. The direction of individual waggle runs (the mean directions are indicated by arrows) is plotted so as to indicate where in the sky the bee expects the e-vector to occur (SM denotes the solar meridian). This is the most simple way to express the bee's waggle dance of orientation, because it is independant of the time of day and directions of feeding stations. The present experiments were performed at noon with a polarization pattern as shown in Fig. 4C. The dotted lines indicate the azimuthal angles of the e-vectors in the real sky. The differences between these angles and the ones inferred by the bees are the orientation errors. Scale: 50 waggle runs.

These behavioral inferences are supported by neurobiological observations. It is well known from anatomical and physiological data that each ommatidium of the POL region contains three polarization sensitive UV photoreceptors. Of the three receptors, two have microvilli orientated parallel to each other, whilst the the third is orientated perpendicularly (10, 16).

The orientation of microvilli varies across the POL region, providing a fan shaped array of crossed polarization analyzers. Optical studies show that the POL regions view a contralateral region of space (10, 16). As a consequence, the microvilli of the "fan-array" rotate from back to front at any given elevation in space. Fig. 6 shows that this rotation resembles in principle the one inferred from the behavioral data. The resemblance is closest in the lateral parts of the eyes, where the orientation of the retinal analyzers varies between the vertical and horizontal, depending on the elevation in space. Note, however, that a complete correspondence of the anatomical and behavioral data is not necessary. Neural convergence and divergence could well transform the retinal array into a neural array that is compatible with the behavioral inferences. We shall come back to this point later.

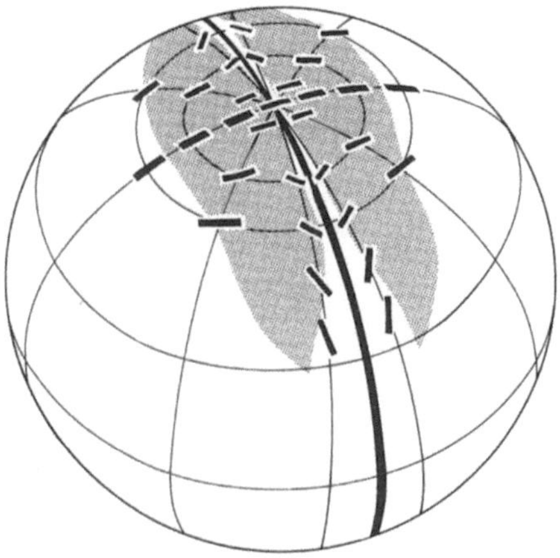

Fig. 6 - The POL regions within the bee's visual field. The meridians marked by the heavy line define the medial plane. The optical axes of all ommatidia contained in the POL region of one eye look contralaterally and occupy a relative small area (grey shading) within the most dorsal part of the visual field. (Note that the effective sampling area of the POL regions extends almost to the horizon. This is because the ommatidia at the dorsal rim of the eyes have extremely large visual fields. The black bars indicate the microvilli directions of polarization sensitive UV receptors. Note that only one type of analyzer is shown. In the real eye each ommatidium is equipped with a set of two perpendicular analyzers. From Sommer (1979).

SCANNING MODEL TESTED

From the data presented so far it is not possible to decide conclusively whether the scanning mechanism proposed has been adopted by the bee. Therefore, we now report experiments designed to test the most basic prediction of the model, namely that polarized light is detected as a modulating signal which the bee obtains by sweeping its analyzer array through the sky (15). Under normal conditions the analyzer array is active when a patch of light is sufficiently polarized. However, in the experiment the signal is generated by an unpolarized patch of light which modulates in intensity as the bee rotates. The model then predicts that the percieved direction of a particular e-vector and the azimuthal angle associated with that e-vector is determined by whatever part of the retina produces the largest response.

Accordingly, the light source is arranged to modulate so that the beam is of peak intensity when it stimulates a predetermined part of the retina. When this is achieved one would expect the bee to orientate as it normally would to the appropriate e-vector in the sky. Before we consider whether the scanning model can be verified by this kind of simulation, we first must mention some technical details (Fig. 7).

As we have seen the array of polarization detectors within the eyes consists of pairs of orthogonally orientated analyzers which we assume to interact so as to compute a differential output (Fig. 3). When presented with polarized light this interaction provides the

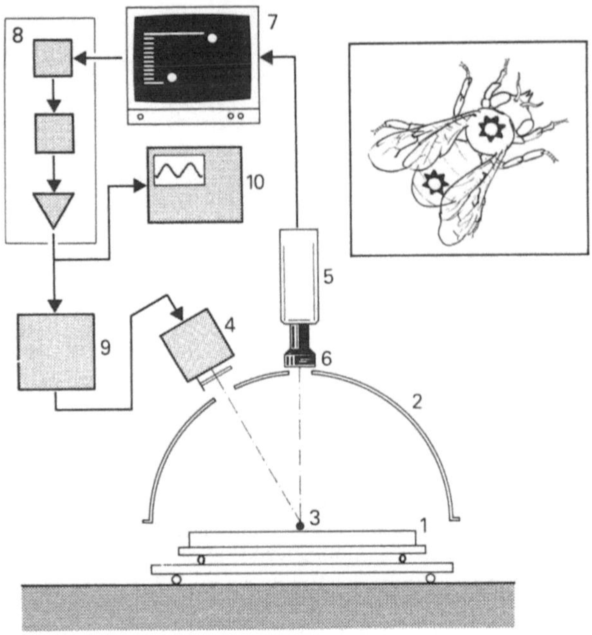

Fig. 7 - Experimental set-up for testing the scanning model. 1 - observation hive with horizontal combs. 2 - Plexiglass dome (radius 33 cm). 3 - dancing bee. The hive can be moved in the x and y direction so as to centre the bee with respect to the Plexiglass dome. 4 - Xenon arc with UV spectral filter. 5 - TV camera. 6 - ring lamp 7 - TV monitor. The two reflectors on the bee's body are visible as bright spots (inset: the circular reflectors are contained in star-shaped plastic tags. The tags have different colors so that each bee can be recognized individually. 8 - Electronic part of the feedback device with line counter, digital to analog converter and amplifier. 9 - Power supply of Xenon arc. 10 - storage oscilloscope. In the experiments the display of 7 and 10 was recorded by a second TV camera (not shown in the figure). From Rossel and Wehner (1986).

bee with a high contrast e-vector signal, because crossed analyzers produce antagonistically modulated response patterns as the bee rotates. This, of course, cannot be achieved by a modulated beam of unpolarized light, which stimulates pairs of crossed analyzers equally and in phase so that the differential output will be zero throughout the modulation cycle. This was in fact shown i.e. the bees danced in the same directions irrespective of whether the beam of unpolarized light was modulated or not (Fig. 8).

At first sight, this seems to rule out any possibility of testing the model directly using modulations of unpolarized light. However, the solution to the problem is to stimulate selectively one of the two crossed receptor arrays on its own. This was achieved by covering the POL regions with a piece of polarizing filter orientated to transmit the set of e-vector planes which contain the transverse axis of the eyes (Fig. 9 A and B). Then, the e-vectors projecting onto the the POL regions of the two eyes rotate from back to the front in the same fashion as do the crossed polarization detectors in the model array. Thus we expect that

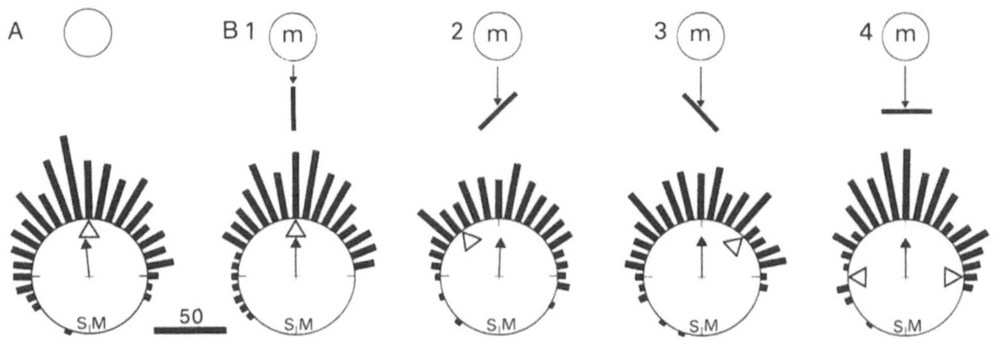

Fig. 8 - Orientation of bees to time-modulated beams of unpolarized light A. In a control experiment the bees are presented with a beam of unpolarized light, non-modulated UV light. The waggle run distributions show the range of azimuthal angles inferred by the bees for such a stimulus (SM, solar meridian). The results confirm the previous finding, that in the bee's internal image of the sky a patch of unpolarized UV light lies anywhere within the antisolar half of the sky (mean direction: antisolar meridian: open arrow). This is indicated in the figure by the large scatter of waggle run directions (for further details see 14). B (1-4). Bees are presented with a modulated beam of light. In the diagrams from left to right the modulations are arranged to simulate the four e-vector directions tested in Fig. 5 (horizontal e-vector, $+45^{o}$ e-vector, -45° e-vector and vertical e-vector). The bars mark the direction of the bee when the modulation (m) within the patch of light reaches a maximum (compare with Fig. 3 for spatial layout of e-vector detectors within the model eyes). The open arrows within the diagrams indicate the azimuthal angles inferred by the bees for the four e-vectors (from Fig. 5). Accordingly, the mean waggle dance directions (solid arrows) should point in these directions if the modulated light source were treated by bees as a patch of polarized light of a given e-vector. Since the eyes have sets of crossed analyzers, the bees did not respond to the intensity modulations, but behaved as in Fig. A.

light is transmitted by the filter so that it stimulates one of the two analyzers in each ommatidium more than the other. To quantify this effect we assume that the photoreceptors of the POL regions have PS values of 10 (ref. 10; the Ps value is defined as the ratio of maximal sensitivity to minimal sensitivity when the e-vector falling within the receptive field of the receptor rotates). Furthermore, in our experiments the intensity of the light source varied by a factor of three as the bee turned about a vertical body axis. In Fig. 9 C we have used these numbers to estimate the effect produced by the overhead polarization filter. Clearly in the real eye the effect will be more complicated than we have allowed it to be here. In particular we did not consider the various adaptation mechanisms which,at least to some extent, could compensate for the effect produced by the filter. However, it is reasonable to assume that at sufficiently low levels of intensity one type of analyzer will cease to respond while the other is still active. When this is achieved we expect that the differential output of the crossed analyzer array will modulate according to the intensity of the unpolarized light source and that this signal will be interpreted by the bee as a beam of polarized light. As a control, some bees were equipped with a filter with its transmission axis orientated at 45° to the transverse axis of the eyes. In this case pairs of crossed analyzers should be stimulated equally so that the differential output should be zero throughout the modulation cycle. Thus no e-vector orientation should occur.

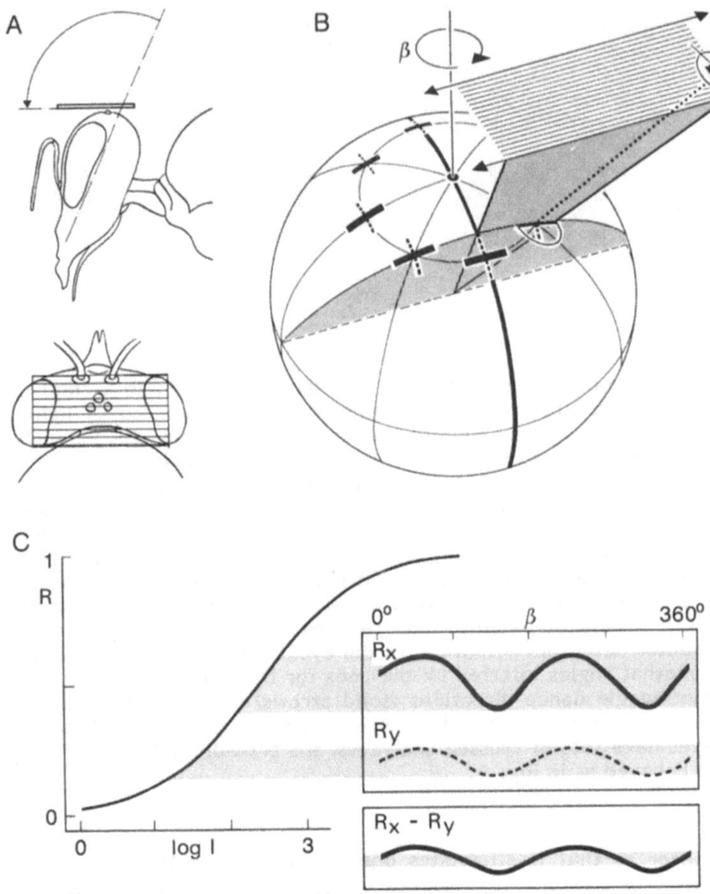

Fig. 9 - Method for stimulating crossed analyzers selectively. A. The bee's head is equipped with a rectangular piece of a polarizing filter. The orientation of the filter on top of the head is defined relative to the posterior margin of the two eyes. The transmission axis of the filter is indicated by the set of parallel lines. B. Model eyes with pairs of crossed analyzers (x and y type) at an elavation of 60°, and part of the polarization filter. Light is transmitted by the filter (one transmission plane is shaded) so that the x-type analyzers are stimulated more than the y-type analyzers. From Rossel and Wehner (1986) C. The intensity/response function (R/log I curve) of photoreceptors and the responses of the x- and y-type analyzers. The transmission axis of the overhead filter is as in Fig. B. The bee rotates through 360°. The differential output of the crossed analyzers is shown in the the lower graph. It should exceed the shaded range which gives the bee's detection threshold for polarized light (degree of polarization: 10%, von Frisch, 1965).

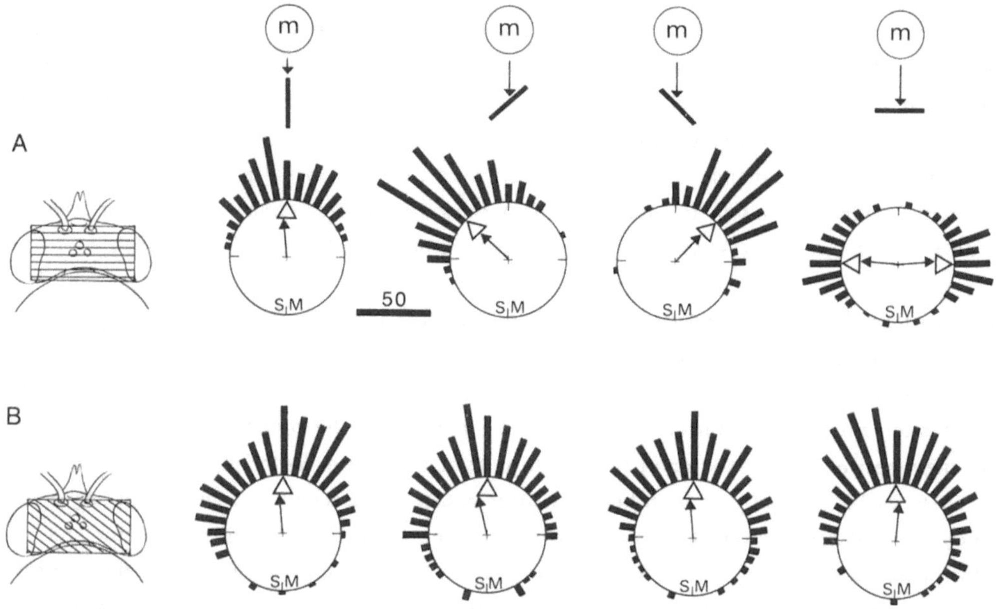

Fig. 10 - E-vector simulation by means of a time-modulated beam of unpolarized light. A. The stimuli conditions are as in Fig. 8B, except that the bees are now equipped with an overhead polarization filter. The transmission axis of the filter is parallel to the transverse axis of the eyes. The waggle dances (the mean directions are marked by solid arrows) point in the same directions as when the bees were presented with a patch of polarized light of a given e-vector (open arrows; compare with data in Fig. 5). B. Same stimuli conditions as in Fig. A, except that the transmission axis of the filter is now 45° from the transverse axis. The bees behave as if they were presented with a beam of unpolarized, non-modulated light (open arrow, compare with Fig. 8 A).

Fig. 10 shows that the bees indeed behaved according to this prediction. With the transmission axis of the filter parallel to the transverse axis of the eyes, dances were orientated in the expected directions*, while with the filter orientated at 45° from this axis, the bees behaved as though they were stimulated by a patch of unpolarized light (15).

* When we started the experiments we failed to simulate a vertical e-vector. Bees treat a patch of vertically polarized light as if it were at right angles to the antisolar meridian. However, the azimuthal angle inferred by the bees for a modulated light source was consistently shifted towards the antisolar meridian by an angle of about 30°. Further experiments showed that this discrepancy was due to the inclination of the overhead filter of the bees tested. Generally, the filter was attached so as to achieve the best fit possible to the topography of the head. In this case the bees kept the filter slightly inclined when they circled around during the waggle dance. Therefore, the filter was readjusted in some bees , so that it was more or less horizontal during the dance. When this was achieved bees behaved as predicted (see Fig. 10). However, only a few of the many dances recorded could be used. This is because light from the overhead ring lamp was strongly reflected by the horizontal polarization filter, so that the experimental feedback loop was frequently interrupted during the dance.

In the experiments described above we used a feedback device to ensure that a patch of unpolarized light optimally stimulated a predetermined retinal region of the dancing bee. Clearly, it is this method which provides the most direct evidence for the scanning model because the dancing bee itself controls the orientation cue. However, the technique is bound to many difficulties, ranging from the preparation of the bees to the proper working of the electronic equipment out in the field. We next show that a less complicated experimental paradigm can be used to test some of the principal predictions of the scanning model.

The idea that the effects produced by the overhead filter should be similar when the bee, in an open-loop experiment, is presented with a patch of polarized light. This can be readily deduced from Fig. 9. Take for instance a patch of light with a vertical e-vector. The transmission axis of the filter on the bee's head is parallel to the transverse axis of the eyes. The angle between the e-vector in the patch of light and the e-vector plane transmitted by the filter varies gradually as both bee and filter rotate. Consequently, light projecting onto the eyes modulates in intensity, rising to a peak in the lateral eye (vertical e-vector and e-vector plane transmitted by the filter are in register) and falling to a trough in the frontal and caudal regions of the eye (e-vector and e-vector plane are at right angles to each other). Similar modulations are produced when the e-vector direction in the patch of light is changed, except that peaks and troughs will now occur in different positions on the retina. Note that any given e-vector maximally stimulates the detectors which are sensitive to that e-vector. Thus bees should orientate as they normally do when presented with polarized light. However, no e-vector orientation is expected to occur when the transmission axis of the filter is at 45° from the transverse axis of the eyes, because in this case pairs of crossed analyzers will be stimulated equally as the bee rotates. The results of an extensive series of experiments in which the bees were presented with different e-vector directions fully confirm these predictions. One example is documented in Fig. 11 A and B.

Based on this finding, the transmission axis of the filter was rotated stepwise through 90°. In one experiment the transmission axis was orientated at 30° from the transverse axis and the bees were presented with a vertical e-vector (Fig. 11 C). As the bee rotated, light transmitted by the filter reached a maximal intensity some 30° from the lateral direction. This means that the vertical e-vector - contary to the experiment in Fig. 11 A - stimulates a retinal region which is sensitive to oblique e-vectors. Thus we expect the bee to orientate as it normally would when presented with an oblique e-vector. The result shows that this is indeed the case. We mention this experiment because it nicely demonstrates that the perceived direction of a given e-vector is determined by which part of the retina generates the largest output. Clearly, this is exactly what our scanning model predicts.

In a second experiment the transmission axis of the filter was orientated 90° from the transverse axis so that the frontal and caudal regions of the eyes were maximally stimulated by the vertical e-vector presented to the bees (Fig. 11 D). To predict the outcome of this

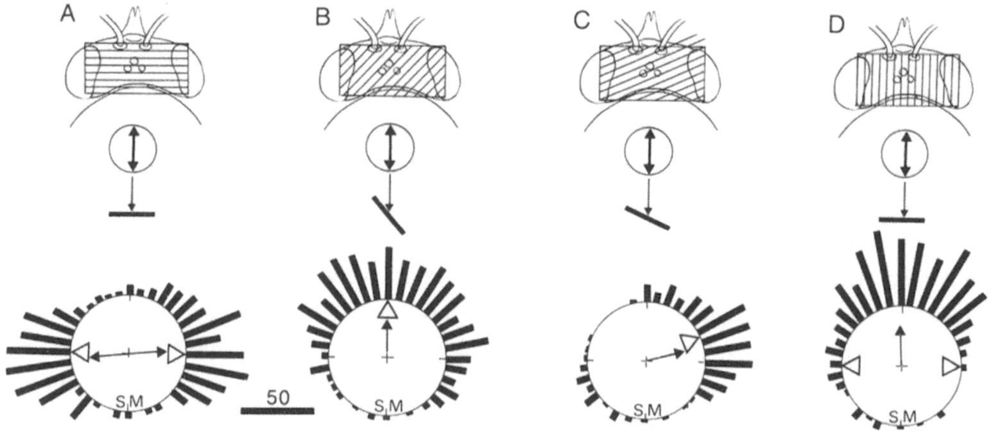

Fig. 11 - E-vector simulation by means of a beam of polarized light transmitted by a polarizer on top of the bee's head. The bees are presented with a patch of light with a vertical e-vector. The bars mark the bee's direction when the light from the patch is maximally transmitted by the overhead filter. Open arrows within the diagrams indicate the expected dance directions if the bees behaved according to the scanning model (Figs. 3 and 9). A and B. The transmission axis of the filter is parallel to the transverse axis (A) and 45° from this axis (B). Accordingly, the bees exhibit e-vector orientation in A, but not in B (compare with data in Fig. 10). C. The transmission axis of the filter deviates by 30° from the transverse axis. The bees behave as though they were presented with an oblique e-vector. D. The transmission axis of the filter is at right angles to the transverse axis. The bees behave as though they were stimulated by a patch of unpolarized light. This contradicts with the predictions derived from the model (but see text).

experiment we must briefly consult the scanning model shown in Fig. 3. In this model we have assumed that the frontal and caudal regions of the eye contain detectors which respond maximally to horizontal e-vectors and minimally to vertical e-vectors (R= -1 for vertical e-vectors; Fig. 3 D lower diagram). Thus in the experimental situation tested we expect the array of detectors to generate a modulating signal which reaches a peak when the patch of light is positioned in the lateral field of view, even though in this position no light is transmitted by the filter (R = 0 for vertical e-vector; Fig. 3 D lower diagram). Therefore the bees should orientate as they normally do when presented with a vertical e-vector because the detectors for this e-vector are positioned in the lateral region of the eyes. Fig. 11 D shows that the bees did not behave according to this prediction, but orientated their waggle dances as though they were presented with a patch of unpolarized light. This contrasts with results obtained from similar experiments in which the bees were presented with one of two oblique e-vector directions. In this case the model perfectly mimicked the bee's behavior. So, why did it fail to do so when the vertical e-vectors were involved?

The answer to this question probably lies in the fact that the spatial layout of analyzers as inferred from behavior is not exactly matched by the orientation of microvilli within the retina (compare Figs 3 and 6). We have already mentioned that major discrepancies seem to exist in the frontal and caudal regions of the eye, where photoreceptors have microvilli orientated in all directions between horizontal and vertical, depending on the elavation in space. This variability is even increased when we consider that the array of detectors in the left and in the right eye are mirror images of each other. Next we note that the visual fields of photoreceptors of the POL regions are extremely large (10), so that the e-vector of a patch of light is sampled by different ommatidia. This has no effect in the lateral regions of the eye where the analyzers are more or less parallel for any given azimuthal angle, so that all detectors generate similar outputs. However, the frontal and caudal detectors would give the bee conflicting information, because each detector involved is optimally sensitive to a different e-vector direction. A simple way to overcome this problem is to sum the differential signals of individual crossed analyzers. The output of the whole retinal region of interest would then correspond to the balanced signal which occurs when a single pair of crossed analyzers is equally stimulated. Note, however, that the summed output will not change, when the e-vector direction in the patch of light is varied. This is because we assume that all possible analyzer directions are involved in the summation process.

With this arguement in mind, we now readily notice that in the experiment of Fig. 11 D a vertical e-vector will have no effect in the frontal and caudal regions of the eye. Similarly, it will have no effect in the lateral regions of the eye because no light is transmitted by the filter. Thus no modulating signal will be generated by the detector array. The situation changes when the bee is presented with an oblique e-vector. To detect such an e-vector the array of analyzers is expected to generate a modulating signal which is balanced between peak and trough when the patch is positioned ahead or behind. Clearly, this expectation is met by both the model and the retinal array. Both arrays also make similar predictions for all other e-vector directions and filter configurations we have tried in the experiments.

CONCLUSIONS

All the above findings argue that the bees rely on a scanning method to detect the plane of polarization of a patch of light. When a patch of light is swept across the eyes, the perceived direction of its e-vector is determined by which analyzers within the array produce the largest response. In addition, the experiments show that e-vector analysis by local detectors exploits antagonistic interactions between orthogonally orientated analyzers. Quite different results would have been found if a simultaneous method of e-vector detection had been used by the bees. Such a method implies that the bee "sees" the same e-vector in the patch of light, irrespective of its horizontal body orientation (Fig. 2). In our experiments, however, the beam of the light source was polarized by the overhead filter so that the e-vectors projecting onto the eyes varied as both bee and and filter rotated (Fig. 9). Clearly this would give a bee using a simultaneous method conflicting compass information. Nevertheless, one might argue that in the "filter" experiments not all e-vectors were equally attractive during a modulation cycle. For instance, the bee could have taken a "snapshot" of the e-vectors projecting onto the eyes when the perceived intensity of the light source reached a maximum. In this case, however, we would have expected the dance behavior to be the same whether the filter was parallel to the transverse axis or orientated obliquely to it. Our data show that this was not the case (Figs. 10 and 11).

We have derived our scanning model by interpreting the orientation errors made by bees when presented with a small patch of polarized light (Figs. 3, 4 and 5). In particular, these errors allowed us to infer the spatial layout of analyzers within the eyes. Our present analysis suggests that this model array correctly describes the spatial representation of e-vectors within the bee's brain. The array provided precise predictions as to how the light source had to modulate temporally and spatially so as to simulate a particular e-vector direction (Figs. 10 A and 11 A). The array also correctly predicted that the e-vector detecting system will be neutralized when the transmission axis of the overhead filter is at 45° from the transverse axis of the eyes (Figs. 10 B and 11 B). Thus we suppose that neuronal convergence and divergence transform the array of retinal analyzers (Fig. 6) into a neuronal array that corresponds to the array inferred from behavior (Fig. 3). The price to be paid for the somewhat disorderly spatial layout of retinal analyzers is then presumably a loss of contrast in the temporally modulating signals which are produced by polarizing light i. e. the modulating signals generated by the retinal array are locally degraded in amplitude. This is indicated by the experiment in Fig. 11 D.

Despite the success of our simulation experiments, it would be premature to conclude that the scanning mechanism is used by bees in all situations. In the experiments described here the bees were presented with small spots of light not larger than 10° in diameter. One might argue that this is a rather special situation, and that the scanning strategy is used by bees merely when confronted with such restricted stimulus conditions. However, we believe that this is not the case. In additional experiments, we examined how bees orientate when presented with large parts of the natural blue sky with many different e-vector directions (13). Even in this case orientation errors occurred. More importantly, these errors were exactly as large as the mean of the errors induced by e-vector alone. This finding is consistent with the idea that the bee rotates sweeping its analyzer array across the sky and sampling the peak responses induced by the range of e-vector directions within the array. In this respect, one type of experiment is very convincing: substantial errors occur, when a large skylight window is displayed to the left (or the right) of the celestial symmetry plane, but none are observed when a similar window is centered about the symmetry plane. Obviously, this is because e-vectors in each celestial half are mirror images of each other (Figs. 1 and 4), so that the error angles induced by e-vectors in the left and right half of the sky are opposite in sign and thus cancel each other out.

The specific spatial layout of analyzers forms the structural basis of the scanning mechanism of e-vector detection. In addition, it closely matches the distribution of the celestial e-vector pattern when the bee is aligned with the solar and antisolar meridian (Fig. 4). To determine the position of these meridians, the bee rotates and detects, when the array of analyzers is maximally active. This suggests that bees use e-vector information merely, or even exclusively, to determine the azimuthal position of the symmetry plane in the sky. Of course, selecting and steering a compass course is more than this. Other kinds of visual (and non-visual) information must be used by bees to determine the compass course relative to the celestial symmetry plane. Nevertheless, it would be premature to exclude the use of e-vector information in any further step of celestial navigation. The e-vector patterns in he sky produce very pronounced patterns in the bee's POL regions (17), and it may well be that the bee exploits these response patterns, in one way or another, to select and/ or stabilize her proper compass course.

References

1) Dyer, F. C., Gould, J. L. 1983. Honey bee navigation. American Scientist 71: 587- 597.

2) Frisch, K. von. 1949. Die polarisation des Himmelslichtes als orientierender Faktor bei den Tänzen der Biene. Experientia 5: 142-148.

3) Frisch, K. von. 1965. Tanzsprache und Orientierung der Bienen. Springer-Verlag, Berlin-Heidelberg-New York.

4) Glas, H. W. van. 1977. Models for unambiguous e-vector navigation in the bee. J. Comp. Physiol. 113: 129-159.

5) Glas, H. W. van. 1980. Orientation of bees, Apis mellifera, to unpolarized colour patterns, simulating the polarized zenith skylight patterns. J. Comp. Physiol. 139: 225-241.

6) Goldsmith, T. H. and Wehner, R. 1977. Restrictions of rotational and translational diffusion of pigment in the membrane of a rhabdomeric photoreceptor. J. Gen. Physiol. 70: 453-490.

7) Helversen, O. von. and Edrich, W. 1974. Der polarisationsempfänger im Bienenauge: ein Ultraviolettrezeptor. J. Comp. Physiol. 94: 33-47.

8) Kirschfeld, K. 1972. Die notwendige Anzahl von Rezeptoren zur Bestimmung des elektrischen Vektors linear polarisierten Lichtes. z. Naturforsch. 27c: 578-579.

9) Kirschfeld, K.; Lindauer, M. and Martin, H. 1975. Problems of menotactic orientation according to the polarized light of the sky. z. Naturforsch. 30c: 88-90.

10) Labhart, T. 1980. Specialized photoreceptors at the dorsal rim of the honey bee's compound eye: polarization and angular sensitivity . J. Comp. Physiol. 141: 19-30.

11) Rossel, S.; Wehner, R.; and Lindauer, M. 1978. E-vector orientation in bees. J. Comp. Physiol. 125: 1-12.

12) Rossel, S. and Wehner, R. 1982. The bee's map of the e-vector pattern in the sky. Proc. Natl. Acad. Sci. USA 79: 4451-4455.

13) Rossel, S. and Wehner, R. 1984a. How bees analyse the polarization patterns in the sky. Experiments and model. J. Comp. Physiol. A. 154: 607-615.

14) Rossel, S. and Wehner, R. 1984b. Celestial orientation in bees: The use of spectral cues. J. Comp. Physiol. A. 155: 605-613.

15) Rossel, S. and Wehner, R. 1986. Polarization vision in the bees. Nature 323: 128-131.

16) Sommer, E. W. 1979. Untersuchungen zur topographischen Anatomie der Retina und zur Sehfeldtopologie im Auge der Honigbiene. Ph. D. Thesis. University of Zürich.

17) Wehner, R. 1982. Himmelsnavigation bei Insekten. Neurophysiologie und Verhalten. Neujahrsbl. Naturf. Ges. Zürich 184: 1-132.

18) Wehner, R. 1983. The perception of polarized light. In: The Biology of Photoreception, eds. D. J. Cosens, D. Vince-Price. Soc. Exp. Biol. Symp. 36: 331-369.

19) Wehner, R. and Rossel, S. 1985. The bee's celestial compass - A case to study in behavioral neurobiology. In Experimental Behavioral Ecology and Sociobiology, eds. B. Hölldobler and M. Lindauer, pp. 11-53. Fischer-Verlag, Stuttgart, New York.

20) Wehner, R. and Strasser, S. 1985. The POL area of insect eyes: behavioral experiments with bees. Physiol. Entomol. 10: 337-349.

Physiological Aspects of Behavior

Texture Sensitivity in the Life of Honeybees

Peter G. Kevan

Department of Environmental Biology, University of Guelph, Guelph, Ontario N1G 2W1, Canada

Abstract. Texture perception is important in the life of honeybees. Larvae of workers and drones use differential textural cues within their cells to orientate with their heads outermost for pupation and emergence. Adult worker bees have a refined sense of texture which they use in building comb and preparing the insides of cells. Also, they can distinguish between flowers of different species of plants and between parts of the same petals by microscopic textural differences. This finding relates to the phenomena of floral constancy and nectar guides, which are important in foraging behavior. Two neurophysiological mechanisms for texture sensitivity are proposed. Phasic-tonic sensilla are suggested to operate in texture sensitivity for substrate preference (TSSP) in which the insects may be almost or entirely stationary whereas phasic sensilla are suggested to operate in texture sensitivity for information processing (TSIP) such as in foraging when insects are moving, often rapidly.

INTRODUCTION

In the lives of insects, mechanical stimuli are involved in more behavioral activities than any other types of external stimulus. The simplest types of mechano-sensitivity is that of the sense of touch. Despite the extensive literature on the physiology and morphology of mechano-receptors in insects (12, 16) there appear to be few studies on the physiology and behaviour of insects using this sensory mode. This is especially true at the level of fine discrimination, or textural discrimination of surfaces.

Surface textures have been shown to be important to various insects, notably for oviposition in Coleoptera (18, 21), Diptera (1, 20) and Lepidoptera (17). Such features may also be important in the discrimination of food by herbivorous insects (19), of resting sites (2), in recognition of nests in bees (2), and perhaps of mates (6) and in pseudocopulation in the pollination of Ophrys (Orchidacea) (13).

TEXTURAL SENSITIVITY IN BEES

Larval Sensitivity

The orientation of the larvae, and especially the pupae, of Hymenoptera in their cells is critical to their emerging successfully. In emerging as adults, they must be directed outwardly. How this is accomplished has not been well studied, but texture has been considered as important in various Hymenoptera e.g. eumenine wasps (4), Osmia (Megachilidae) (7) and honeybees (Apis mellifera L.) (8, 9). Jay investigated this problem by using artificial cells (gelatin capsules) in which to rear the larvae of the three castes. With the capsules, he used natural cappings from honeybee cells, paper tissues, surgical gauze, capsule lids with fine holes punctured inwardly, and fine plastic mesh. He also experimented with the gross shapes, concave and convex, of the ends of the "cells", and with the effects of gravity, ventilation, and length of cells. He concluded that the anterior-posterior orientation of larvae of workers and drones is controlled by texture and that, for workers, the shape of the end walls of the cell is of secondary importance. For the larvae of queens, gravity seems to be the most important cue in their vertically oriented cells; the rough texture of the cacoon may also be involved. Neither Jay (8, 9) nor Cooper (4) discuss the mechanism by which the textural cues are sensed by the larvae they studied. Dorso-ventral orientation is presumably mediated through the dorsal sense organs as described by Lukoschus (14) (see also 5).

Adult Sensitivity in the Hive

With the texture of the cells having been shown to be important to the orientation of larvae, it is logical to suppose that cells should be built with the appropriate smooth textures on the bottom and walls. It would be difficult for cell building insects to create a smooth inner surface for the lid or plug (cf. eumenines, Osmia, Apis mellifera mentioned above). Honeybees build comb in which the bottoms and walls are smooth and non-porous, whereas the cappings, which are made up of aggregates of wax particles, are porous and rough. Martin and Lindauer (15) have explored the sensory physiological components of comb-building, including the angular orientation of the cells and the thickness and texture of the walls, in honeybees. The tips of the antennae have special groups of mechano-sensory sensilla trichodea which are involved in the honeybeeś abilitÿ to finely control the thickness of the cell wall and to check for smoothness. Normally, honeybee workers produce cells with a wall thickness of about 73 um, but when their antennae have been amputated or mutilated they produce cells with a cell wall of up to more than twice as thick as usual.

Adult sensitivity in foraging

In that the texture sensitivity of honeybees has been shown to be important within the hive, one may suppose that this sensory ability should be used in foraging. The functional significance of the textural characteristics of floral surfaces has not been investigated, except as mentioned above (13) or in relation to visual cues caused by the textures creating coloured optical interference patterns (3). However, Kevan and Lane (10, 11) reasoned that the microtextural patterns on the petals of flowers may be important to bees in floral recognition and foraging orientation because i) the microtextural patterns on the petals of flowers can be used as diagnostic taxonomic characters (i.e. they are not plastic characters), ii) they are in the same size range and scale as the sensilla on bees antennae, and iii) bees tap flower petals with their antennae when landing on them.

Kevan and Lane (10,11) used dried and gold coated ray florets of Helianthus annuus (L.) and Xylorhiza wrightii (A. Gray) E. Greene (Asteraceae) as training objects for honeybees. The drying and gold coating removed intrinsic color and odour cues which may have been present on the florets, yet allowed the texture of the surface of the floret to remain. The bees were trained in a Y maze to distiguish between the two species, between florets of H. annuus in normal orientation (adaxial surface uppermost, distal end of the floret at the entrance of the choice chamber) and upside down, and normal and back-to-front (reversed end to end). The Y maze was designed so that as the bees entered the choice chamber they encountered a different item of texture on each antenna. In these experiments the honeybees were well able to distinguish the widely different patterns between H. annuus in its normal orientation versus upside down and versus X. wrightii. They also distinguished the normal from the reversed florets of H. annuus, but failed to distinguish between two normally oriented florets of H. annuus presented together. Their ability to discern normal from reversed florets may be important in orientation on the flowers and finding the reward. The textural differences and pattern direction may act as nectar guides.

A second experiment relied on the bees being trained to extend the proboscis when presented with a prepared floret of H. annuus in normal orientation. They were rewarded with sugar syrup for responses to florets of H. annuus, but not to those of X. wrightii. Although numerous bees were subjected to the experiment, only 8 could be trained. Those that could not be trained failed to respond by extendind their proboscides to any stimulus. The 8 trained bees responded erroneously only 10 % of the time (26 errors in 268 presentations) and then mostly (18 errors in 150 presentations) as extensions of the proboscis to the non-rewarding texture. These errors may have been the bees' exploratory tests of the experimenters reliability (11).

The ability of honeybees, and presumably other insects to learn to distinguish flowers on the basis of microscopic textural differences was hitherto unrecognized and is of considerable interest to botanists and animal ethologists and physiologists. For the botanists, the taxonomic characters on floral petals have been shown to be biologically functional. For animal physiologists textural discrimination has been shown to operate on a much finer scale than previously considered and for ethologists a new modality for learning (through texture) has been demonstrated in invertebrates.

Neurophysiology

Mechanosensory sensilla trichodea in insects fall into two catagories; those which respond to steady deformation (phasic-tonic) and those which respond rapidly upon being deflected (phasic). Both types may be involved in texture sensitivity, but, as far as I am aware, no neurophysiological studies have been made. Therefore, I present the following tentative ideas as to how insects percieve texture.

Sensilla which respond in a tonic or phasic-tonic manner are presumably involved in the detection of movement (as in flight), of the relative positions of the body part (e.g. the hair plates of the neck of honeybees; these relay information on the position of the bee's head in the building of the comb (15) and in other activities) and of the position of the body (e.g. in the dorso-ventral orientation of larvae in their cells (5, 14). On a roughly textured surface, an insect would have adjacent sensilla differently deformed: one on a ridge of the surface would be deflected more than one in a depression. On a smooth surface, adjacent sensilla would be similarly deflected and differential deflection would reflect the contours of the insect's body and different lengths of trichodea. The sensilla trichodea involved in this type of texture sensing for substrate preference must act in concert with one another so that the differential stimuli can be neurally integrated to provide the insect with an appreciation of the topographic nature of the substrate upon which it finds itself.

Phasic responses in texture sensitivity must be involved in rapidly moving insects. Again, the sensilla trichodea must act in concert so that the stimulus caused by the texture can be interpreted. The "sensillenkombination" on the tips of the antennae of honeybees is a good example of how the sensilla may be combined (15). Presumably, as any group of trichodea is rattled or swept over the textured surfaces, the rapid, phasic, responses from the individual setae make for a signal which is characteristic of the topographic pattern of the texture being felt. One may also assume that the degree of rugosity of the surface can also be interpreted by the insect as a result of differential deformation in individual, and adjacent, sensilla as the pass from crest into trough of the surface. Patterning in textured surfaces (such as found on petals) may be sensed by regularity in the deflection of individual and groups of sensilla as they pass over the surface being felt. The neural processes involved in this type of texture sensing for information processing must be complex as honeybees have been shown to discriminate and learn to recognize microscopic texture differences (10, 11).

CONCLUSION

Mechanoreception, especially as related to the sense of touch, seems to have been little studied. Perhaps that is because other sensory systems, even in mechanoreception, appear to be more complex and interesting; the sense of touch is thought to be the most primitive of the senses. However, I think that I have shown that the sense of touch in insects is a fertile area for research. Types of tactile sensitivity (texture sensing for substrate preference <u>versus</u>

texture sensing for information processing) need investigation and studies on neural intergration of information from groups of sensilla should give exciting results. The degree of resolution of textural sensitivity in insects is clearly fine, at least in honeybees, and research on this aspect of the subject may lead to new insights into various facets of insect behavior.

Acknowledgements. I am grateful to C. Schisler for her comments on this manuscript and discussions on the problem of texture sensitivity. R. Menzel kindly made possible the publication of these considerations.

REFERENCES

(1) Atkinson, W. D. 1983. Gregarious oviposition in Drosophila melanogaster is explained by surface texture. Aust. J. Zool. 31: 925-929.

(2) Berthold, R. 1967. Behavior of the german cockroach, Blatella (L.), in response to surface textures. J. New York ent. Soc. 75: 148-153.

(3) Brehm, B. G. and Krell, D. 1975. Flavonoid localization in epidermal papillae of flower petals: a specialized adaptation for ultraviolet absorption. Science (Washington) 190: 1221-1223.

(4) Cooper, K. W. 1957. Biology of Euminine wasps. I Digital communication in wasps. J. exp. Biol. 134: 469-509.

(5) Gontarski, H. 1957. Die Orientierung der Larve von Apis mellifera in der geschlossenen Zelle. I. Dorso-ventrale Orientierung. Z. Bienenforschung 3: 216-220.

(6) Gwynn, D. T. and Rentz, D. C. F. 1983. Beetles on the bottle: male buprestids mistake stubbies for females (Coleoptera). J. Aust. ent. Soc. 22: 79-80.

(7) Hirashima, Y. 1958. Comparative studies on the cacoon spinning habits of Osmia excavata Alfken and Osmia pedicornis Cockerell (Hymenoptera: Megachilidae). Scient. Bull. Fac. Agricult. Kyushu 16: 481-497.

(8) Jay, S. C. 1961. The longitudinal orientation of larval honeybees (Apis mellifera L.) within cells. Anim. Behav. 9: 3-4.

(9) Jay, S. C. 1963. The longitudinal orientation of larval honeybees (Apis mellifera) in their cells. Can. J. Zool. 41: 717-723.

(10) Kevan, P. G. and Lane, M. L. 1985. Flower petal microtexture is a tactile cue for bees. Proc. Nat. Acad. Sciences U. S. A.

(11) Kevan, P. G. and Lane, M. L. 1986. Bees can distinguish flowers of different plant species by microscopic textural features on petals. Honeybee Science (in press).

(12) Kiel, T. A. and Steinbrecht, R. A. 1984. Mechanosensitive and olfactory sensilla of insects. In: Insect Ultrastructure (Vol.2), eds. R. C. King and Akai, pp. 477-516. Plenum Publ. Corp.

(13) Lullenberg, B. 1961. Studies in Ophrys pollination. Zoolog. Bidrag Uppsala 34: 1-340 + plates.

(14) Lukoschus, F. 1955. Uber Hautsinnesorgane der Bienenlarve (Apis mellifera). Z. Bienenforschung 3: 85-87.

(15) Martin, H. and Lindauer, M. 1966. Sinnesphysiologische Leistungen beim Wabenbau der Honigbiene. Z. vergl. Physiol. 53: 372-404.

(16) McIver, S. B. 1975. Structure of cuticular mechanoreceptors of arthropods. Ann. Rev. Entomol. 20: 381-397.

(17) Pedigo, L. P. 1971. Ovipositional response of Plathypena scabra (Lepidoptera:Noctuidae) to selected surfaces. Annls. ent. Soc. Amer. 64: 647-665.

(18) Poston, F. L.; Whitworth, R. J.; Loera, J.; Safford, H. B. 1979. Effects of substrate characteristics on the ovipositional bahavior of the Southwestern Corn Borer. Annls. ent. Soc. Amer. 72: 47-50.

(19) Radkevich, V. A. and Bakaeva, G. Z. 1968. Peculiarities of the texture of leaves as an index of their palatability for leaf-eating insects. Zhurnal Obshchei Biologii 29: 723-730.

(20) Russo, R. 1978. Substrate texture as an oviposition stimulus for Aedes vexans (Diptera: Culicidae). J. med. Ent. 15: 17-20.

(21) Takahashi, F. and H. Mizuno. 1982. Infestation of rice weevils in rice grain in relation to drying procedures after harvest and the form of the grain at different stages in the milling process. Environ. Control Biol. 20: 9-16.

(22) Tepedino, V. J.; Loar, J. M.; Stanton, N. L. 1979. Experimental trapnesting: notes on nest recognition in three species of megachilid bees (Hymenoptera: Megachilidae). Pan Pacific Entomol. 55: 195-198.

Thermoregulation by Individual Honeybees

Bernd Heinrich

Department of Zoology, University of Vermont, Burlington, Vermont 05405, USA

Abstract. Honeybee workers warm up by shivering prior to flight until thoracic temperature (T_{th}) reaches near 35°C. Patterns and levels of endothermy of bees not in flight depend on tasks, caste and apparently motivation. External vibrations of the thorax are not always evident during shivering, but the indirect flight muscles are mechanically active during heat production whether the bees are in flight or not. There is little or no thermoregulation during flight until high (greater than 35°C) air temperatures when evaporative cooling from the head withdraws heat from the working flight muscles in the thorax. Thermoregulation by individual bees appears to involve a lower set-point (near 35°C) in the thorax that regulates the onset of heat production, and a higher set-point (near 44°C) in the head that regulates the onset of heat loss. The circulatory system contains loops in the petiole that conform to a counter-current heat exchanger that should aid to conserve heat in the thorax. Other hypotheses for the functions of these loops are presented. Indirect evidence suggests that drones have different patterns of endothermy and different mechanisms of heat loss than workers. However, this remains to be explored.

INTRODUCTION

Few aspects of insect thermoregulation have been so long and so well explored as the colony-level thermoregulation by honeybees. Recent studies have focussed on the physiology and behavior of thermoregulation by individual bees. However, this knowledge has not been consolidated. I here provide an overview of our present knowledge of thermoregulation by individual bees and point out puzzles that remain to be elucidated.

HEAT PRODUCTION

Warm-up

Like other insects with myogenic flight muscles (31), honeybees produce heat in the thorax prior to flight (9). Heat production is caused by contractions of the flight muscles, and the mechanics of this process have been of some interest. Esch (10) measured the relationships between temperature, action potentials and thoracic movements, and observed that increases in muscle temperature were always correlated with action potentials. External vibrations of the thorax, however, were often not measurable during heat production.

Subsequently, more detailed analyses of the mechanical activity of the indirect flight muscles (3, 12) showed that the dorso-ventral (DV) flight muscles shorten with individual twitches in response to normal excitation during heat production prior to flight. At high spike frequencies the muscles contract in an isotonic contraction with 1.6 u shortening for each Hz increase of action potential frequency up to at least 10 Hz. A spike frequency of 10 Hz causes enough heat production to increase thoracic temperature at a rate of 2.3°C per minute (12). The electrical activity of the dorsal longitudinal (DL) muscles is apparently no different than that of the DV; electrical activity of the DL follows that of the DV, although there are no preferred phase relationships in the timing of activation between the two muscle groups. During warm-up, the two sets of activated muscles stretch against each other to produce the isotonic contraction; a stop in electrical activity releases the tension and the heat production stops.

Flight

The action potential specific rate of oxygen consumption (and presumably heat production) is constant between warm-up and flight, averaging 1.16 and 1.14 ul/g/min respectively (3). During flight, however, there are approximately 10 muscle contractions per action potential, and the timing of action potentials is favored near the middle of the wing cycle (12). Wingbeat frequency (muscle contraction frequency) is, in part, a function of action potential frequency (12).

Since both the frequency and shape of the action potentials are similar during warm-up and during flight (12), it was of interest to determine why the muscles were used to produce isotonic contractions, on the one hand, while alternating their contractions to move the wings, on the other. The change from the warm-up to the flight mode is not well understood. However, 50-120 msec before mechanical oscillations of the muscles (wingbeats) occur, there is a transient increase in action potentials in both the DV and DL muscles (12). As a result, the DV shortens 20-40 u. The DL muscle is apparently stretched by the opposing DV muscles at the same time that it is caused to contract by the electrical activity it receives, and as a result of the two opposing forces, it increases in tension but it does not increase significantly in length. As in bumblebee flight muscles (4), the increased tension of the muscles (probably in conjunction with other muscles that regulate wing opening) is necessary to start the contraction oscillating of the myogenic wingbeat (28).

The action potential frequency (and associated muscle tension) could not in itself be the reason for the switch-over from the non-oscillating mode during warm-up to the oscillating during flight. Esch and Bastian (12) suggest that the momentary high action potential frequency of both the DV and DL muscles is the command to start the oscillations. However, the role of the direct flight muscles and the role of the articulations of the wings that would allow them to beat, and hence allow the alternate contractions and stretching of the indirect muscles, is so far not well understood.

Aerodynamic power (and heat production) of the honeybee flight system is positively correlated with action potential frequencies of the indirect flight muscles (13). However, with increasing muscle temperature, wingbeat frequencies can increase from 120 Hz to 190 Hz, lift can more than double, and flight velocity triple, while the action potential frequency does not change significantly (11). The large increase in power output under constant neural activation is likely due to increases of efficiency of the flight muscles when they are at a higher temperature. At low muscle temperature, the contractions of the antagonistic upstroke and downstroke muscles are of long duration (5) and the two sets of muscles, in part, contract against each other before they have fully relaxed. In order to get rapid alternate contractions so that full power is available for flight, honeybees, like many other insects, raise their thoracic temperature before initiating flight and stop flight to shiver if they are cooled by convection.

Before the significance of thermoregulation was understood, an insect's stopping in flight was often interpreted as a rest. For example, honeybees need more time to return from a feeder than for the flight out to it, and von Frisch (15) supposed "That is connected with the fact that with their burden they do not infrequently stop to rest." Bees leaving the hive start out with thoracic temperature near 36°C (19), while those at a feeder 600 m from the hive (at ambient temperature T_a = 17-20°C) have a thoracic temperature of 19 to 28°C (9). Presumably bees returning from a feeder often stop (at low T_a) to shiver after cooling convectively. If so, it can be predicted that return time shortens at higher T_a.

The mechanical properties of bumblebee indirect flight muscles (4) appear to be similar to those of the honeybee, and the limited amount of comparative data in bumblebees so far (20) is largely consistent with the model worked out for honeybees by Esch and his associates.

Variability of thoracic temperature

Honeybees have a preferred body temperature near 35°C (6), and bees within the core of a swarm cluster, within the brood nest, and around freshly built honeycomb maintain a body temperature within 1°C of 35°C (24, 27). The thermal stability of the large mass of thousands of bees is a product of the combined endothermy of the individuals. However, individuals by themselves who are not in flight show a highly variable T_{th}, with T_{th} often fluctuating 10°C over 2 minutes or less (24), presumably due to on-off shivering (3).

Individual bees within the hive, such as drones (6), could potentially be passive with regard to thermoregulation and still experience near optimal temperatures. However, if the workers all adopted the same passive strategy, then sub-optimum hive temperatures might result. Very little is understood relative to what extent the individuals attempt to regulate hive temperature, and to what extent they regulate their own body temperature and then secondarily affect hive temperature. A considerable amount, but by no means all, of the observed thermoregulation of honeybee swarms can be explained in terms of bees regulating their own body temperatures (24, 25), while other data show that individual bees are willing to put themselves in thermal stress to help regulate hive temperature (34). The extent to which hive thermoregulation can be explained in terms of thermoregulation of individuals has been discussed (25). Since young bees have considerably less thermogenic ability than older bees (1), it is likely that the younger bees tend to be more "parasitic" in the hive microclimate while the older bees are more active in regulating their own, and subsequently also the hive's temperature.

Aside from age polyethism in thermoregulation within the hive, task polyethism also results in thermoregulatory differences. Cena and Clark (7), using a thermal imaging camera, showed that darker bees in a wind tunnel running at 0.5 m s^{-1} and exposed to a radiant flux used to simulate sunshine, were about 1°C warmer than light bees. Esch (9), using infrared thermal photography, was able to follow the body temperature of dancing honeybees who were not hindered by thermocouple leads. He showed that bees in an open hive (at 30.5°C on the open comb) maintained T_{th} of 29-32°C, while the dancers next to them maintained T_{th} of 32-43°C. Round dancers had T_{th} = 40.5°C ± 2.3°C, while waggle dancers had T_{th} 32-38°C. When the dancer stopped to feed a follower, its T_{th} dropped by 1°C, while that of the follower simultaneously increased to that of the dancer. The T_{th} varied near 0.8°C within any one waggle dance, falling during the straight run and then again rising during the circle run before the next straight run. It is possible, however, that the energy expended is the same, with some of the energy during the straight run appearing as kinetic energy of buzzing, rather than as heat. Similarly, the bees that leave the hive also have T_{th} elevated to 36 - 38°C, while bees returning to the hive (at T_a of 7 to 23°C) have T_{th} lower than that of bees within the hive (19). Furthermore, of the bees leaving the hive, those engaged in nest defence have higher T_{th} than those leaving to forage, as do the bees of a swarm just prior to take-off (23). It appears, therefore, that the level of motivation (such as that related to retrieve food, to move to a new domicile or to attack enemies) affects T_{th}, which in turn affects flight speed.

A bee in the hive, or one otherwise not in flight, has the option of shivering or not shivering and thus quickly varying T_{th}. However, once flight is initiated, heat is produced uninterruptedly. At least until there is danger of overheating from the flight metabolism (at T_a is greater than 35°C), T_{th} appears to be a passive function of rates of convection and flight metabolism. At T_a = 10°C the bees cool rapidly and are unable to remain in continuous flight, whereas at T_a from 15°C to 30°C, T_{th} is near 15°C above T_a (19).

Bees departing from the hive show a T_{th} independent of T_a (8, 19) presumably because the internal hive temperature is stable and independent of T_a. However, bees returning to the hive (over a wide range of T_a) show a wide range of T_{th} (8). Nevertheless, bees returning at T_a near 12°C have a T_{th} near 35°C, even though they are unable to remain in continuous flight (in a temperature-controlled room) at that temperature (19). During continuous flight at 15°C, T_{th} is only 30°C, the minimum for flight. These observations suggest that the high T_{th} (35°C) observed in bees returning to the hive is most likely achieved by periodically stopping flight to reduce convective heat loss and to shiver before resuming flight. Indeed, under some conditions, bees may leave the hive to forage even at 4.5°C, although they then stop flight approximately every 10 sec to warm up (H. Esch, personal communication).

HEAT LOSS

The circulatory system

In some insects the circulatory system serves a primary function in thermoregulation by redistributing heat from the working thoracic muscles (16, 17). In bumblebees, the circulatory anatomy and physiology function to facultatively transfer heat to the abdomen both when brood is incubated (with the abdomen) and when heat must be dissipated from the thorax during flight at high air temperatures (20). At low air temperatures, however, the bees conserve heat to maintain T_{th} sufficiently elevated for flight, and the anatomy in the petiole area conforms to a counter-current heat exchanger which should help conserve heat in the thorax. The key to physiologically transferring heat into the abdomen depends on shunting blood quickly through the petiole before counter-current heat exchange has taken place. Conversely, for efficient heat exchange between the cool blood from the abdomen and the hot blood from the thorax, it is necessary to reduce blood flow, to slow the blood down, as well as to provide a large area for heat exchange.

The anatomy of the honeybees' circulatory system is notably unlike that of bumblebees, and the reason for this unique anatomy has long been of speculation. It was first noted by Pissarew (32, as quoted by (14)) that the aorta in honeybees, unlike those in wasps, hornets, leafcutter bees and bumblebees, is highly convoluted in the petiole area. Pissarew noted nine loops that appeared to be attached to each other and enclosed in a membrane. These observations were confirmed by Freudenstein (14) in his detailed study of the honeybee circulation. Various hypotheses have been presented to account for the functional significance of the loops. Pissarew (32) alluded that they might act in a pulsatile fashion, amplifying the pumping action of the heart. Arnhart (2) suggested instead that they function to provide resistance to the blood, so that during expansion of the heart in the abdomen, blood would enter the lateral valves of the heart rather than being sucked back from the head and thorax. Zander (37) concluded that they provided the slack so that the heart attached to the thoracic phragma would not tear during the rapid vibrations of the thoracic muscles during flight.

Freudenstein (14) provided data and rationale against all of the above hypotheses and presented an alternate hypothesis. He noted large numbers of trachae in the petiole area near the loops and suggested that the convolutions acted analogously to the lungs of vertebrates in providing a large surface area for helping to aerate the blood and to carry oxygen to the thoracic muscles. However, the oxygen carrying capacity of insect blood lacking respiratory pigments is probably minimal, and Freudenstein's hypothesis is also unsubstantiated.

One possibility is that the loops function in thermoregulation. According to Freudenstein (14), blood from the thorax flows over and around the loops before returning to the abdomen. Since the honeybee's thorax is heated by endogenous heat production, this blood is necessarily hot. On the other hand, the blood flowing through the coils from the unheated abdomen (22) is necessarily cool. The coils could function in three ways to promote counter-current heat exchange. First, they would obliterate discrete pulses of blood that could be quickly shuttled through the petiole, as occurs in bumblebees when they dump heat into the abdomen (17). Secondly, the loops would create a large surface area for possible counter-current heat exchange. Lastly, they would provide resistance and slow down the blood so that there is more time for counter-current heat exchange.

As predicted by the above hypothesis, honeybees do not transfer excess heat from the thorax to the abdomen (22). However, the carpenter bees, Xylocopa veripuncta, who also have a series of aortal loops in the petiole area, transfer considerable amounts of heat to the abdomen from the thorax (26). It remains to be determined whether or not the loops in Xylocopa also act as a counter-current heat exchanger. Perhaps they can in some way be reduced in their effectiveness when the bee needs to dump heat into the abdomen.

The contrast in physiologies of temperature regulation of honeybees and bumblebees is probably, in part, a result of the difference in body size. Because of their larger size, bumblebees may often face a potential problem of overheating, whereas honeybees, because of smaller size (and less insulation), face the problem of keeping heated up. So far all of the work has been restricted to workers. However, drone honeybees weighing near 200 mg, are as large and larger than most bumblebee workers. In addition, unlike bumblebee and honeybee workers, drones normally fly continuously rather than stopping and starting at flowers like workers do. Drone flights average 33 minutes, but can last an hour or more (36). Furthermore, drones leave the hive presumable carrying concentrated honey (rather than dilute nectar) so that they may not have the option to cool evaporatively (discussed later) as workers do. One might predict that drones would need to dissipate excess heat during flight, and that since the circulatory anatomy is the same as in workers (14), that they do something different than workers. So far, however, thermoregulation by honeybee drones is a mystery that has not yet been explored.

Evaporative Cooling

Lindauer (29) showed that a colony of honeybees can cool itself by evaporative cooling. During colony over-heating the hive bees selectively accept dilute nectar or water, and the colony's preferred foraging for sugar changes to water. Individual bees regurgitate dilute nectar, or water, hold it on the tongue, and deposit it on the combs. Esch (11) observed that bees in flight at high air temperatures also regurgitate fluid from the honeycrop, and they work it with their mouthparts and sometimes spread it over the underside of their thorax with their legs, presumably for evaporative cooling.

Laboratory experiments (18, 20, 21) directly confirmed the hypothesis that honeybee workers stabilize thoracic temperature during flight by evaporative cooling using regurgitated honeycrop contents. During free flight at T_a from 15°C to 25°C, honeybee workers did not regulate T_{th}; thoracic temperature varied directly with T_a, but some 15°C above it (19). However, at T_a greater than 42°C thoracic temperature was reduced to within 0.5°C of T_a (22) even though the rate of heat production during flight was relatively independent of T_a from 20°C to 42°C (22).

The ability to dissipate heat from the thorax was due primarily to evaporative cooling from the head. All bees who could fly at T_a greater than 40°C had an extruded droplet of fluid at the mouth, and their head temperatures were on the average 2°C below T_a (21). A detailed analysis of water economy of the honeybee during various kinds of activity revealed directly that evaporative water loss rises sharply when water is extruded from the mouth (30), rising from 17 mg $g^{-1}h^{-1}$ at T_{th} = 30°C to 139 mg $g^{-1}h^{-1}$ at T_{th} = 45°C. When the mouth parts were sealed with a wax-resin mixture, the evaporated water loss rose from 10 mg $g^{-1}h^{-1}$ to 61 mg $g^{-1}h^{-1}$ over the same temperature range. Evaporative cooling from the tracheal system has been briefly investigated (22) and so far its significance has not been shown to be of primary importance.

The transfer of heat between the thorax, where it is produced by the flight muscles, and the head, where it is lost evaporatively, occurs by both passive and active processes. The isolated head of a honeybee cools three times as fast as the thorax. However, in intact live as well as dead bees, head temperature closely tracks T_{th} due to conductive heat flow (21). Dead bees with water on their tongue show a rapid drop in T_{th} that is followed within seconds by a decline in head temperature.

The circulatory system probably aids in heat transfer. Heating of the head results in large amplitude pulsations of the aorta in the thorax, although heating of the thorax usually does not result in significant changes in the pumping of the thoracic aorta or the abdominal heart. These results are consistent with the observation that the abdomen does not serve as a major heat sink for excess heat from the thorax, and they contrast strongly with those of bumblebees (17) and sphinx moths (16) who use the abdomen as a radiator for excess heat and in whom the pumping of the abdominal heart is strongly dependent on thoracic temperature.

The physiological model of thermoregulation in honeybees that emerges is that head temperature is regulated, but only by defending an upper set-point. Thoracic temperature is tightly coupled to head temperature, and T_{th} is maintained less than 46°C secondarily, since heating of the thorax to near lethal temperatures by itself elicits neither the regurgitation of cooling liquid nor the associated response of the aorta. However, the thorax appears to contain a set-point (near 36°C) below which the bee shivers and above which it does not. At these (lower) temperatures, head temperature is a passive function of T_{th}.

Cooper et al. (8) confirmed that honeybees regulate head and thoracic temperature at high T_a by regurgitating droplets of honey stomach contents which are then evaporated. Furthermore, they extended the observations to provide an ecological perspective of honeybees foraging in the Sonoran desert at high air temperatures. Bees were foraging for nectar (but no pollen) at T_a above 40°C, and the proportion of bees returning to the hive who carried a fluid droplet on the tongue increased from essentially none at 20°C to 40% at 40°C. Pollen foragers, who on the average carry only 1.3 ul of fluid (in comparison to a mean content of 7.9 ul in other bees) decreased their activity at high T_a, but those pollen foragers who were foraging at high T_a almost never regurgitated fluid, and they had significantly higher T_{th} than the nectar foragers at the same T_a (8). Some of the pollen foragers had T_{th} exceeding 50°C, near their lethal limit.

A heat budget of foraging bees revealed that bees could fly for 45 s at T_a = 40°C before T_{th} would increase from 40 to 50°C; evaporation of 1.58 mg H_2O over the 45 s flight would prevent any increase in body temperature. Pollen foraging may be limited at high T_a (although many flowers also stop producing pollen during the hottest parts of the day).

Water foragers who specifically ferry water into the hive for hive thermoregulation may airlift 52 mg of water, or 65% of their body mass. These water carriers experience very high metabolic demands (30) which could potentially cause greater thoracic heating. However, heavily loaded honeybees at high T_a, in general, have lower T_{th} than those with low wing-loading (8), suggesting that they use more water for evaporative cooling.

It is possible that the above results on honeybee workers do not apply to drones. As already indicated, drones, because of their larger mass and their long continuous flights (36), may have a greater need to dissipate excess heat during flight than workers. However, they do not have access to sources of water, such as dilute nectar, and they presumably rely on honey from the hive as an energy source. This raises the question of whether or not they use evaporative cooling.

There is probably more known about the thermoregulatory physiology of honeybees than about any other insect. Both heat production and heat loss mechanisms have been examined in terms of physiology and in their ecological contexts. However, there are still numerous questions to be explored.

Acknowledgements. I thank Harald Esch for helpful comments on a draft of the manuscript.

REFERENCES

(1) Allen, M.D. 1955. Respiration rates of worker honeybees of different ages and at different temperatures. J. exp. Biol. 36: 92-101.

(2) Arnhart, L. 1906. Die Bedeutung der Aortenschlangenwindungen des Bienenherzens. Zoolog. Anzeiger 30: 721-722.

(3) Bastian, J., and Esch, H. 1970. The nervous control of the flight muscles of the honey bee. Z. vergl. Physiol. 67: 307-324.

(4) Boettiger, E.G. 1957. Triggering of the contractile process in insect fibrillar muscle. In Physiological Triggers, ed. T.H. Bullock, pp. 103-106. Washington: American Physiol. Soc.

(5) Buchthal, F.; Weis-Fogh, T.; and Rosenfalk, P. 1957. Twitch contractions of isolated flight muscles of locusts. Acta physiol. scand. 39: 246-276.

(6) Cahill, K., and Lustick, S. 1976. Oxygen consumption and thermoregulation in Apis mellifera workers and drones. Comp. Biochem. Physiol. 55A: 355-357.

(7) Cena, K., and Clark, J.A. 1972. Effect of solar radiation on temperatures of working honey bees. Nature 236: 222-223.

(8) Cooper, P.; Schaffer, W.M.; and Buchmann, S.L. 1985. Temperature regulation of honey bees (Apis mellifera) foraging in the Sonoran desert. J. exp. Biol. 114: 1-15.

(9) Esch, H. 1960. Über die Körpertemperaturen und den Wärmhaushalt von Apis mellifica. Z. vergl. Physiol. 43: 305-335.

(10) Esch, H. 1964. Über den Zusammenhang zwischen Temperatur, Aktionspotentialen und Thoraxbewegungen bei der Honigbiene (Apis mellifica L.) Z. vergl. Physiol. 48: 547-551.

(11) Esch, H. 1976. Body temperature and flight performance of honey bees in a servo-mechanically controlled wind tunnel. J. comp. Physiol. 109: 265-277.

(12) Esch, H., and Bastian, J. 1968. Mechanical and electrical activity in the indirect flight muscles of the honey bee. Z. vergl. Physiol. 58: 429-440.

(13) Esch, H.; Nactigall, W.; and Kogge, S.N. 1975. Correlations between aerodynamic output, electrical activity in the indirect flight muscles and wing positions of bees flying in a servomechanically controlled wind tunnel. J. comp. Physiol. 100: 147-159.

(14) Freudenstein, K. 1928. Das Herz und das Zirkulationssystem der Honigbiene (Apis mellifica L.) Z. Wiss. Zool. 132: 404-475.

(15) Frisch, K.v. 1967. The Dance Language and Orientation of Bees. Cambridge, Mass.: Harvard University Press.

(16) Heinrich, B. 1971. Temperature regulation in the sphinx moth, Manduca sexta. II. Regulation of heat loss by control of blood circulation. J. exp. Biol. 54: 153-166.

(17) Heinrich, B. 1976. Heat exchange in relation to blood flow between thorax and abdomen in bumblebees. J. exp. Biol. 54: 561-585.

(18) Heinrich, B. 1979a. Keeping a cool head: honeybee thermoregulation. Science 205: 1269-1271.

(19) Heinrich, B. 1979b. Thermoregulation of African and European honeybees during foraging, attack, and hive exits and returns. J. exp. Biol. 80: 217-229.

(20) Heinrich, B. 1979c. Bumblebee Economics. Cambridge, Mass.: Harvard University Press.

(21) Heinrich, B. 1980a. Mechanisms of body-temperature regulation in honeybees, Apis mellifera. I. Regulation of head temperature. J. exp. Biol. 85: 61-72.

(22) Heinrich, B. 1980b. Mechanisms of body-temperature regulation in honeybees, Apis mellifera. II. Regulation of thoracic temperature at high air temperatures. J. exp. Biol. 85: 73-87.

(23) Heinrich, B. 1981a. Energetics of honeybees swarm thermoregulation. Science 212: 565-566.

(24) Heinrich, B. 1981b. The mechanisms and energetics of honeybee swarm temperature regulation. J. exp. Biol. 91: 25-55.

(25) Heinrich, B. 1984. The social physiology of temperature regulation in honeybees. In Fortschritte der Zoologie, eds. B. Hölldobler and M. Lindauer, Vol. 31, pp. 393-406. Stuttgart, New York: G. Fischer Verlag.

(26) Heinrich, B., and Buchmann, S. 1986. Thermoregulatory physiology of the carpenter bee, Xylocopa varipuncta. J. comp. Physiol. B., in press.

(27) Himmer, A. 1927. Der soziale Wärmhaushalt der Honigbiene. II. Die Wärme der Bienenbrut. Erlanger Tb. Bienenkd. 5: 1-32.

(28) Kammer, A.E., and Heinrich, B. 1978. Insect flight metabolism. In Advances in Insect Physiology, eds. J.W.L. Beament, J.E. Treherne, and V.B. Wigglesworth, Vol. 13, pp. 133-228. London, New York: Academic Press.

(29) Lindauer, M. 1954. Temperaturregulierung und Wasserhaushalt im Bienenstaat. Z. vergl. Physiol. 36: 391-432.

(30) Louw, G., and Hadley, N. 1985. Water economy of the honeybee: a stoichiometric accounting. J. exp. Zool. 235: 147-150.

(31) Machin, K.E.; Pringle, J.W.S.; and Tamasige, M. 1962. The physiology of insect fibrillar muscle. IV. The effect of temperature on a beetle flight muscle. Proc. Roy. Soc. B. 155: 493-499.

(32) Pissarew, W.J. 1898. Das Herz der Biene (Apis mellifera L.). Zoolog. Anzeiger 21: 282-283.

(33) Schmaranzer, S. 1983. Thermovision bei trinkenden und tanzenden Honigbienen (Apis mellifera carnica). Verh. Dtsch. Zool. Ges. 1983: 319.

(34) Snodgrass, R.E. 1956. Anatomy of the Honey Bee. Ithaca, N.Y.: Comstock Publishing Associates, Cornell University Press.

(35) Vogt, F.D., and Heinrich, B. 1985. The response of workers to thermal stress in honeybee colony thermoregulation. Am. Zool. 25: Abstract No. 65.

(36) Witherell, P.C. 1971. Duration of flight and of interflight time in drone honey bees, Apis mellifera. Ann. Ent. Soc. Amer. 64: 609-612.

(37) Zander, E. 1911. Der Bau der Biene. Stuttgart: Verlag Eugen Ulmer.

Sleep Research on Honeybees: Neurophysiology and Behavior

Walter Kaiser and Jana Steiner-Kaiser

Zoologisches Institut der Technischen Hochschule Darmstadt, Schnittspahnstr. 3, D-6100 Darmstadt, FRG

Abstract. Observations and experiments on forager honeybees under various conditions have revealed that, when these insects rest at night, they exhibit phenomena which are strongly reminiscent of several features characteristically accompanying sleep in humans and mammals. In an observation hive at night, large numbers of bees remain stationary for long periods of time. These bees are not actively engaged in maintenance of hive temperature. In the laboratory (under various conditions), individual forager bees show daily or circadian rest-activity rhythms. At night, the following phenomena have been observed in intact bees: isolated, individual animals remain at one location for extensive periods of time during which only sporadic overt activity (e.g., grooming) can be observed; thoracic temperature falls to the prevailing environmental level (25 °C); the threshold for elicitation of a behavioral reaction rises; antennal motility gradually declines and the antennae assume characteristic positions which are also seen in resting hive bees, at night. Long-term recordings from visual interneurons in bees revealed the following features: the sensitivity of neurons in the lobula to visual stimuli (moving patterns) declines at night but can be transiently restored by mechanical or strong visual stimulation. Neuronal sensitivity and spontaneous activity fluctuate with a circadian rhythm. Electromyographic activity recorded from the bee's neck muscle 42 over several days show a progressive reduction in amplitude during the night. The corresponding overt expression of this decrease in neck-muscle tone is the gradual increase in the inclination of the head. The results obtained to date support our hypothesis that forager bees do, in fact, sleep at night.

INTRODUCTION

Hans Berger's discovery (2) of the electroencephalogram (EEG) in humans marked the start of modern, experimental sleep research. Since sleep in man involves changes in the state of consciousness, sleep researchers were initially reluctant to apply the term sleep to non-human species. Many entomologists who worked in the first half of this century apparently did not share this fear of being anthropocentrically biased. They published numerous descriptions of sleep behavior in insects, mainly Hymenoptera (6, 17). Lindauer (14), in contrast, was more cautious and described the behavior of bees which were resting as "idling".

Nowadays, it is generally accepted that some of the daily, regularly recurring inactivity (rest) seen in mammals and birds is comparable to human sleep. This inference is based on the many similarites between sleep signs in humans and the phenomena accompanying rest in birds and mammals. Sleep signs are behavioral and physiological parameters which are used to objectively define the state we call sleep (20). Recently, we have accumulated evidence which, in our opinion, justifies using the term sleep for forager honeybees as well.

EVIDENCE FOR THE PRESENCE OF SLEEP IN FORAGER HONEYBEES

Only a brief outline of the various methods which have been employed will be presented here. Detailed information is available elsewhere (10, 11, 12, 13).

Observations under natural conditions

The natural behavior of bees at night was studied in an observation hive. Observations were made for brief periods under dim incandescent illumination. A thermovision camera with display screen was kindly put at our disposal for one night. We saw that large numbers of bees were sitting still at the edges of the comb, where brood is absent, as well as on the wooden walls of the hive and on the glass panes. Only a small number of bees could be seen resting in empty cells, although these were available in large numbers. Those bees which rested on the horizontal lower comb-frames which had not yet been covered with comb-cells yielded the first indication of the existence of a sleep-like state: the bodies of several of these bees had sunken down so close to the substrate that the mandibles made contact with the latter. The tone in the leg muscles had obviously decreased. The antennae of these animals were observed to occupy an unusual position. This postural constellation was subsequently also observed in the laboratory and examined there in detail (12). The same antennal position could be seen in many of the bees which rested on vertical surfaces in the hive. The stationary bees showed very few or no movements of the head, body or legs; the antennae were seen to move more frequently.

Viewing the comb with the thermovision camera ruled out the possibility that the resting animals were producing heat with their thoracic muscles - motionless bees were indistinguishable from the dark background. The only bright patch on the screen was the brood area. Direct observation revealed that most of the active bees on the comb were, in fact, moving over the brood area. These finding are in agreement with the results obtained by Esch (5) who measured the thoracic temperature of single bees in a hive.

Time lapse video observations on individual, unrestrained forager bees in the laboratory

In order to make uninterrupted observations on resting bees at night, we put individual foragers into a lucite chamber and monitored their behavior continuously with video equipment. Total darkness at night was achieved by using a video camera sensitive to infrared radiation and short wavelength infrared illumination (see (12) for details). Ambient temperature was held constant at 25°C.

The analysis of the video tapes yielded the following results: There was a clear day/night difference in the behavior of the bees. During the day, the animals constantly moved around in the chamber, making only brief interruptions for feeding and grooming. At night, bees remained in one and the same location for extensive periods of time. Detailed observations of their overt behavior during such times showed clearly that these resting animals were by no means immobile. Figure 1 represents the fifth night of a long-term video observation.

These data are a typical example of all the results obtained to date in this experimental situation. Figure 1A shows that the amount of time in which both body and head are motionless increases progressively during the night, reaches a maximum late at night and then decrease until locomotor activity begins. Antennal movements can be observed even when all head and body movements are absent. Thus movements of the antennae or absence thereof seem to be a more sensitive behavioral indicator than head/body movements for the

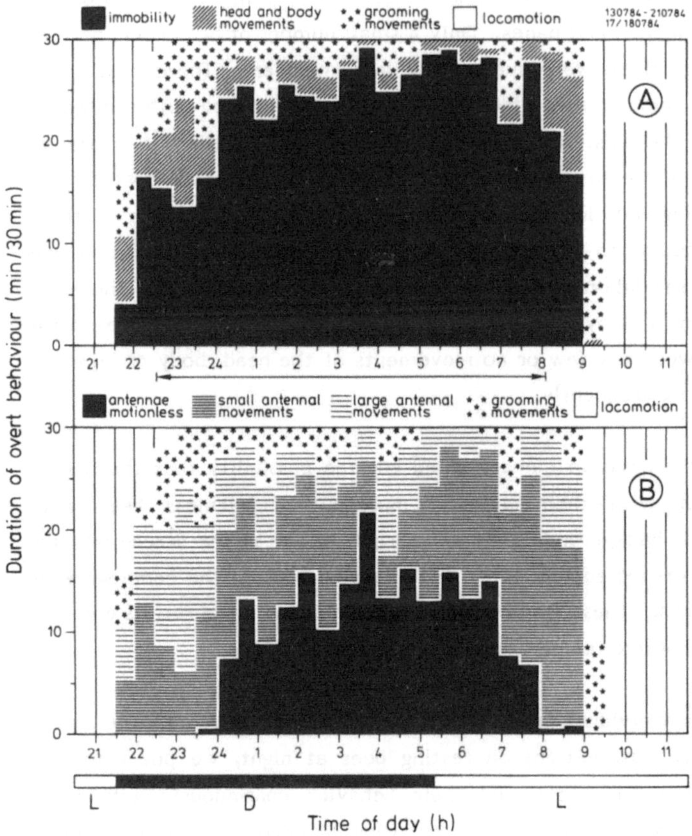

Fig. 1 - The motility of an individual bee maintained in a lucite chamber. Resolution in time for both diagrams is 2 s. The category "antennae motionless" includes spasmodic movements of very small amplitude. The interval between the arrowheads indicates the period of time for which the bee remained stationary in one and the same location (right chamber wall, head pointing upwards). L, D: light and dark phases, respectively, of the daily illumination cycle. Animal from an outdoor hive. July 1984. (From (12).)

level of central nervous excitation. Figure 1B is a reanalysis of the data from the video recording in which only antennal movements were scored. As expected, the black area in Figure 1B (antennae motionless) is much smaller than the black area in Figure 1A (absence of all head and body movements). The total amount of time occupied by each of the overt behaviors scored is as follows: immobility of body and head, 8.8 h; head and body movements, 1.2 h; antennae motionless, 3.5 h; small antennal movements, 4.1 h; large antennal movements, 2.4 h. Grooming movements constitute an independent category whose duration is 1.1 h.

Tobler (19) has used the presence of complete behavioral immobility as a measure of sleep time in cockroaches. This would correspond to the category "antennae motionless" in our data and yield a total sleep time of 3.5 h. The cockroach was found to have a total sleep time of 14 h. However, Tobler only scored the presence or absence of large antennal movements on her video tapes. On the basis of our detailed analysis of antennal motility and position, we believe that, at the very least, the small antennal movements belong to the state of sleep (antennae motionless). Thus a conservative estimate of the total sleep time for this bee (which is a typical example) is 7.6 h. The duration of "immobility" is probably an even more appropriate estimate of the bee's total sleep time. The bees' antennae also display a progressive decrease in motility at night; the peak of antennal immobility (Fig. 1B) coincides with that of body immobility (Fig. 1A).

In man, motility has been shown to be an adequate indicator of the depth of sleep (21). Motility is minimal during deep sleep (stages 3 and 4 of human non-rapid-eye-movement sleep). In contrast to humans, it appears that bees experience their deepest sleep late at night.

The threshold for the elicitation of grooming movements

Stimulation of the antennae with pulses of infrared radiation proved to be a very good method for eliciting grooming movements. Following a thermal stimulus of sufficient intensity, a bee will sweep over its head and antennae with its forelegs. Thermal stimuli elicit grooming movements ("Wärmeputzen" (9)) in many insect species. This reaction has not been described, to date, in honeybees. The threshold for the grooming reaction was determined during relatively long pauses in locomotor activity. During such pauses, and also during inactivity at night, the thoracic temperature fell to the prevailing environmental level (25°C). In Figure 2, the curve with the unfilled circles and dashed lines shows the typical daily course of the reaction threshold. During the day, the threshold values are low, but they increase during the night to a maximum of about 3 times the daytime values. Threshold measurements were always performed during video observation of the bees. Higher thresholds were associated with more pronounced downward tilting of the head and reduced antennal activity.

In humans, an increase of reaction threshold is a reliable sleep sign. A comprehensive review of threshold determinations during sleep in mammals can be found in (3). High thresholds for responses to sensory stimulation in "sleeping" insects have been described qualitatively by a number of authors (1, 6, 7, 8).

Inclination of the bee's head during the day and the night

The observed correlation between high reaction threshold and increased inclination of the head at night was investigated in more detail. The angle of inclination of the head, alpha , of a bee which was mounted above a treadwheel was measured once every 10 min on the video monitor. (The video tapes contained real-time information). Figure 2 (filled circles, continuous line) shows a typical daily course of alpha. During the night, the bee's head displays varying degrees of downward tilt (negative alpha values). Particularly low values occur late at night. In contrast, during the day, almost all alpha values are positive: the head is held raised. The transitions between activity and rest are characterized by gradual changes in alpha. At "light-on", the bee only briefly raises its head. Thereafter, alpha remains within the range of values typical for the night for quite some time before gradually increasing to its daytime level.

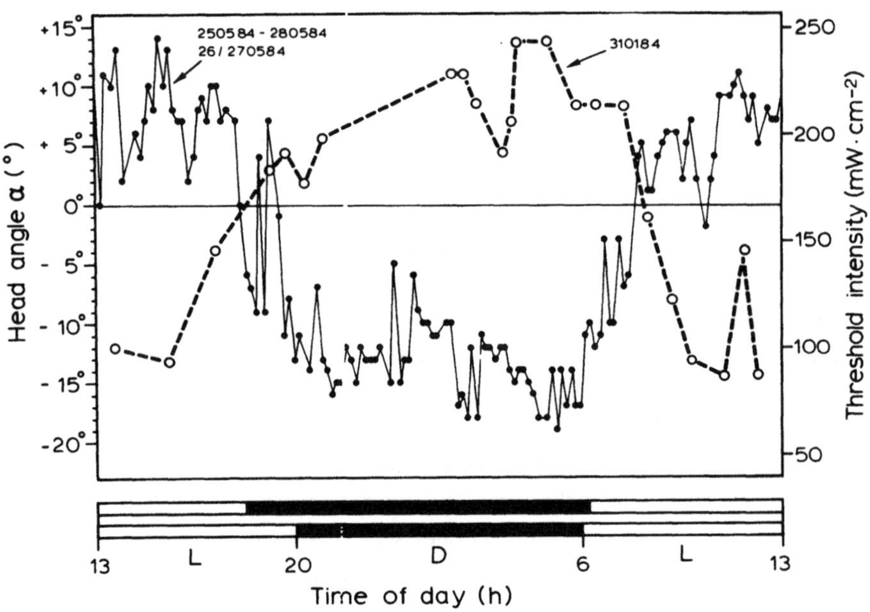

Fig. 2 - Dashed line: Time course of the threshold intensity of infrared radiation (ordinate on the right) which elicits grooming of the head and antennae. These results were obtained during the second experimental day. The upper bar underneath the time-axis indicates the corresponding LD-cycle. Animal from a winter flight-room. January 1984. Continuous line: Time course of the angle of inclination of the head (ordinate on the left). Alpha is defined as the angle between the vertical plane (direction of the force of gravity) and the line which passes through the base of an antenna and the anterior edge of the ipsilateral mandible. Negative alpha values correspond to the bee's "chin" coming close to the "chest". Second day of a 3-day experiment. The LD-cycle of this experiment is represented in the lower bar under the time-axis. The bee came from an outdoor hive. May 1985. The bees were mounted above a treadwheel in both experiments (From (12).)

The two curves in Figure 2 are surprisingly similar despite the fact that they represent different data from different animals: the reaction threshold curve is almost a mirror-image of the head-angle curve. There is a gradual day/night transition in both curves. These results clearly demonstrate that particular postural constellations of the head and antennae are correlated with particular threshold values.

A reduction of tone in the neck muscles is a reliable sleep sign in mammals (16). It seemed reasonable to suppose that the increased downward tilt of the bee's head at night was due to a reduction in the tone of the neck muscles. This was confirmed by the results of the experiments described below.

Electromyography of neck muscle 42

Muscle 42 (18) raises the bee's head and can also participate in turning it. The electromyogram (EMG) of this muscle was recorded over several 24-h cycles. Activity was sampled for 20 s at 5-min intervals. The amplitude of the EMG is time-dependent. Largest amplitudes occur during the day. Late at night, only small-amplitude potentials are present. On the basis of the amplitudes of the dominant potentials, the EMGs can be assigned to one of four classes. Level 4 corresponds to the waking level; level 1 is equal to about twice the noise level of the recordings. Figure 3 shows the course of the EMG level over one 24-h cycle. "Light-on" produces only a transient effect.

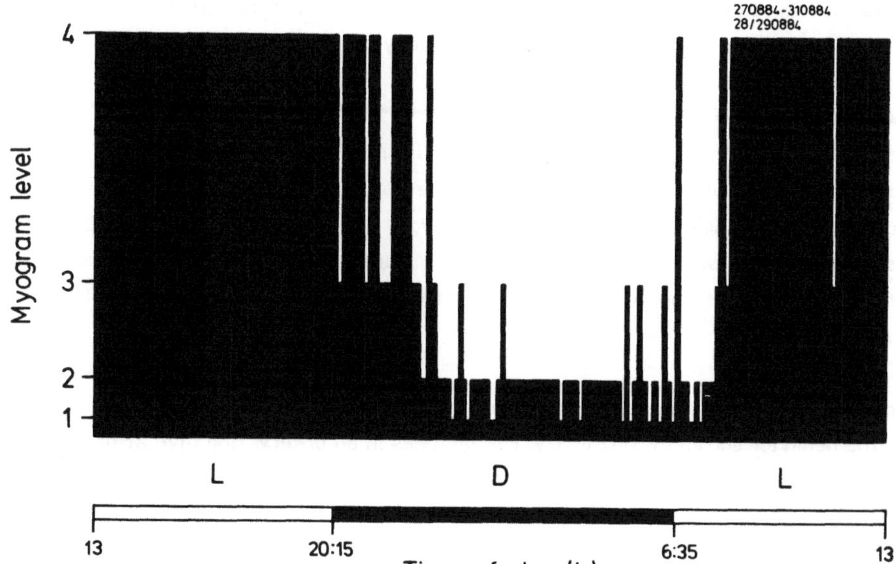

Fig. 3 - Myogram level of neck muscle 42 as a function of the time of day. The height of each level on the ordinate reflects the relative amplitude of the respective EMG. Results from the second day of a 4-day recording. Bee from an outdoor hive. August 1984. (From (12).)

The four sleep signs described above - reduction in motility, increased reaction threshold, decreased thoracic temperature and reduced neck-muscle tone - are, in themselves, very strong evidence in support of the hypothesis that bees experience sleep at night.

Results from long-term neurophysiological experiments

We also have important neurophysiological data which favor the idea that bees do, in fact, sleep. During the course of electrophysiological recordings from single, higher-order interneurons in the third optic ganglion (lobula) of the honeybee's brain (10, 13) the presence of a circadian oscillation in their sensitivity to a visual stimulus (a moving, striped pattern) was revealed. The neurons are more sensitive during the subjective day than during the subjective night. The spontaneous activity of these visual interneurons also fluctuates in a circadian fashion. These circadian rhythms are of particular interest since it has been recently demonstrated that circadian processes play a central role in sleep regulation (4).

The key result of the electrophysiological experiments was that, during the time of reduced neuronal responsiveness at night, the sensitivity of the neurons could be rapidly, albeit temporarily, restored by mechanical or strong visual stimulation of the animals. These data were surprisingly similar to results obtained by Livingstone and Hubel (15) during the course of investigations of visual interneurons in the lateral geniculate body and visual cortex of cats. During slow-wave sleep, the sensitivity of the cats' neurons to visual stimuli was lower than during waking. Acoustic and tactile stimulation of sleeping cats induced an immediate return to higher levels of neuronal sensitivity. A comparison of our data with those from the cat yields strong support for the existence of sleep in honeybees.

CONCLUSIONS

The data presented here strongly support the hypothesis that sleep occurs in bees. With the exception of the observations made on bees in an observation hive at night, all the results have been obtained from single forager bees, isolated from their normal surroundings. Despite the various experimental situations, the results are surprisingly uniform: the stage of profoundest sleep at night is approached gradually; it occurs late at night and the return to wakefulness is also gradual.

The sleeping behavior shown by individual bees in the laboratory was similar, in many respects, to the behavior shown by stationary, resting bees in an observation hive at night. We are therefore confident that we are not dealing with an artefact.

Despite the enormous progress made in experimental sleep research during the last 60 years, we still understand relatively little about the biological purpose of sleep and the mechanisms which control it, particularly at the cellular level. We believe that the bee represents a model system with many advantages for comparative sleep research. Despite the fact that they are systematically so far removed from man, forager worker bees have several features in common with mature humans: they are social, have a highly developed communication system and learning capacity, are diurnally active, spend their resting phases in sheltered surroundings and have one main bout of sleep, at night, every 24 h. We hope that further study of the cellular processes occurring during sleep in bees will reveal general principles which are common to a wide variety of animals and which have been conserved in the course of evolution.

Acknowledgements. Generous financial support has been provided by the Deutsche Forschungsgemeinschaft under the program SFB 45.

REFERENCES

(1) Andersen, F.O. 1968. Sleep in moths and its dependence on the frequency of stimulation in Anagasta kuehniella. Opusc. Ent. 33: 15-24.

(2) Berger, H. 1929. Über das Elektrenkephalogramm des Menschen. I. Arch. Psychiat. Nervenkr. 87: 527-570.

(3) Bonnet, M. 1982. Performance during sleep. In Biological Rhythms, Sleep and Performance, ed. W.B. Webb, pp. 205-237. Chichester, New York: John Wiley and Sons.

(4) Daan, S.; Beersma, D.G.M.; and Borbély, A.A. 1984. Timing of human sleep: Recovery processes gated by a circadian pacemaker. Amer. J. Physiol. 246: R161-R178.

(5) Esch, H. 1960. Über die Körpertemperaturen und den Wärmehaushalt von Apis mellifica. Z. Vergl. Physiol. 43: 305-335.

(6) Fiebrig, K. 1912. Schlafende Insekten. Jena. Z. Naturwiss. 48 (NF41): 315-364.

(7) Frisch, K.v. 1918. Beitrag zur Kenntnis sozialer Instinkte bei solitären Bienen. Biol. Zbl. 38: 183-188.

(8) Haufe, W.O. 1963. Ethological and statistical aspects of a quantal response in mosquitoes to environmental stimuli. Behaviour 20: 221-241.

(9) Herter, K. 1953. Der Temperatursinn der Insekten. Berlin: Duncker & Humblot.

(10) Kaiser, W. 1983. Effects of non-visual and circadian inputs to visual interneurones in the honey bee. In Multimodal Convergences in Sensory Systems, ed. E. Horn (Fortschr. Zool. 28), pp. 149-166. Stuttgart, New York: Gustav Fischer Verlag.

(11) Kaiser, W. 1985. Comparative neurobiology of sleep - the honey bee model. In Sleep '84, eds. W. P. Koella, E. Rüther and H. Schulz, pp. 225-227. Stuttgart, New York: Gustav Fischer Verlag.

(12) Kaiser, W. in press. Busy bees need rest, too. - Behavioural and electromyographical sleep signs in honey bees. J. Comp. Physiol.

(13) Kaiser, W., and Steiner-Kaiser, J. 1983. Neuronal correlates of sleep, wakefulness and arousal in a diurnal insect. Nature 301: 707-709.

(14) Lindauer, M. 1952. Ein Beitrag zur Frage der Arbeitsteilung im Bienenstaat. Z. Vergl. Physiol. 34: 299-345.

(15) Livingstone, M.S., and Hubel, D.H. 1981. Effects of sleep and arousal on the processing of visual information in the cat. Nature 291: 554-561.

(16) Morrison, A.R. 1983. A window on the sleeping brain. Sci. Amer. 248: 86-94.

(17) Rau, P., and Rau, N. 1916. The sleep of insects; an ecological study. Ann. Entomol. Soc. Amer. 9: 227-274.

(18) Snodgrass, R.E. 1956. Anatomy of the Honey Bee. Ithaca, London: Comstock Publishing Associates.

(19) Tobler, I. 1983. Effect of forced locomotion on the rest-activity cycle of the cockroach. Behav. Brain Res. 8: 351-360.

(20) Tobler, I. 1984. Evolution of the sleep process: A phylogenetic approach. In Sleep Mechanisms, eds. A.A. Borbély and J.-L. Valatx (Exp. Brain Res. Suppl. 8), pp. 207-226. Berlin, Heidelberg, New York, Tokyo: Springer-Verlag.

(21) Wilde-Frenz, J., and Schulz, H. 1983. Rate and distribution of body movements during sleep in humans. Percept. Mot. Skills 56: 275-283.

Behavioral and Pharmacological Analysis of the Stinging Response in Africanized and Italian Bees

N. Balderrama[1], H. Díaz[1], A. Sequeda[1], J. Núnez[2] and H. Maldonado[2]

[1]Lab. Fisiol. Insectos, Instituto de Zoología Agrícola, Facultad de Agronomía (UCV), Apartado 4579, Maracay 2101, Edo. Aragua. Venezuela

[2]Departamento de Biología, FCEN (UNBA), Buenos Aires, Argentina

Abstract. Sensitivity to a noxious stimulus was determined for the stinging response of Africanized and Italian bees. The more "aggressive" Africanized bees proved to be less sensitive (i.e., they responded with fewer stinging responses) than the more "gentle" Italian bees to the same nociceptive stimulation. Italian bees showed positive correlation of sensitivity with nectar flow during the year and the same seems to be true for Africanized bees during the day. Results obtained after morphine and naloxone + morphine treatment on bees suggest the existence of an endorphinic system for pain modulation, but its implication for the observed sensitivity changes is not yet known.

INTRODUCTION

Hive defensive behavior is primarily elicited by some external stimuli, but subsequently it is enhanced by recruitment stimuli (i.e., alarm pheromones). The defensive response thresholds to these stimuli probably determine the intensity of the collective behavior (6). The social defensive responsiveness ("aggressiveness") depends on genetic factors of the line of bees (13), but it seems to be regulated by both internal and external factors of the hive (2). Methods for assessing "aggressiveness" of whole hives in order to diagnose pure and inbred lines (1, 14) proved to be neither precise enough nor reproducible enough; therefore, assays using a small number of bees were recommended and therewith utilized (5).

Individual defensive reactions to a noxious stimulus have been measured on shrimp (7), honeybees (11), and praying mantises (15) to analyse behavioral changes in intact animals injected with opiates. With honeybees (11), the individual defensive reaction considered in the assays was the stinging response, which is a culminating behavior displayed by alarmed bees defending the hive (4).

It was considered relevant to analyse the reliability of the stinging response method to quantify the social defensive responsiveness of certain lines of bees. This article summarizes a pharmacological one investigation of the stinging response (11).

RESULTS

Behavioral Analysis

Africanized honeybees (A) and Italian honeybees (I) were captured when foraging at artificial food sources (50% w/w sucrose solution). Each bee was chilled at $0^{o}C$ for 3-4 min and placed in a holder designed to ensure that the bee came into close contact with 2 electrodes plates, one positioned at the neck and the other positioned at the penduncle between the thorax and the abdomen. Using conductive gel, the measured resistance between the electrodes was 80-90 K . After 15 min in the holder, bees were given five electrical stimuli (AC-60 Hz current) of 2 sec duration and increasing voltage intensity (1, 2, 3, 4 and 5 volts), with inter-trial intervals of 1 min. The reactions registered were all or none full-stinging responses (i.e., when the sting chamber was wholly opened, the shaft turned down and the lancets completely protracted during the entire trial of 2 sec) (11).

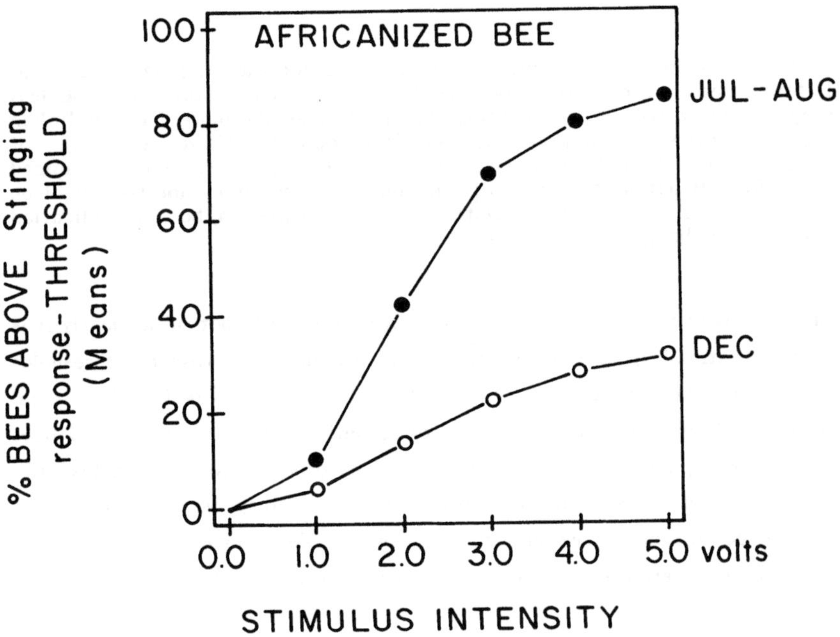

Fig. 1 - Percentage of Africanized bees (means) that, by increasing voltage on successive trials, attained the stinging response threshold. 17 groups of 10 bees in July-August and 22 groups of 10 bees in December.

The percentage of bees giving a full-stinging response increased with stimulus intensity up to 4 volts. A slight decrease in the values was observed with a stimulus intensity of 5 volts. Results obtained with 144 groups of 10 Africanized bees give the following % means ($\pm$ s.e.): 8 ($\pm$ 1); 23 ($\pm$ 2); 37 ($\pm$ 2); 44 ($\pm$ 1); and 39 ($\pm$ 2) for the corresponding stimulus intensities : 1; 2; 3; 4; and 5 volts.

Figure 1 represents the percentage of Africanized bees that, by increasing stimulus intensity on successive trials, attained the stinging response threshold. Results are the means of 17 groups of 10 bees tested in July-August and 22 groups of 10 bees tested in December. In July-August 85.0% ($\pm$ 0.1%) of the bees attained the stinging response threshold in the range of stimulus intensity used (1 to 5 volts); on the other hand, only 31% ($\pm$ 0.5%) of the bees reached that threshold in December.

An estimation of the sensitivity of bees to the noxious stimulus was obtained by ranking the bee's responses according to the lowest stimulus intensity eliciting a full-stinging response. The scores, or sensitivity index values, were: 1.0 when the stinging response was already apparent at 1 volt stimulation; 0.8 when at 2 volts; 0.6 at 3 volts; 0.4 at 4 volts; 0.2 at 5 volts; and 0.0 (zero) when no stinging response was observed.

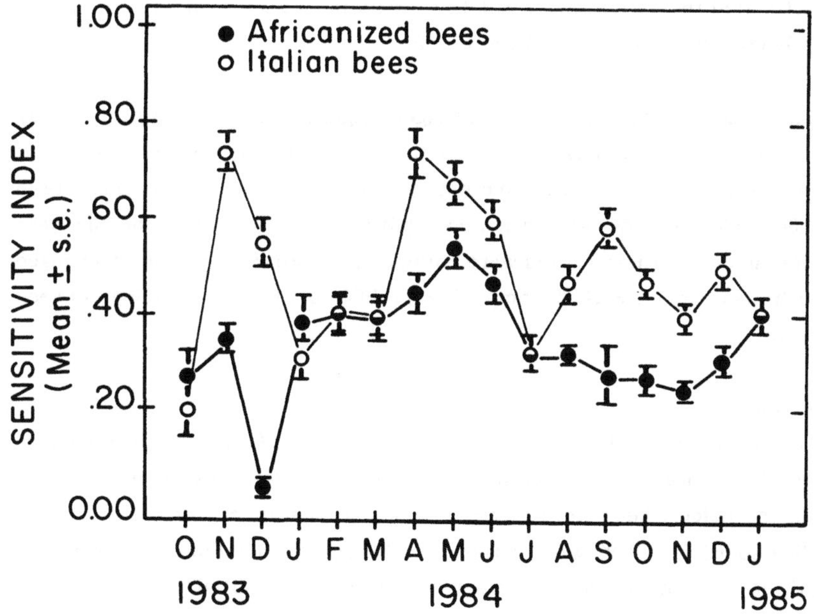

Fig. 2 - Sensitivity index variation during the period Oct. 1983 to Jan. 1985 for Africanized and Italian bees.

When comparing the July-August bee performances with those of December (Fig. 1) by different evaluation procedures, the following ratios were obtained: a) 85/31 = 2.74 (from maximal responsiveness attained for the 1-5 volts range); b) 7.5/2.25 = 3.33 (from the ratio of slopes of the linear part of the logistic curves); and c) 0.55/0.19 = 2.89 (from the sensitivity index values); all approximately similiar ratios.

Sensitivity index values were estimated for successive months of the period from October 1984 to January 1985 for Africanized and Italian bees randomly sampled in the course of the day. Figure 2 shows significant changes in the values of the sensitivity index during the course of the year, both for Italian and Africanized bees. The majority of the sensitivity index-monthly values were significantly greater for the Italian than the Africanized bees. Estimation of total mean values gave 0.47 ± 0.01 (n = 3460) and 0.33 ± 0.01 (n = 3382), respectively for the Italian and Africanized bees (Student t-value = 19.24; p is less than 0.001).

The density of bees foraging at an artificial food source with a constant sugar flow has been taken to be proportional to the rate of nectar output by the natural unknown food sources. This value was called foraging pressure (10). Foraging pressure of Africanized and Italian bees was estimated during the course of the year with an artificial food source of constant sugar flow (i.e., 11 ul/min - 50% w/w sucrose solution). A positive correlation was obtained between sensitive index-monthly values (Y) and foraging pressure-monthly values (x) for the Italian bees. The estimated regression line $Y = 0.23 + 0.02\ x$ ($r^2 = 0.55$) evinces a significant correlation at p = 0.05 (Student t-value = 2.18 and 11 DF).

With the Africanized bees, the sensitivity changed significantly (ANOVA, one-way classification, F = 3.48 with 11, 1548 DF; p is less than 0.001) in the course of the day, showing two maximal values, one early in the morning (hr: 8:00-9:00) and another one late in the evening (hr. 17:00-19:00). On the other hand, no significant changes during the day were observed with the Italian bees. These results were obtained in February-June for Africanized bees (n = 1549) and Italian bees (n = 1488) sampled from 7:00 to 19:00 h, including between 100-130 bees per hour.

Pharmacological analysis

The experimental procedure utilized has been described elsewhere (11) and was similar to that described in the behavioral analysis section but with two differences: a) immediately after being fixed in the holder, bees were given a 2 ul injection of one of the following: distilled water, saline solution (0.9 % w/v), different solutions of morphine-HCl, morphine HCl + naloxone-ClH, or solutions of enkephalin and related peptides. b) after 15 min in the holder, bees were given three electrical stimuli of the same voltage intensity (i.e., equivalent to 2 volts as compared with the previous method). Each result was the mean ± s.e. corresponding to a group of 40 Africanized bees.

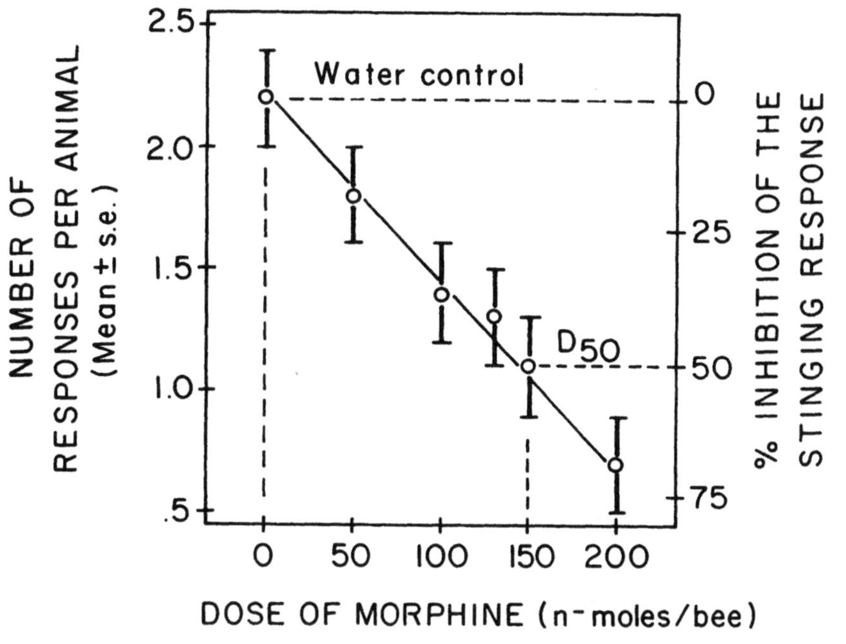

Fig. 3 - Dose-response curve for the inhibition of the stinging response by morphine.

The number of stinging responses per animal (mean ± s.e.) obtained with bees injected with distilled water (2.2 ± 0.2), with saline solution (2.1 ± 0.2) or without any injection (2.1 ± 0.2) were statistically all the same. However, as is shown in Figure 3, bees injected with different doses of morphine-HCl, (i.e., 50, 100, 130, 150 and 200 n-moles/bee, showed a decrement in responsiveness in comparison with the distilled water control (0.0 n-moles/bee of morphine-HCl). The number of responses per animal (Y) decreases linearly with morphine dose (x): regression line Y = 2.2 - 0.007 x; r^2 = 0.99. A 50% inhibition of the stinging response (D_{50}) was found with 150 n-moles of morphine-HCl/bee.

The inhibitory effect of morphine on the stinging response was reduced and completely blocked by simultaneous administration of naloxone. Figure 4 shows the effect on the stinging response of different doses of naloxone-HCl (i.e., 0.1, 0.2, 0.4, 0.7, 0.9, 1.4, 1.8 and 3.5 n-moles/bee) given in conjunction with the D_{50} of morphine-HCl (150 n-moles/bee). Naloxone blockade of morphine D_{50} increased almost linearly with log naloxone dose up to 0.9 n-moles/bee, and then a decreasing tendency was evident with higher naloxone doses. In fact, with doses higher than 0.1 n-moles naloxone-HCl/bee, the number of responses per animal was significantly greater than that obtained with a D_{50} dose of morphine, and, with doses higher than 0.4 n-moles/bee, response was not significantly different from that obtained with the distilled water control.

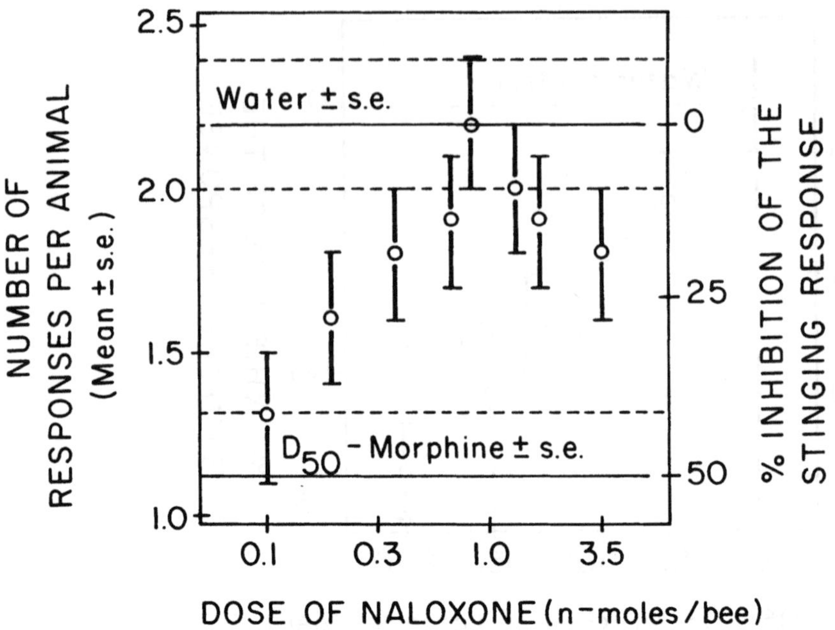

Fig. 4 - Effect of different doses of Naloxone (log scale) given in conjuction with the D_{50} of Morphine (150 n-moles/bee) on the stinging response.

Injection of met-enkephalin, leu-enkephalin, kyotorphin and (D-Ala^2) methionine-enkephalinamide, given in doses of 200 n-moles/bee, an amount greater than that of the morphine D_{50}, exhibited no effect on the stinging response.

DISCUSSION

The fact that the sensitivity index was higher for Italian than for Africanized bees could be considered a rather surprising result since the "aggressive" behavior of Italian bees is known to be lower than that of Africanized bees (3, 12).

Italian bees showed an increase in sensitivity index with the decrease of the natural food supply during the year (i.e., increase of the foraging pressure at the controlled food source). However, the Africanized bees did not present such a correlation. Furthermore, the foraging pressure of the Italian bees reached higher values than that of the Africanized bees. These results could be explained by the fact that the Africanized bees, unlike the Italian bees, are prone to abscond when the rate of nectar flow drops (8).

Italian bees did not show significant changes of sensitivity index during the day. Africanized bees showed maximal values early in the morning and late in the evening, that is when nectar flow is reported to be at its highest (9). Thus, sensitivity index for Africanized bees seems to be directly correlated with nectar flow during the day. The same correlation proved to be significant with Italian bees; however, this was during the year.

Morphine (50 to 200 n-moles/bee) produces a dose-dependent inhibition of the honeybee response to the electrical stimulus and this effect is antagonized by naloxone. These findings indicate the occurrence of opiate receptors in the honeybee and suggest the existence of endogenous opiates (i.e., an endorphinic system for pain perception modulation). However, two facts have to taken into account. First, even though the doses of naloxone that antagonize morphine are similar for bees and vertebrates, the D_{50} of morphine for honeybees (927 ug/g) was found to be far greater than that reported for behavioral tests in vertebrates (0.30 - 10.0 ug/g), and 3 to 10 times higher than that reported in other arthropods (7, 11, 15). Second, bees injected with enkephalins and related peptides at a dose of 200 n-moles/bee did not exhibit the effect of the same dose of morphine.

The results obtained by the morphine experiments suggest that an endorphinic system is responsible for pain modulation in bees. To what degree this system could be responsible for some of the changes in sensitivity to noxious stimulation observed on foraging bees over the course of the year or during the day can only be elicited by future experiments.

Acknowledgements. This work was partially supported by Grant A-12-1/80 to N. Balderrama from the Consejo de Desarrollo Científico y Humanístico, UCV, Venezuela.

REFERENCES

(1) Boch, R., and Rothenbuhler, W.C. 1974. Defensive behaviour and production of alarm pheromone in honeybees. J. Apic. Res. 13: 217-221.

(2) Brandeburgo, M.A.M.; Goncalves, L.S.; and Kerr, W.E. 1976. Nota sobre o estudo do efeito das condicoes climáticas sobre a agressividade das abelhas africanizadas. Cienc. Cult. Sao Paulo 28: 276-277.

(3) Collins, A.M.; Rinderer, Th.E.; Harbo, J.R.; and Bolten, A.B. 1982. Colony defense by africanized and european honeybees. Science 218: 72-74.

(4) Collins, A.M.; Rinderer, Th.E.; Tucker, K.W.; Sylvester, H.A.; and Lackett, J.J. 1980. A model of honeybee defensive behaviour. J. Apic. Res. 19: 224-231.

(5) Collins, A.M., and Rothenbuhler, W.C. 1978. Laboratory test of the response to an alarm chemical, isopentyl acetate, by Apis mellifera. Ann. Entomol. Soc. Amer. 71: 906-909.

(6) Fletcher, J.C. 1978. The African bee, Apis mellifera adansonii, in Africa. Ann. Rev. Entomol. 23: 151-171.

(7) Maldonado, H., and Miralto, A. 1982. Effect of morphine and naloxone on a defensive response of the mantis shrimp (Squilla mantis). J. Comp. Physiol. 147: 455-459.

(8) Michener, C.D. 1975. The Brazilian bee problem. Ann. Rev. Entomol. 20: 399-416.

(9) Núnez, J.A. 1977. Circadian variation of flight activity in colonies of Apis mellifera ligustica. J. Insect Physiol. 23: 387-392.

(10) Núnez, J.A. 1982. Foraging pressure and its annual variation. J. Apic. Res. 21: 134-138.

(11) Núnez, J.A.; Maldonado, H.; Miralto, A.; and Balderrama, N. 1983. The stinging response of the honeybee: effects of morphine, naloxone and some opioid peptides. Pharmacol. Biochem. Behav. 19: 921-924.

(12) Padilla, A.G. 1985. Variacion anual en respuestas evocadas por feromonas de alarma en Apis mellifera. M.Sc. Thesis, UCV, Maracay-Venezeula.

(13) Rothenbuhler, W.C. 1960. A technique for studying genetics of colony behavior in honey bees. Am. Bee J. 100: 176-198.

(14) Stort, A.C. 1970. Metodologia para o estudo da genética da aggressividade de Apis mellifera. Anais 1º Congr. Bras. Apic. Florianopolis.SC: 36-51.

(15) Zabala, N.A.; Miralto, A.; Maldonado, H.; Núnez, J.A.; Jaffé, K.; and Calderón, L.de C. 1984. Opiate receptor in praying mantis: effect of morphine and naloxone. Pharmacol. Biochem. Behav. 20: 683-687.

Visual System

The Structural Basis of Information Processing in the Visual System of the Bee

Willi A. Ribi

Max-Planck-Institut für Biologische Kybernetik, Spemannstrasse 38, D-7400 Tübingen, FRG

Abstract. The optic lobes of the bees are composed of three ganglia. From the periphery inward, the three regions are known as the lamina, the medulla and the lobula. The three optical ganglia are connected to each other by the outer chiasma which connects the lamina with the medulla and the inner chiasma which connects the medulla with the lobula (Fig. 1). The first optic ganglion, the lamina, is a neuropil zone consisting of thousands of cylindrical units, the optical cartridges, which receive the inputs of the receptor cell axons (RCA's). The nine RCA's emerging from the ommatidium, project in one bundle either as short visual fibers (svf) or long visual fibers (lvf) to the cartridge below. In addition to the RCA's and the four different L-neurons in each cartridge an unknown number of tangential, centrifugal, and horizontal fiber elememts are found. The medulla, like the retina and lamina, shows in its distal layers a highly regular arrangement of axon bundles. The visual information reaches the medulla through at least seven channels either directly from the retina via the three long visual fibers or after relay from the six short visual fibers via the four L-fiber types. The main neuronal elements in the medulla are the transmedullary cells and an unknown number of tangential and amacrine cells. Y- and T- cells link the medulla with the third optic ganglion. The lobula is a multi-stratified, spherical-shaped ganglion. The three outermost strata contain endings of the transmedullary cells and those of the shallow endings of Y- and T-cells. The neuronal endings leave the ganglion in several fibre bundles and project to the posterior or anterior protocerebrum.

Retina

The morphological visual unit in the bee's compound eye is the ommatidium which is - with the exception of the dorsal rim - composed of eight long and one short-, proximal retinula cells. All nine retinula cells contribute their photomembranes, the microvilli, to a central light gathering and absorbing structure, the fused rhabdom (Fig. 2a). The eight long visual receptors donate microvilli, to two more or less mutually perpendicular arranged sets of microvilli. The ninth cell is inserted into the rhabdomeric unit as the long receptor cell withdraws to leave the retina as an axon. In the region of the dorsal rim, all nine receptor

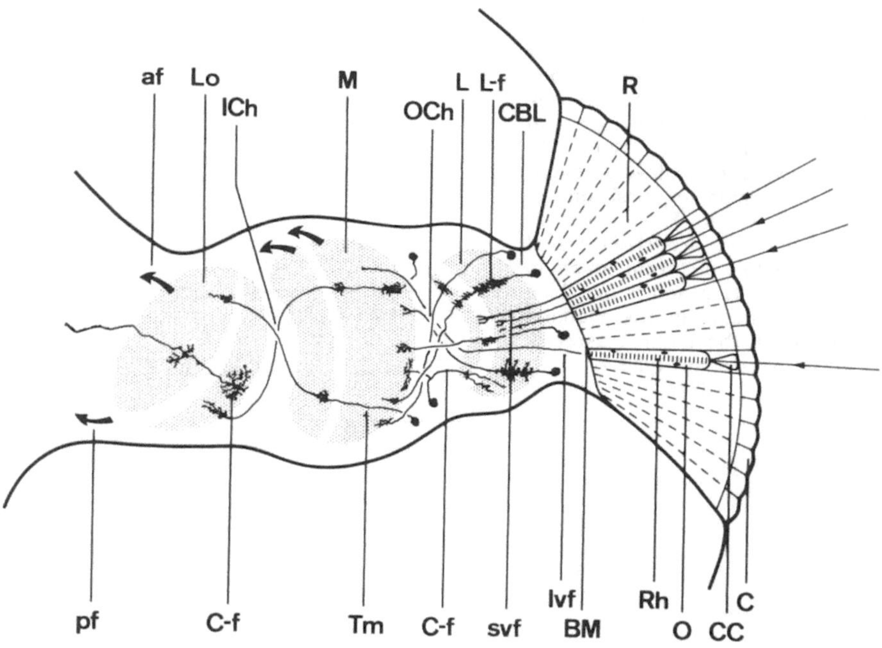

Fig. 1 - Horizontal cross-section through the compound eye of the worker honey bee (right eye). af anterior focus, BM basement membrane, C cornea, CBL cell body layer, CC crystalline cone, C-f centrifugal fibre, Ich inner chiasma, L lamina gangionaris, L-f L-fiber, Lo Lobula, lvf long visual fiber, M medulla, O ommatidium, OCh outer chiasma, pf posterior focus, R retina, Rh rhabdom, svf short visual fiber, Tm transmedullary fiber, Y Y-cell.

cells extend over the whole length of the ommatidium, from the crystalline cone to the basement membrane (8, 12).

Retina-lamina projection

Each ommatidium grades into an axon bundle 5-10 um distal to the basement membrane. The nine receptor cell axons (RCA) of each ommatidium run together in a unit which is called a pseudocartridge. Each pseudocartridge consists of a circle formed by the six short visual fibers (svf types 1-3) surrounding the three long visual fibers (lvf 1-3) (Figs. 1, 2b). At the level of the monopolar cell body layer, the pseudocartridges become cartridges as a consequence of the appearence of second order fibers (L-fibers) which join the retinula-axon bundle. The L-fibers take up characteristic positions within the cartridge (Fig. 3).

Serial sections from the level of the ommatidia down to the lamina show that axon bundles do not mix and do not permutate the receptor mosaic. All axons from one ommatidium retain their neighbourhood relationships within the bundlefrom the level of the basement membrane into the lamina.

Fig. 2 a, b - a) Spatial arrangement of the nine rhabdomeras within the ommatidium of the compound eye of the worker bee (median eye region). b) Illustration relating retinula cells (RC) and their spectral sensitivity (SS; G green, B blue, UV ultraviolet) to types of retinula-cell axons (RCA) and their corresponding positions in the pseudocartridge (PC). The axons of retinula cells 2-4 and 6-8 are short visual fibers (svf) ending at two different levels in the lamina (La). Cells 1, 5 and 9 are long visual fibers (Lvf) ending in the medulla (Me). A, B, C strata in the lamina, asterisk indicates the male-specific svf type 4.

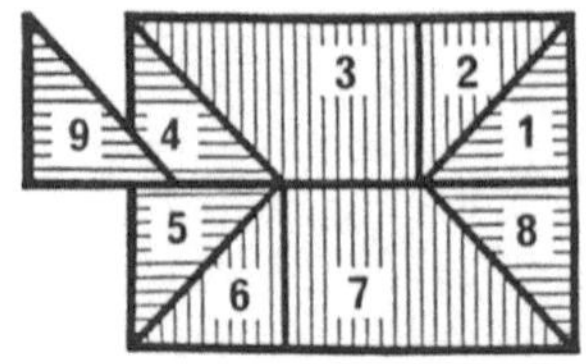

a

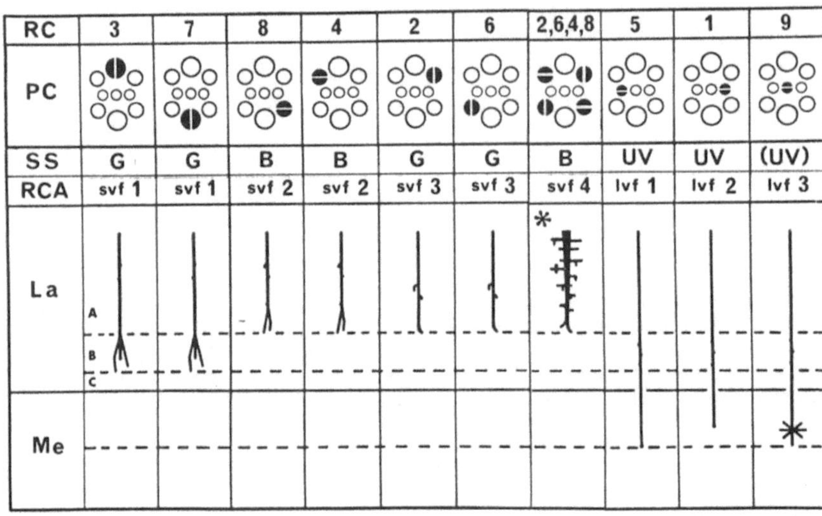

b

Lamina

The lamina neuropil is the first synaptic region where contacts between receptor cell axons and first order interneurons take place. Its region extends from the monopolar cell body layer proximally to the outer chiasma. The three strata labelled from distal to proximal as A, B, and C are the results of the homogeneous neuropil structure arising from the different levels of svf endings, the presence of horizontal fiber layers and the distinctive branching pattern of the monopolar fibers (Figs. 1-4).

Whereas the six svf end at two different levels (strata A and B) in the lamina, the three lvf project across the first optic chiasma to the second optic ganglion, the medulla. They run in parallel with, and as part of a coherent bundle, with the first order interneurons (L-fibers) that derive their information from optically equivalent short receptors (Figs. 1, 2b).

The monopolar cells (L-fibers) have their origin in the so-called cell-body layer (CBL) proximal to the tracheal region and distal to the neuropil of the lamina ganlionaris (Fig. 1). The axon of each type of L-fiber projects through the first synaptic region, across the outer

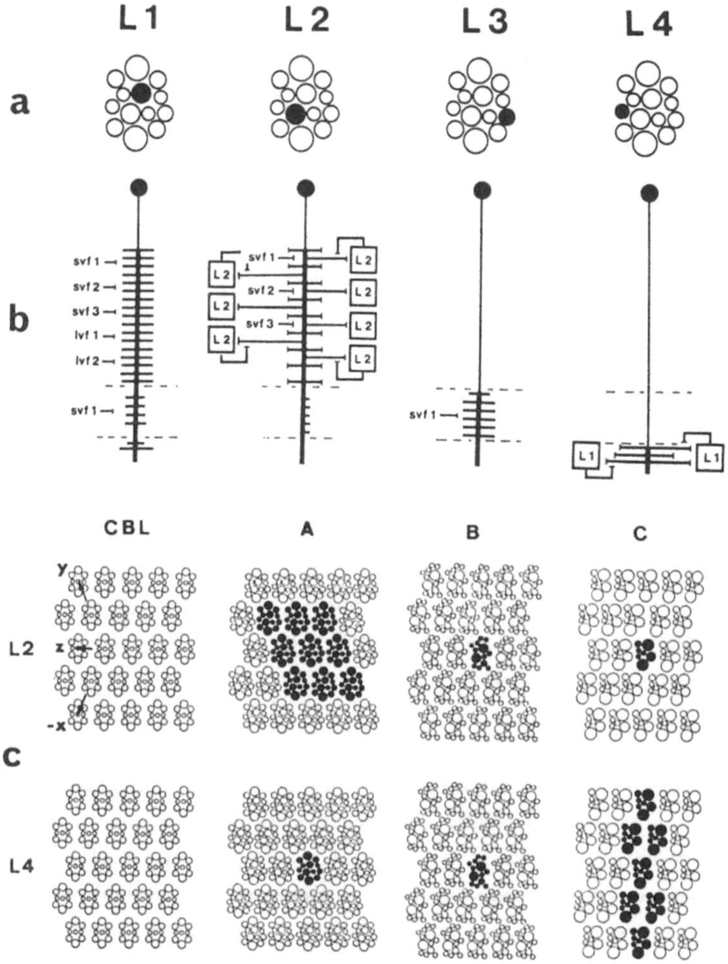

Fig. 3 - Connectivity patterns of the four L-neurons L-1 to L-4. a) Schematic illustrations of cross sections through a cartridge at the level of the distal stratum A. The black dots represent the position of the four L-fibers within the cartridge. b) Schematic illustration of the four L-fiber types in longitudinal view showing their synaptic inputs. c) The long collaterals of L-2 and L-4 fibers innervate seven or six neighbouring cartridges, respectively; L-2 in stratum A, L-4 in stratum C. y, -x, z eye axes.

optic chiasma, and ends in the medulla. The L-fibers in each lamina cartridge can be classified into four different categories - L1, L2, L3, and L4. The clear stratification in the first synaptic region provides the best criterion for a morphological and functional classification of the four L-fiber types (Fig. 1, 3).

In addition to the lateral branching patterns within the parent cartridge, two of the four fiber types (L-2 and L-4) have long collaterals innervating neighbouring cartridges; L-2 in stratum A and L-4 in stratum C (Fig. 3b, c). In contrast to the fibers, RCA's have few, if any, collateral branches, and these do not penetrate neighbouring cartridges (Fig. 2b). The spatial arrangement of RCA's and the L-fibers within a cartridge remains constant throughout the depth of the lamina. All neuronal elements in the optical cartridge are surrounded and separated from other neural elements by cytoplasmic extensions of glial cells.

The following synaptic connectivity patterns, including chemical and electrical synapses, were found between RCA's, L-fibers and accessory fibers within and between neighbouring cartridges. Sites of synaptic contacts were localized between adjacent axonal trunks, between adjacent dendritic branches (knots and spines), or between dendritic specializations and axonal elements (9).

The L-1 fiber recieves multiple synaptic inputs from all short visual fibers (svf 1-3) and a few from the long visual fibers, lvf 1 and 2. These observations correlate well with the electrophysiological findings of Menzel (5) on dark adapted monopolar cells in the lamina of the worker bee. The spectral sensitivities of these cells have their maxima at 482 nm and a broad band shoulder around 550 nm, suggesting that they receive inputs from more than one color type, and that the green and blue receptors are positive inputs. As the spectral sensitivity of these fibers displays a small UV response at 360 nm, it seems very likely that besides the green and blue receptors, UV receptors in the form of lvf 1 and 2 may also supply synaptic inputs to the L-1 neuron (Figs. 2b, 3a, b).

The short lateral branches of the L-2 fiber within the cartridge receive inputs from all three svf types and thus from the green and blue receptors. No UV inputs from lvf were observed. In contrast to L-1, L-2 has both pre- and postsynaptic structures opposing svf elements either having excitatory or inhibitory characteristics in the form of spherical (excitatory) or oval shaped (inhibitory) synaptic vesicles respectively (9). Thus, this area of the neuropil may be responsible for self-inhibition. As svf 1 and 3 are believed to belong to green receptors (2, 7) and are postsynaptic to L-2, L-2 may act as a color opponent cell, similar to those found in the lobula of the bee (3). The L-2 fiber may therefore inhibit the inputs from the green receptors and act as a narrow-band neuron with a maximal spectral sensitivity in the blue.

The cartridges are connected to each other by fibers, the most regular of which are the collateral branches of the L-2 and the L-4 neurons. It has been suggested that the long collaterals interconnecting L-2 fibers in seven neighbouring cartridges may play a central role in the lateral inhibition (Fig. 3b, c). In the dark-adapted retina the spectral light information may pass through each of the seven L-2 fiber collaterals. All available RCA inputs would, therefore, be summed in neighbouring L-2 neurons to provide the maximum possible light signal. In this case, the inhibitory synapses of the collaterals connecting the axis fibers of neighbouring L-2 neurons must be inactive. During light adaption there may be a change in input signals resulting from threshold effects and intensity-dependent feed-back and feed-foreward circuits; in this case, the inhibitory synapses may prevent information cross-talk between neighbouring L-2 fibers.

The L-3 neuron shows a lateral branching pattern that interconnects postsynaptically with the end-arborisation of the svf type 1, at the level of stratum B (Fig. 3b). Since the two type 1 svf's are derived from green receptors (7), the L-3 neuron is probably a green monochromatic small band neuron.

The collaterals of L-4 fibers provide, in addition to the L-2 neurons, the most extensive cross-cartridge extensions. They span neighbouring cartridges over the entire lamina and are orientated along all three eye axes (Fig. 3c). The L-4 provides a pathway between its own cartridge and L-1 fiber elements of six adjacent cartridges (Fig. 3b). It seems likely that the L-4 cells modify the outputs of L-1 fibers in neighbouring cartridges in response to sudden intensity fluctuations mediated by short and long visual fiber elements.

If the influence of the six neighbouring L-4 elements on the central one is exicatatory e. g. under dim light, the effectiveness of light will be increased, and one must expect a wider visual field for this central neuron. If the surrounding L-4 elements have an inhibitory influence (inhibitory synapses active), the "visual field" of the L-4 cell will be narrower.

In summary, the anatomical results suggest that four physiological types of L-fibers are present in the lamina: broad-band neurons (L-1); spectrally opponent neurons with inputs either from green or blue receptors (L-2); and small-band neurons with synaptic inputs from just one receptor type (L-3). A regular network of collaterals interconnects the L-2 neurons and connects the L-4 fibers with the broad-band L-1 neurons.

In the median region of the eye the two long visual fibers lvf 1 and 2, which derive from UV-sensitive receptor cells (6), are synaptically connected to the L-1 neuron in stratum A. The most probable candidates for polarization sensitivity coding and afferent information pathway are the three UV-cells (RC 1, 5 and 9) in the dorsal rim area (4). It has been suggested that these fibres, like the lvf 3 in the remaining eye area, project through the lamina without any synaptic contacts to either L-neurons or neighbouring RCA's.

The svf 1, 3 and lvf 1, 2 of the same ommatidium are connected with each other in the lamina by gap junctions (9). Whether or not these anatomical specializations represent low resistant electrical couplings requires further physiological analysis.

The topography of the bee lamina suggests that in addition to the monopolar neurons accessory fibers maintain synaptic contacts with the fiber elements within and between different cartridges. Although a great number of different accessory fiber types can be identified at the light microscope level, we have concentrated on four types of centrifugally arranged fibers.

All four cell types originate in the outer chiasma; they have an efferent end-branch in the lamina and an afferent branch terminating in the distal region of the second optic ganglion, the medulla. These interneurons are referred to as (i) Garland-cells: The efferent fibre has on its tangential branch numerous centripetal side branches, so called "garlands", which synapse with RCA's and L-fibres. (ii) Y-cells: The lamina branch bifurcates before entering the lamina. It innervates two neighbouring cartridges. Synaptic contacts can be seen in the two laminar strata (A and C) where bottle-brush-like collaterals occurred. (iii) Single bottle-brush cells: The efferent part of the cell has only one centrifugal branch, which can be compared morphologically and in terms of synaptology with those of the Y-cell. (iv) Triptych-cells: The lamina component innervates three neighbouring cartridges at the three different laminar layers (A and B) interconnecting different first- and second- order visual neurons (10) (Fig. 4).

The structural studies provide suffficient ground for the supposition that the RCA's and L-fibers maintain numerous synaptic contacts with horizontally extended fiber elements. The laterally arranged interconnections of the garland cells, Y-cells and triptych cells are of great interest because they are (besides the L-2 and L-4 fibers) the most peripheral cross-connections in the visual system of the bee. They span short distances along the vertical axis of the eye.

It is suggested that the centrifugal fiber types provide local intergration within the first synaptic region together with efferent control of RCA's and L-fibers. The separate areas of dendritic spread of the garland cells, Y-cells and triptych cells within the lamina and the medulla could well act as local circuits.

The study of the lamina of the bee has revealed a complexity of synaptic inter-connections that is not found in other insects. In particular, the variety of inputs and their frequency, together with the clear stratification of the neuropil (strata A, B, C), represent an extremely highly evolved system.

Outer chiasma

The majority of the neuronal fibers that leave the lamina to project into the medulla are involved in a single horizontal crossover. Fibers from the anterior region of the lamina, usually in bundles, project posteriorly to the medulla, whereas fibres arising posteriorly project into the anterior region of the medulla. Thus the linear array of fibers in the horizontal plane in the lamina is reversed in the medulla.

Medulla

The medulla can be subdivided into several strata in planes parallel to its proximal and distal surfaces. These layers consist of horizontal cell populations and lateral branching patterns of transmedullary (Tm), amacrine (am), T- and Y-fibres (Fig.1). The medulla, like the retina and lamina, shows at its distal surface a highly regular arrangement of axon bundles.

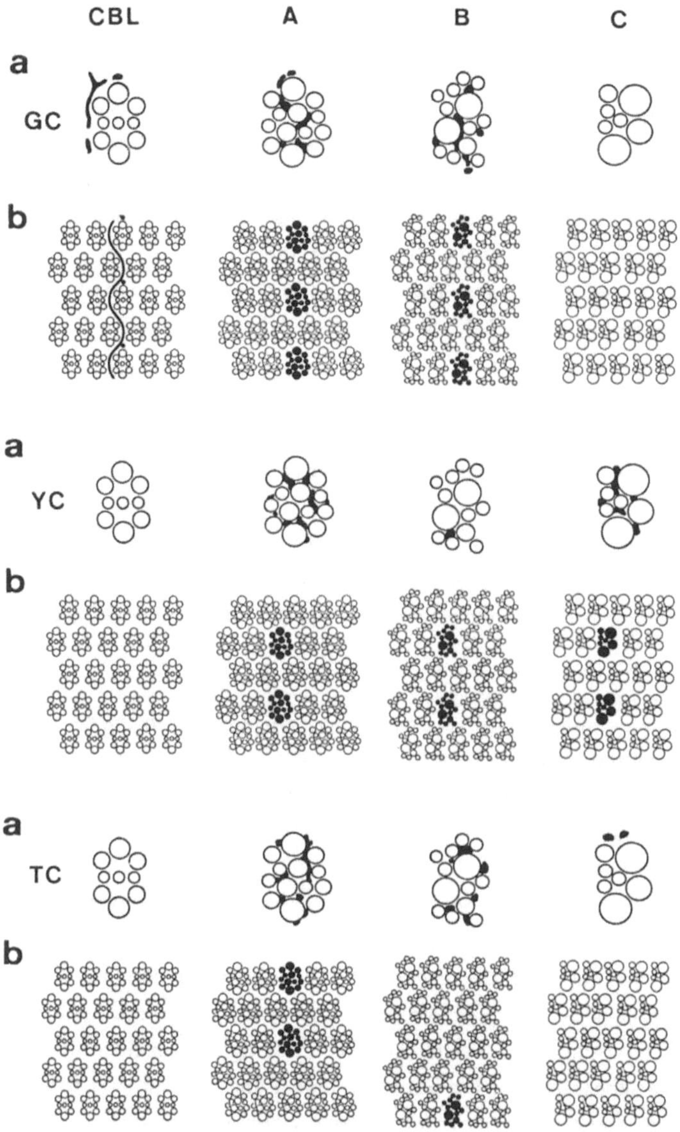

Fig. 4 - a) Semischematic diagram of tangentially cut laminar cartridges at the four horizontal strata CBL, A, B, C. For the three centrifugal fiber elements, GC garland cell, YC Y-cell and TC triptych-cell, in addition to the axial fibre, those of the intercartridge collaterals are shown. b) The pattern of black cross sections represents the set of cartridges that receives collaterals of the same fibre elements which innervate neighbouring cartridges.

Visual information reaches the medulla through at least seven channels, L-fibres 1-4 and lvf1-3, either directly from the retina via lvf or, after relay from svf, via L-fibers. The three lvf provide a direct projection from the ommatidium to the distal strata of the medulla where they terminate in characteristic forms. The four L-fiber types are characterised by their different depths of penetration in the medulla and by their end-arborisations. L-fibers and lvf end in the medullar stratum 1 or 2.

Neuronal elements in the medulla are third order interneurons, so-called transmedullary-Tm-cells. The axon fibers of Tm-cells transverse all the medullary strata, some even leaving its inner face to enter the lobula (Fig.1). Their cell bodies are situated above the medulla in the cell body cortex, which surrounds the outer chiasma. Tm-cells can be classified according to their stratification in the medulla. The most commonly observed cell type possesses dendritic pinnaform arborisations in different strata. Abundant rami, in a fine comb-like grouping, and the correspondence of their form and orientation with those of the lvf and L-fiber endings distinguish these fibers in the first medullar strata. The lateral branching pattern of the Tm-cells is confined to the specific medullar strata 1-3 and 5, 6.

Some L-fibers and lvf terminals establish contacts with different medullary interneurons, whereas others converge onto the same medullary interneurons. The information, therefore, is transferred either from or to the lobula, protocerebrum or even lamina via the axons of the Tm-cells, centrifugal fiber elements and others. The tangential small-field neurons, which are common in the distal strata of the medulla, have a restricted lateral spread and thus interact with a smaller number of cartridges. On the other hand, some diffuse, wide-field elements and multistratified tangential elements invest more than one stratum and connect a greater number of cartridges.

The term amacrine defines a nerve cell having processes in only one ganglion. In the bee such cells are present in all of the medullary strata. They usually possess a fine descending axon, which originates from the perikaryal layer surrounding the optic ganglia and penetrates into the plexiform zone of the medulla. A characteristic of such elements is that the end aborisation is confined to particular strata.

Inner chiasma

The inner chiasma connects each column of the medulla to corresponding columns in the lobula. Hence, each visual neuropil can be interpreted as an anatomical map of the mosaic of sampling stations in the ipsilateral visual field. Due to the fibre crossing in both the outer and the inner chiasms, this map is horizontally inverted between lamina and medulla and rotated again between medulla and lobula. The retinotopic order, however, remains unchanged.

Lobula

Unlike the dipterans, coleopterans and lepidopterans, the third optic ganglion of the honeybee is not divided into two parts (a lobula and a lobula plate). The ovoid- to spherical-shaped lobula has approxiametely the same volume as the lamina. It is a complex stratified ganglion with six clearly distinct layers. The three outermost strata contain endings of the Tm-cells and those of the shallow endings of Y- and T- cells. The lobula receives and sends elements from or to the protocerebrum. The neuronal axons of the lobula leave the ganglion in several fiber bundles and project to dicrete and characteristic optic foci in the posterior or anterior protocerebrum.

Sexual dimorphism

The regional differences in the compound eyes of the drone bee shows that in the dorso-frontal portion of the eye - instead of the svf types 2 and 3 - a sex-dimorphic receptor cell ending (svf type 4) exists; this cell type is not found in the other regions of the eye or in the compound eye of the worker bee (11)(Fig. 2b). All four svf type 4 cells are synaptically interconnected with L-fibers of the same cartridge. The simplest hypothesis according to the general morphology and synaptic patterns suggests a summation process of all the svf type 4 cells in one and the same cartridge, and that all of these cells contain the same photopigment. In contrast to the worker bee where tri-chromatic vision is expected (7, see Backhaus et al. in this volume), the dorso-frontal portion of the drone bee retina has only UV and blue sensitive photoreceptors (1). Because the scattered light from the clear sky is predominantly blue and UV, the short-wavelength receptor sensitivity maximises target contrast against the sky (13). Thus, the UV and blue sensitivity of the dorso-frontal retina in the drone bee can be thought of as a cut off filter that selects the part of the visual spectrum containing the strongest signal. The special type of svf in this region may be involved in the control of flight behaviour to fix queens. This region apparently has a particularly high angular resolution suggesting an important role in mating behaviour.

Acknowledgements

The work was supported by the Swiss National Science Foundation (Grant 3.081-0.84).

References

(1) Autrum, H., and Zwehl, V. v. 1964. Die spektrale Empfindlichkeit einzelner Sehzellen des Bienenauges. Z. vergl. Physiol. 48: 357-384.

(2) Gribakin, F. G. 1969. Types of photoreceptor cells in the compound eye of the worker honey bee relative to their spectral sensitivity. Cytologie (Tokyo) 11: 309-314.

(3) Kien, J., and Menzel, R. 1977. Chromatic properties of interneurons in the optic lobes of the bee. II Narrow band and color opponent neurons. J. Comp. Physiol. 113: 35-53.

(4) Labhart, T. 1980. Specialized photoreceptorsat the dorsal rim of the honey bee's compound eye: Polarizational and angular sensitivity. J. Comp. Physiol. 141: 19-30.

(5) Menzel, R. 1974. Spectral sensitivity of monopolar cells in the bee lamina. J. Comp. Physiol. 93: 337-346.

(6) Menzel, R., and Snyder A. W. 1974. Polarized light detection in the bee, Apis mellifera. J. Comp. Physiol. 88: 247-270.

(7) Menzel, R., and Blakers, M. 1976. Color receptors in the bee eye morphology and spectral sensitivity. J. Comp. Physiol. 108: 11-33.

(8) Meyer, E. P. 1984. Retrograde labelling of photoreceptors in different regions of the compound eye of bees and ants. J. Neurocytol. 13: 825-836.

(9) Ribi, W. A. 1981. The first optic ganglion of the bee. IV. Synaptology of receptor cell axons and first order interneurons (a Golgi-EM study). Cell Tiss. Res. 215: 443-464.

(10) Ribi, W. A. 1984. The first optic ganglion of the bee. V. Structural and functional characterization of centrifugally arranged interneurons. Cell. Tiss. Res. 236: 577-584.

(11) Ribi, W. A. 1985. The first optic ganglion of the bee. VI. A sexually dimorphic receptor-cell axon. Cell Tiss. Res. 240: 27-33.

(12) Schinz, R. H. 1975. Structural specialisation in the dorsal retina of the bee, Apis mellifera. Cell Tiss. Res. 162: 23-34.

(13) Shaw, S. J. 1969. Interreceptor coupling in ommatidia of drone honey bee and locust compound eye. Vision Res. 9: 999-1029.

Processing of Visual Information in the Honeybee Brain

Horst Hertel and Ulrike Maronde

Institut für Tierphysiologie, Neurobiologie, Freie Universität Berlin, Königin-Luise-Str. 28–33, D-1000 Berlin 33, FRG

Abstract. Knowledge about processing of visual information in the bee brain mainly comes from investigations on higher order interneurons. The first set of interneurons, the monopolar cells of the lamina, is almost unexplored. The second stage, the medulla, is involved in coding spatial and color contrast, and in detecting directionally unselective movement. In the third optic neuropile, the lobula, the direction of movement of a stimulus is coded. This information is transferred to descending interneurons in the ventro-lateral protocerebrum. Some widefield extrinsic medulla neurons display color coding properties with an opponent reaction to green and UV-light stimuli.

INTRODUCTION

Neuroanatomical and electrophysiological techniques are considered to be a fruitful combination for analyzing neural networks. Nevertheless, obtaining sufficient results by using both methods on a central nervous system like a bee brain, which consists of 850,000 cells (half of which are included in the optic lobes (19)), is difficult because most of the neurons within the brain are extremely small and densely packed. Therefore, one has to be aware of the fact that such an analysis is restricted to relatively thick neurons, many of which are assembled in specific tracts within the bee brain (Fig. 1). However, because the visual system, at least in its peripheral part (retina, lamina, medulla and distal lobula), consists of thousands of parallel and identical channels, the investigation of only a few neurons may provide an understanding of visual information processing to the central brain.

Lamina

The first step of signal processing is in the lamina. Here, the axons of the retinula cells are connected to first order interneurons. While the neuroanatomy of the lamina neuropile is well established (Ribi, this volume), knowledge of its function is still very limited. The few successful recordings from monopolar cells (8) indicate an input from more than one photoreceptor type; their spectral sensitivity covers a part of the light spectrum that is much wider than that of a single receptor. It should be noticed that in all cases where dye

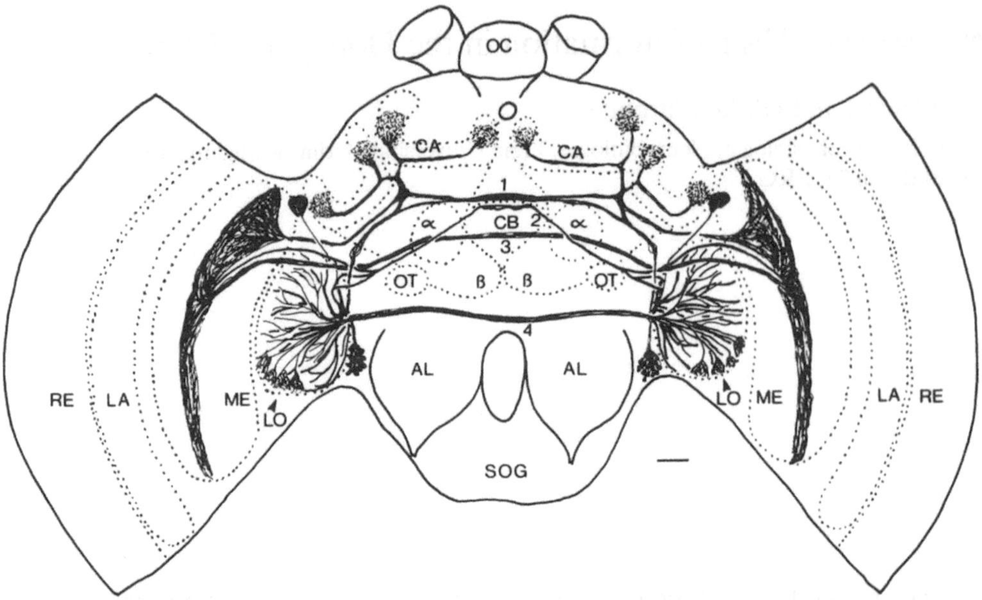

Fig. 1 - Frontal view of the bee brain. The positions of the main visual commissures, indicated with no. 1 - 4, and their dendritic branchings in the optic lobes are schematically inserted according to cobalt stainings. The outlines of prominent neuropiles are indicated with dotted lines. Scale = 100 µm.

1. The anterior optic commmissure (AOC), consisting of about 3200 neurons, gathers cells from the medulla and lobula. The axons project to the contralateral optic lobe or to the calyces of the mushroom bodies crossing the protocerebrum dorsally to the central body.
2. The serpentine optic commissure (SOC) consists of four cells which each interconnect both the medullae and lobulae, the axons crossing the protocerebrum in a serpentine shaped manner.
3. The 200 cells of the posterior optic commissure (POC) connect both medullae, the axons run along the posterior side of the protocerebrum.
4. The inferior optic commissure (IOC), consisting of about 210 neurons, links both lobulae together, their axons pass through the brain close to the oesophagus.

Abbreviations for all figures: AL = antennal lobe; substructures of the mushroom bodies are αL = alpha lobe, ß = beta lobe, and CA = calyx; C = neck connective; CB = central body; CH 1 = first optic chiasma; La = lamina; LO = lobula; ME = medulla; OC = ocelli; OES = oesophagus; OT = optic tubercle; RE = retina; SOG = suboesophageal ganglion. The numbers in the figures indicate the depth of the neuron relative to the frontal or dorsal brain surface.

injections are missing, the classification has to be taken cautiously because the recording site is solely estimated from landmarks on the brain surface. Recent investigations on monopolar cells combining electrophysiology and histology (de Souza, unpublished) confirmed earlier findings (8) that in bees the value of the hyperpolarizing response to a light stimulus is lower than that of the depolarization in the receptor cells. The hyperpolarization shows both a phasic and a tonic component which saturate with increasing light intensity at about 20 and 10 mV respectively; the depolarizing receptor potential, however, reaches more than twice these values. This finding is in contrary to the high amplification properties of the signal input which is characteristic for monopolar cells in diptera (7). Most results come from the

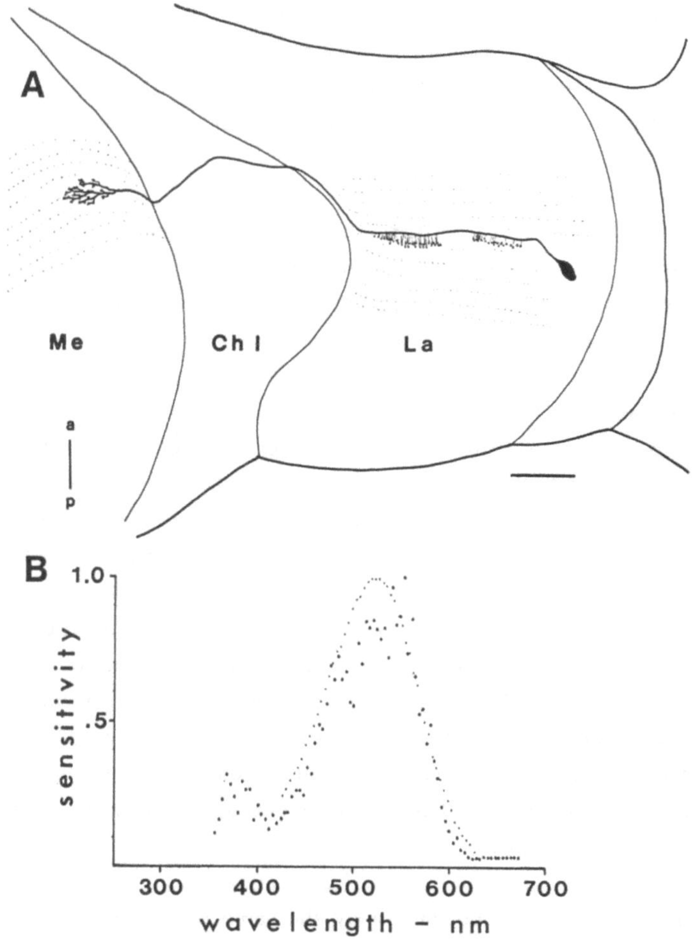

Fig. 2 - Lamina monopolar cell. A. Horizontal reconstruction. In the lamina spine processes indicate the input region of the cell. The axon passes through the first optic chiasma and terminates in the distal medulla. The anterior (a) to posterior (p) direction is given. Scale = 50 µm. B. The spectral sensitivity function of the cell (thick dots) has its maximum at 540 nm. The shape is almost identical with that of a green sensitive photoreceptor and corresponds to the theoretical absorption curve for photopigments (Dartnall nomogram, fine dots). Courtesy of J. M. de Souza.

lamina monopolar cell type 2 (14), a neuron which has spines along its axon in the lamina and wide terminal ramifications in the medulla (Fig. 2). The spectral sensitivity of this type of neuron, as measured with a fast spectral scanning method (9), is similar to that of the green receptors. This points to a connection to only this receptor type. The present results do not yet explain the function of these cells at this first stage of signal processing. The possible role of anaxial elements, to which the inputs of different ommatidia converge, is unknown since no physiological data are yet available .

In addition to these lamina neurons transmitting the information from the retina to the central brain, some centrifugal fibers (10, 18) are known to come from the protocerebrum and to have wide dendritic branchings in a shallow anaxial layer (C-layer, (13)). These neurons probably control the sensitivity of the compound eye at the first link of the pathway.

Medulla

The second optic ganglion, the medulla, receives information from elements crossing the first optic chiasma where the axons of the three UV-cells of each ommatidium and the four corresponding lamina monopolar cells are arranged in distinct "cartridges", thus maintaining the topographic structure of the compound eye within the medulla neuropile (15).

The columnar organization of the medulla results from the parallel arrangement of medulla monopolar cells whose cell bodies are located in the first optic chiasma and which extend to the third optic ganglion, the lobula. Due to the small fiber-diameter of these cells (approx. 1 um), only a few have been identified by dye injection and tested for their response to light stimuli. As one would expect from their anatomy, these neurons receive their input from only a small array of ommatidia which have a receptive field of about 20 ^{o} in diameter. Responses to stationary light flashes are dominant, but some of the small field elements show additional responses to a moving light stimulus without any preference to the direction of the movement. They exhibit a broad-band spectral sensitivity, and show a slight enhancement in sensitivity for green light (3). Nevertheless, it must be mentioned that the amount of data concerning these columnar cells is still too small to make any valid statements about whether or not color coding mechanisms, as will be described below, occur in these axial elements at this early stage of visual information processing.

Tangentially extending amacrine cells of the medulla display the same properties to light stimuli as observed for columnar cells. Their spectral sensitivity is broad- or narrow-band, and they respond to stationary light or movement without preference to the direction. Some of the amacrine cells with wide dendritic fields, are specialized with respect to the substructure of their receptive fields: the wavelength dependence of the response is not equally distributed over the whole input area, but may show a local separation for long and short wavelength sensitivity (3).

Centrifugal input into the medulla is delivered by commissures (see below) that transfer the visual information to the contralateral optic lobe, as well as by small extrinsic cells which are restricted to one brain hemisphere. The neuron in Fig. 3 represents an example of an extrinsic fibre which has a small dendritic field in the distal half of the medulla and which displays spectrally broad-band characteristics. The neuron gives a phasic ON-OFF response to a stationary light, and responds to movement without any directional preference. The receptive field of the cell covers both eyes, the sensitivity to a contralateral stimulus (CO) being much higher than that of an ipsilateral stimulus. The reponsiveness and the widefield

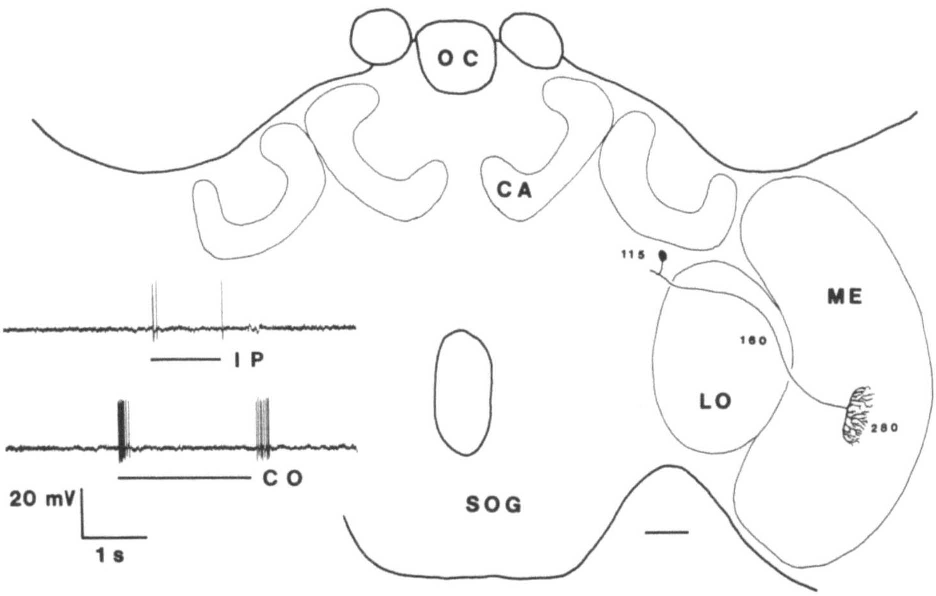

Fig. 3 - Extrinsic cell of the medulla. Its narrow dendritic field is located distally to the serpentine layer. Scale = 100 µm. The neuron is sensitive to the movement of a target without showing directional preference. A light stimulus (540 nm) applied to the ipsilateral eye (IP) gives only a weak ON-OFF response, while the same stimulus to the contralateral side (CO) causes a very strong phasic answer.

sensitivity suggests a probable contralateral input via a neuron of the serpentine optic commissure (SOC), which shows very similar response characteristics (see below).

In the medulla some neurons show wavelength-specific coding mechanisms. These cells display a response pattern whose quality only depends on the wavelength of the light stimulus and which is not influenced by the intensity of the light stimulus. This can be expressed in a phasic response, where long wavelength light gives an excitation to light OFF, while UV light elicits an additional excitation at the beginning of a light stimulus (3). Functionally, these phasic neurons may be involved in the enhancement of color contrast; a phasic UV signal in a green world will cause an additional burst in such a cell. Phasic ON/Off neurons, however, cannot discriminate whether a light is turned on or off, because they only react to the change in contrast of a stimulus, regardless of the direction of change. Therefore, the evaluation of these responses by afferent neuronal networks is ambiguous, and parallel tonic elements are necessary for a clear analysis. A more striking wavelength dependent opponency concerning the response of a neuron is the modulation of its discharge around a spontaneous activity. Such neurons have been described frequently (6, 16). Two marked cells of this type are given in Fig. 4. These cells change the sign of their discharge, one of them (B) gives a pronounced excitation to long wavelength light stimuli and is inhibited by short wavelength light, whilst theother cell (A) shows the same spectral opponency but less distinctly and in a reversed

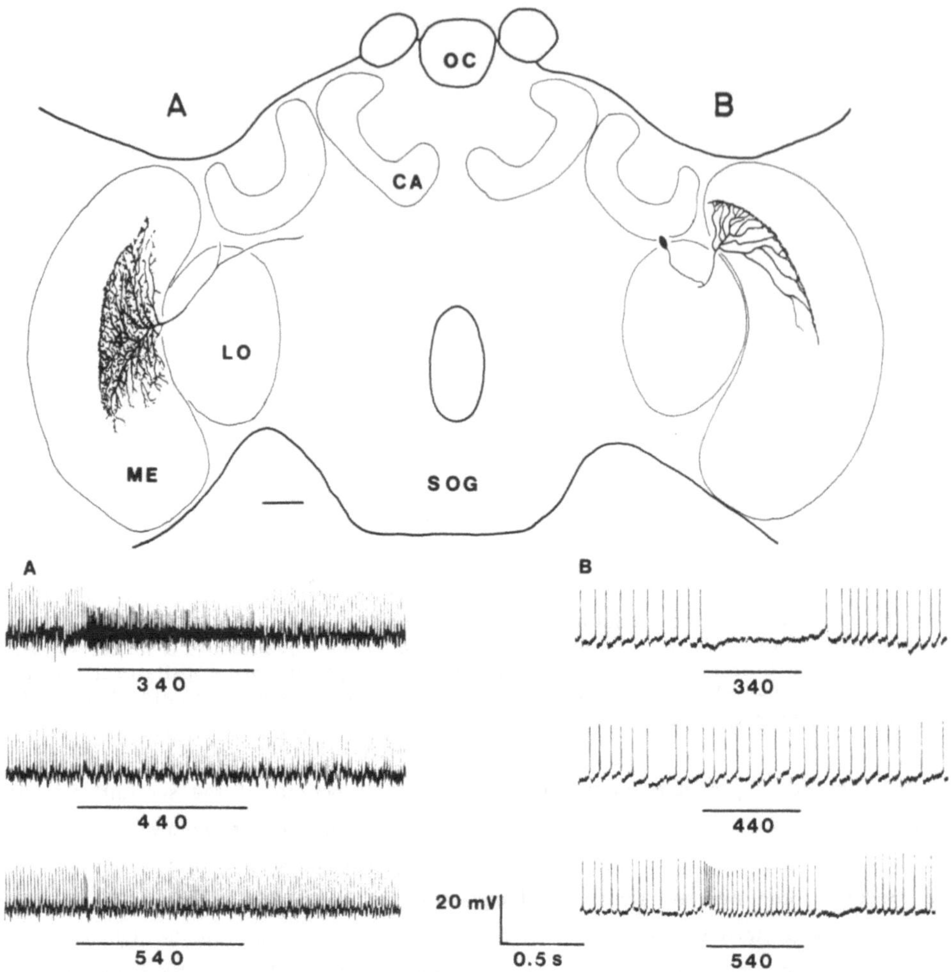

Fig. 4 - Neurons, presumably of the AOC, each with a dendritic branching in a single anaxial stratum close to the serpentine layer of the medulla. Scale = 100 µm. Both cells display a spectrally opponent response: A. Green light stimuli elicit an ON-inhibition, UV light an excitation. B. Green light (1 sec) leads to a tonic excitation, UV light to an inhibition (recorded by Schäfer, (17)). In both cells, blue light gives no response.

fashion. There is no response to blue light in both cases. The dendritic ramifications of these neurons invade a single tangential medulla stratum in the serpentine layer.

The medulla is connected to the protocerebrum either via the lobula or directly by extrinsic neurons, in which case their axons leave this neuropile anteriorly. From there, they project into three different commissures: the serpentine optic commissure (SOC), which will be discussed later together with lobula neurons, the posterior optic commissure (POC), and the anterior optic commissure (AOC) (Fig. 1).

The AOC, which consists of about 3200 neurons, crosses the brain dorsally to the central body. Its axons connect either both optic lobes or one optic lobe with the calyces of the mushroom bodies and run in bundles anteriorly and posteriorly to the pedunculus of the mushroom bodies (12): Each medulla neuron of the AOC collects information from single anaxial medulla layers with wide dendritic fields. There is some evidence to suggest that neurons in this bundle are involved in color coding . A few AOC neurons with similar dendritic branchings in the dorsal medulla, as is the case with the neurons in Fig. 4, respond preferentially to UV and may be involved in the analysis of polarization patterns in the sky.

The POC consists of about 200 neurons which interconnect the medullae of both brain hemispheres. It invades each medulla from the anterior and branches from here into numerous arborizations extending throughout the whole serpentine layer. The axons cross the brain near its posterior surface ventral to the protocerebral bridge. As the structure of these neurons implies, they may receive input from either one or both eyes. They are strongly involved in the localization of visual objects without showing movement sensitivity, and give a spatially opponent tonic response, the sign of which depends on the position of the light stimulus in the receptive field (Fig. 5). In many of these neurons, the mode of the antagonistic response is split between both eyes. Furthermore, they seem to be involved in the orientation of the animal with respect to a stationary target, e. g. a flower: the localization "left" or "right" is discriminated by the sign of the response, but as soon as the bee begins to turn in order to approach the flower, this target is shifted in the bee's binocular field. Both receptive fields of the cell are now equally stimulated and, therefore, the spike frequency approximates the spontaneous activity of the cell (its neutral point). Physiologically receptive fields among different POC-cells may vary: whilst there are some neurons which have receptive fields with left-to-right eye opponency, there are others which have a small receptive field of approximately 60 ^{o}. The latter give the opposite response within a homogeneous wide field that covers one eye or both.

From the medulla to the midbrain, the POC is accompanied by neurons that terminate in the posterior median protocerebrum. They show similar properties as the POC cells, but a peculiar combination of spatial and color opponency can also be observed. In one example, green light always caused inhibition of a spontaneous spike discharge in the binocular receptive field. UV-light, however, elicited the same inhibition only on the right eye, but always gave a strong excitation on the left eye. Such a cell is suited for a gross localization of colors: excitatory signals indicated UV on the left, and turning the animal to this stimulus reduced the response, since the zero-point for UV is in the binocular field of this cell. However, the color contrast analysis remains ambiguous as maximum inhibition occurs under UV-right plus green-left conditions, and also under wide field green light. An unequivocal color contrast analysis was performed by double opponent cells as will be described below.

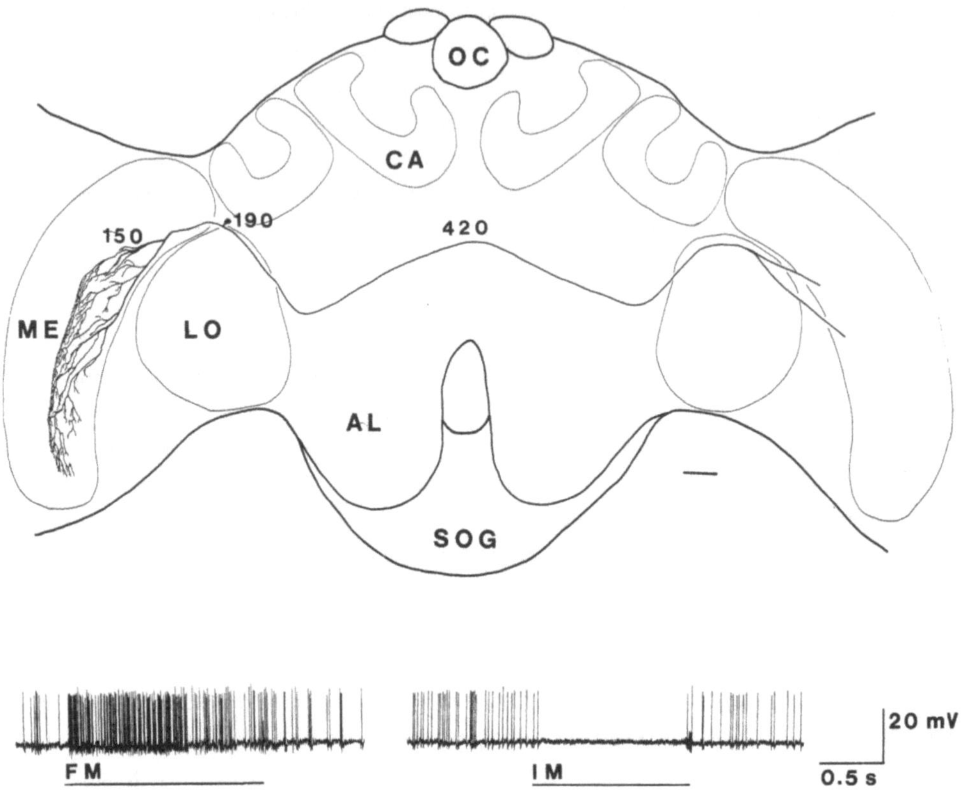

Fig. 5 - Neuron of the POC. In this spatially opponent cell the sign of the response depends on the position of a visual stimulus in its receptive field. Scale = 100 μm. A light presented in the frontal median (FM) region causes strong excitation; the same light shone onto the median part of the eye ipsilateral to the side of the soma (IM) leads to a complete suppression of the spike activity that is registered in the dark.

Lobula

In the third optic neuropile, the lobula, the columnar stratification is preserved in its distal part, whilst the proximal part is characterized by an irregular substructure. In the distal lobula, the retinal mosaic is maintained by the medulla monopolar cells, which terminate here. The information is transferred onto lobula intrinsic cells, e.g. the lobula amacrines, and onto extrinsic fibers that leave this neuropile and project into the protocerebrum. In the latter, the retinotopic structure is still preserved by neurons of the lobula-to-optic tubercle tract (anterior optic tubercle tract of Mobbs, (12)), which are axially arranged and leave the lobula at its posterior side. From here, they bend anteriorly and terminate in the optic tubercle. Other lobula neurons project into the AOC, the inferior optic commissure (IOC), and the SOC; many neurons extend to different regions of the protocerebrum via small tracts which are not particularly striking in histological investigation, and therefore have no specific nomenclature.

Nothing is known about lobula intrinsic cells, and no information exists concerning the function of neurons in the lobula-to-optic tubercle tract. All knowledge concerning the processing of visual information in the lobula comes from investigations on other extrinsic lobula cells. The results shown below indicate that the lobula is the center for the analysis of moving visual stimuli in the bee brain.

The nerve cells that probably have the most extensive ramifications in the bee brain are the serpentine neurons (2,4,17). There are only two pairs, and these form the serpentine optic commissure (SOC), each pair interlinking the medullae and lobulae of both hemispheres (Fig. 6). The neurites leaving the medulla and lobula of one optic lobe join in the lateral protocerebrum and form a serpentine shaped axon that crosses the brain posteriorly to the mushroom bodies and anterior-dorsally to the central body.

The receptive field of a serpentine neuron covers one eye only, although the arborizations extend throughout both the lobulae and medullae. The neuron responds to a stationary flash of light with a short phasic ON and OFF excitation, and is highly sensitive to a moving stimulus irrespective of its direction; it does not, however, habituate to repeated stimulations (Fig. 6).

The symmetrical shape of the SOC suggests a possible involvement in navigation: during a straight forward flight, the whole visual world moves symmetrical relative to the mosaic of the two eyes. This stimulus exists in all serpentine cells equally, and a deviation from this situation (e.g. approaching an object, turning) leads to an asymmetry in their responses and permits processing.

A prominent commissure gathering the axons of cells with arborizations in the distal lobula neuropile is the inferior optic commissure (IOC). These neurons interconnect both lobulae by running as a commissure straight through the brain just above the oesophagus. About 210 of these axons have been counted. The IOC is accompanied by lobula neurons which either project to the contralateral protocerebrum or terminate ipsilaterally; some have both connections. All of these cells are very sensitive to the direction of a moving visual stimulus. In most examples, this selectivity is expressed by antagonistic responses i. e. a movement in one direction leads to tonic excitation, whilst a movement in the opposite direction causes inhibition of spontaneous discharge (Fig. 7). This opponency can be restricted to one eye but may also cover the entire visual field. Furthermore, the excitatory response increases with an enlargement of the visual angle of a target in the frontal visual field (which is equivalent to the approach of an object), whilst an inhibitory response increases with its diminuation.

Only a few of the neurons that connect both lobulae via the anterior optic commissure (AOC) have been analyzed at this present time. They have wide branchings in both optic ganglia and also show the lobula-typic movement sensitivity with a preference for one direction.

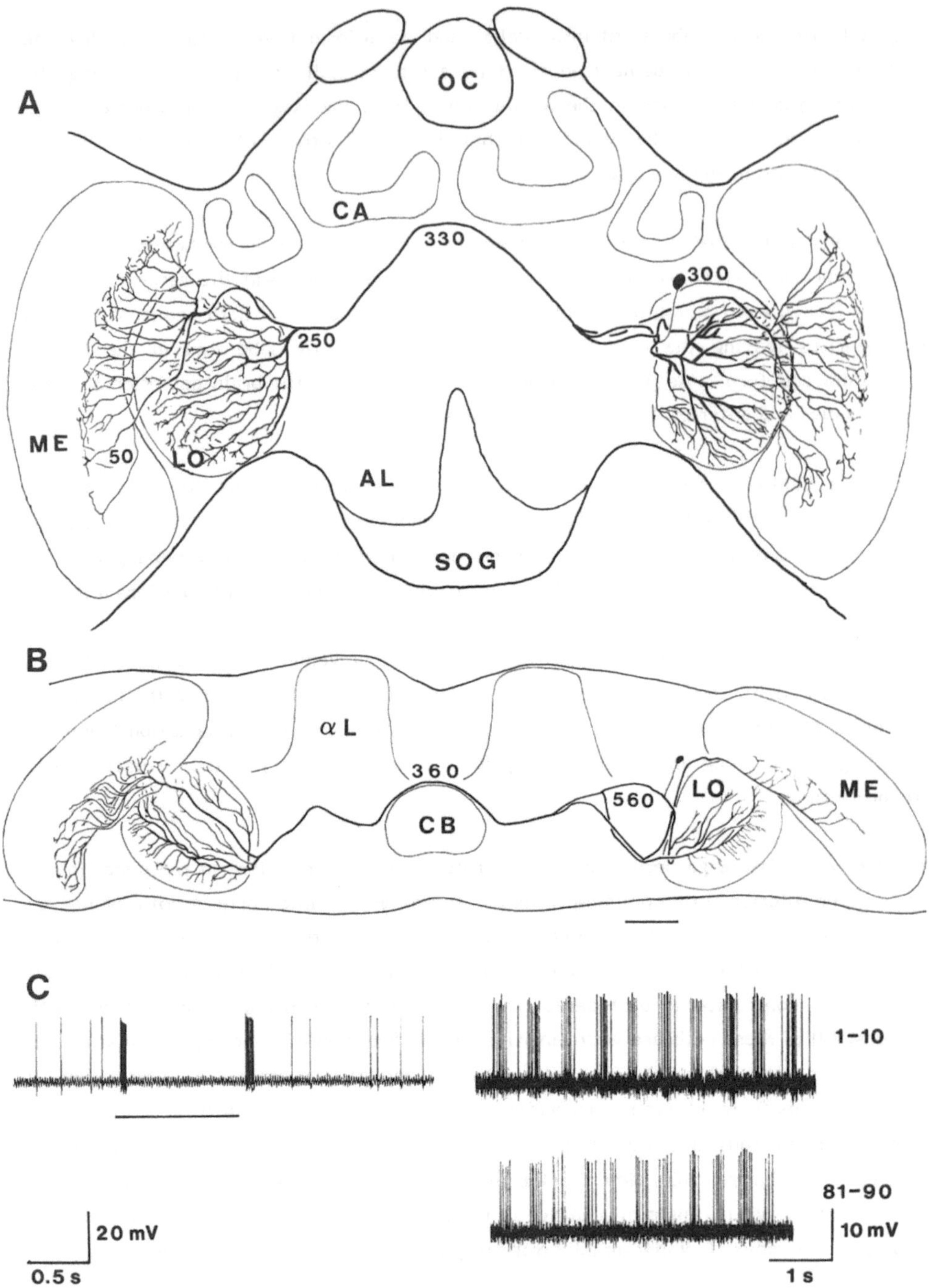

Fig. 6 - Structure and function of a serpentine neuron. A. Frontal view of the cell, B gives a horizontal view. Scale = 100 µm. C. A stationary light elicits short phasic ON and OFF responses. A moved pattern causes bursts of action potentials. A continuous repetition of this stimulus does not reduce the responsiveness of the cell. Here the responses to stimuli No. 1 - 10 and 81 - 90 are shown.

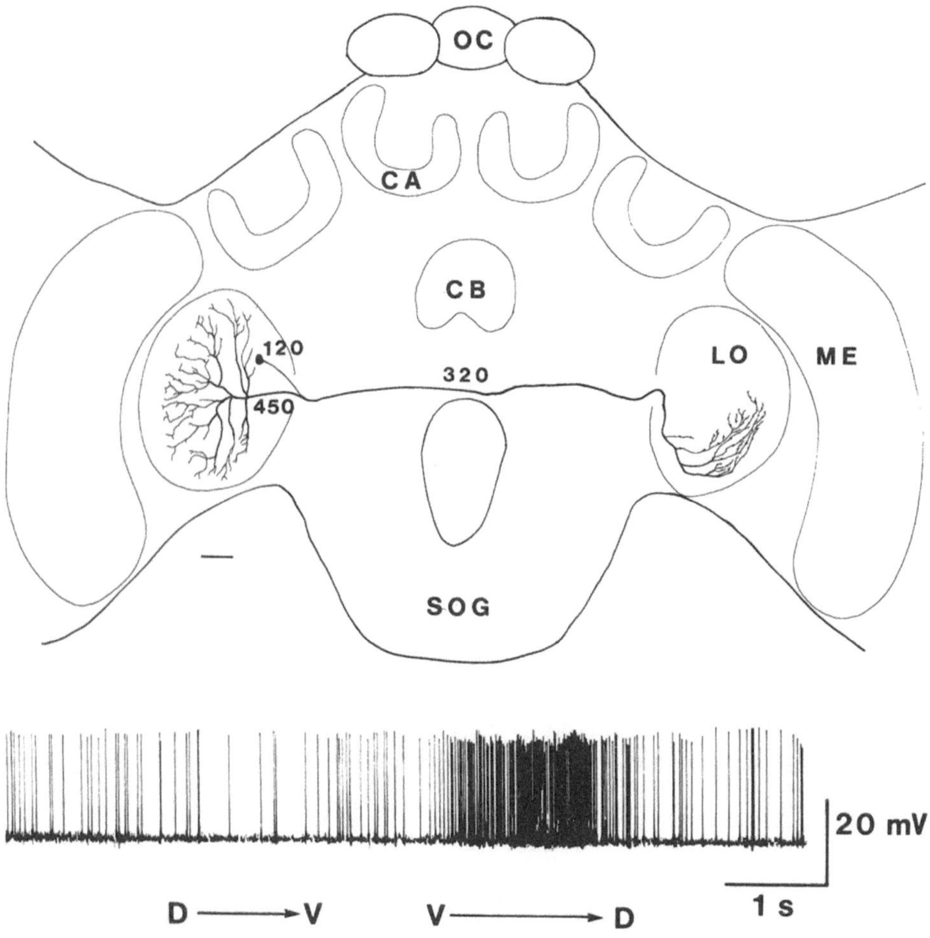

Fig. 7 - The dendritic field of this IOC neuron extends into the middle part of a posterior lobula layer; its axon projects to the contralateral side and there invades the ventral lobula with fine terminal endings. Scale = 100 μm. The neuron displays a distinct sensitivity for the direction of movement: a dorso-to-ventral (D-V) movement decreases, and the opposite direction (V-D) increases the spontaneous activity of this cell.

In extrinsic lobula neurons that have wide field arborizations in a single lobula and terminate in the lateral protocerebrum, the location of the cell does not always correspond to the side of visual input. This indicates centrifugal connections onto those extrinsic elements, probably via IOC or AOC neurons. Other horizontal movement sensitive neurons have been described by DeVoe et al.(1).

As far as wavelength dependence is concerned, most of the movement sensitive neurons are dominated by a green photoreceptor input. This is in good agreement with behavioral results which have shown that the optomotor response is triggered by the inputs of green sensitive photoreceptors (5).

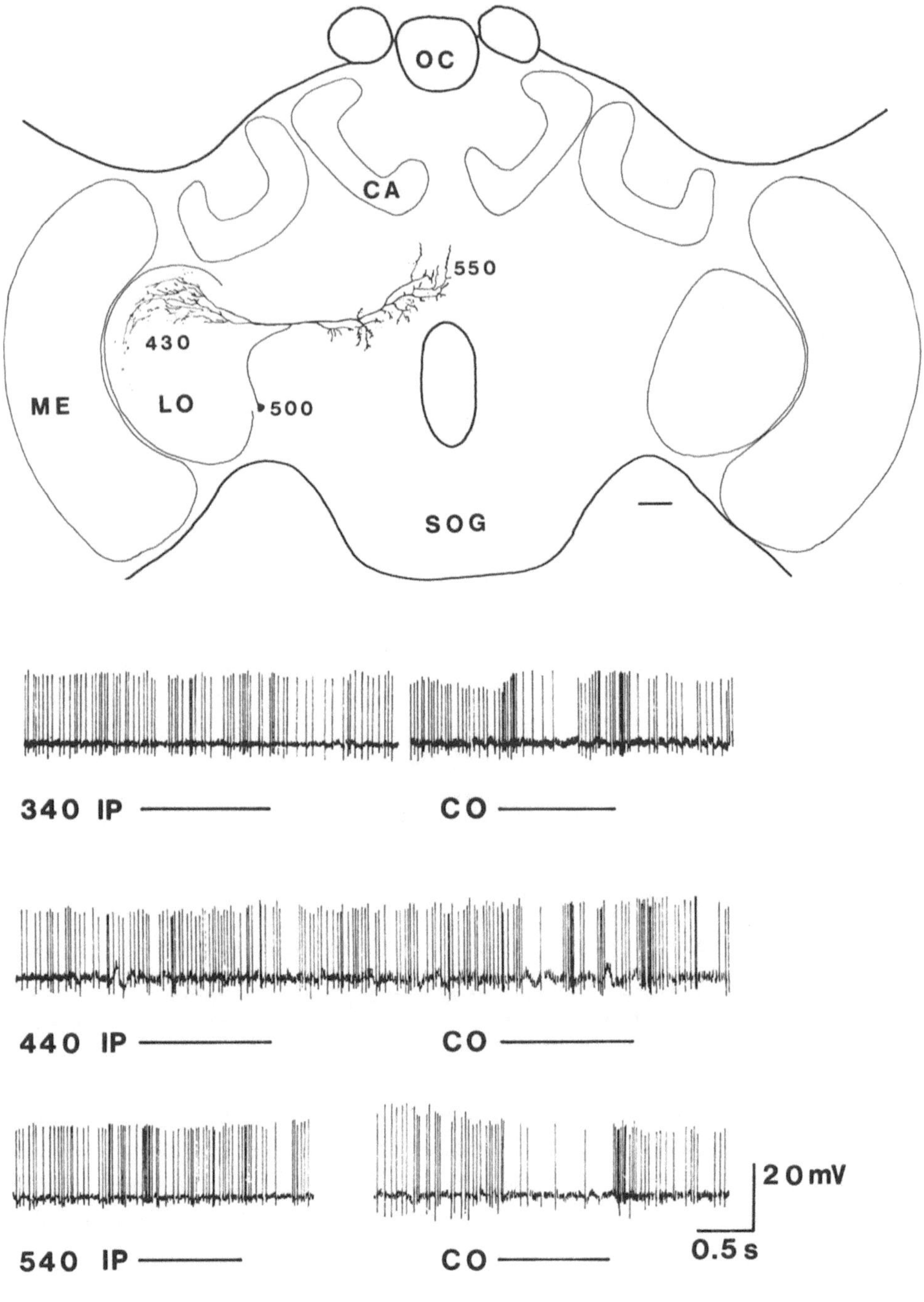

Fig. 8 - Double-opponent neuron with smooth dendritic arborizations in the dorsal lobula and varicous dendrites close to the oesophagus. Scale = 100 µm. Presenting light of equal quanta, the sign of the response depends on the position and the color of the stimulus: on the ipsilateral eye, UV light causes a short inhibition, whilst green light leads to excitation. On the contralateral eye the responses are opposite to those described above.

In the medulla, neurons have been found with either spectrally opponent (presumably in the AOC) or spatially opponent (POC) characteristics. Among lobula extrinsic fibers, however, there are cells which show both opponencies at the same time. An example of these double opponent cells is given in Fig. 8. This neuron is located at the most posterior side of the brain. One arborization is located in the dorsal lobula, and the second ramification with obvious blebs lies in the median protocerebrum close to the oesophagus. This widefield cell responds to an ipsilateral UV-light stimulus with an ON inhibition; green light, however, causes an ON excitation. Similar light stimuli, presented to the contralateral eye, lead to antagonistic responses: green light inhibits the cell, whilst UV light elicits an ON excitation.

The dual opponency of this cell is due to its connection to antagonistically responding UV-to-green opponent cells of both eyes, and these cells may play an important role in color discrimination. Optimal responses are elicited by the presentation of two adjacent colors simultaneously, and in this example, maximum inhibition is due to wide-field ipsilateral UV and contralateral green light, whilst the strongest excitation occurs under the reverse conditions. A stronger saturation of the colors results in a higher color contrast and this in turn leads to a stronger response. It is also interesting to note that these cells are almost insensitive to a monochromatic surrounding. Narrow field double opponent cells with a center-surround organization, as described in the visual cortex of vertebrates (11), have not yet been found.

Lobula fibers that branch laterally to the oesophagus may transfer information, without much processing, to local interneurons which arborize in the neuropile next to the oesophagus. Here again, as has been described before, directional selectivity to a moving target is well established.

The descending interneurons are the next step in the processing of movement detection (Fig. 9; see also Goodman, this volume). They show the same response characteristics i.e. weak responses to stationary light, but strong ones to moving gratings. It is also worth mentioning that they are the most proximal efferent elements which respond to a constant repetition of the same stimulus with a gradually decrease of the discharge frequency. Furthermore, the broad-band sensitivity with enhanced sensitivity to green light is still found at this stage in processing of movement information.

Mushroom body

The mushroom bodies receive visual input mainly via neurons from the medulla and lobula that run as the anterior superior optic tract (2,12) within the anterior optic commissure and branch in the collar region of the calyces ipsi-and contralaterally in the brain. Visual information can be faintly detected in extrinsic neurons at the alpha-lobe. It is possible that it is concealed by a high threshold in these neurons to visual input. It has been demonstrated that after applying a depolarizing current during intracellular recording, the previously weak

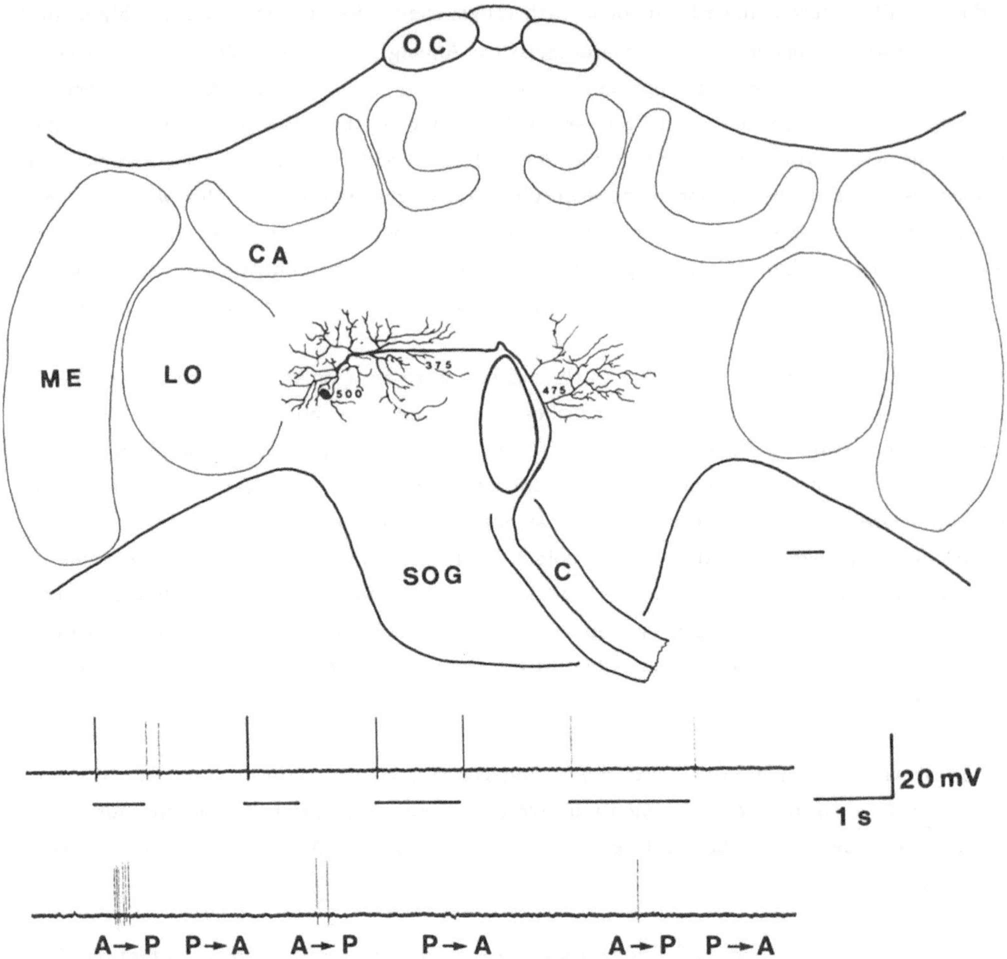

Fig. 9 - Descending interneuron with dendritic fields at the proximal lobula and close to the contralateral side of the oesophagus. The axon leaves the brain via the neck connective. Scale = 100 µm. A stationary light stimulus (upper trace) elicits an ON and OFF response. Movement of a grating gives a directional selective answer (lower trace): only a movement from anterior (A) to posterior (P) causes action potentials, their number being reduced by the repetition of the stimulus.

response was turned into a very prominent directional selective response to movement. This may indicate a high threshold that can be overcome with additional sensory input, probably of a different modality, or by internal threshold control of unknown origin.

Optic tubercle

The role of the optic tubercle in signal analysis still remains unknown, and the fibers of the lobula-to-optic tubercle tract and the inter-optic tubercle commissure have not yet been recorded. Some cells connecting the optic tubercle with the posterior protocerebrum have been analyzed. They either show a directional unselective movement sensitivity in a binocular receptive field, or, whilst only slightly responding to light stimuli, give indications for additional input from mechanoreceptors of the head or the abdomen (4).

Central complex

According to Homberg (4), most elements of the central complex are not or only weakly sensitive to visual stimuli. The protocerebral bridge, however, seems to be an important structure for the central analysis of visual information, with a high sensitivity for moving objects. The central body is connected to various sensory organs. In its fan-shaped dorsal part, the cells recorded so far have not shown any distinct responses to visual, olfactory or mechanical stimuli (4). An exception is shown in Figure 10. This neuron shows a strong motion sensitivity with a preference for the direction of movement. In the ventral part of the central complex, the ellipsoid body, movement sensitivity is more prominent. Here, the cells often display a directional selectivity by opponent responses, similar to the neurons of the IOC (see above). This was also demonstrated by Homberg (4).

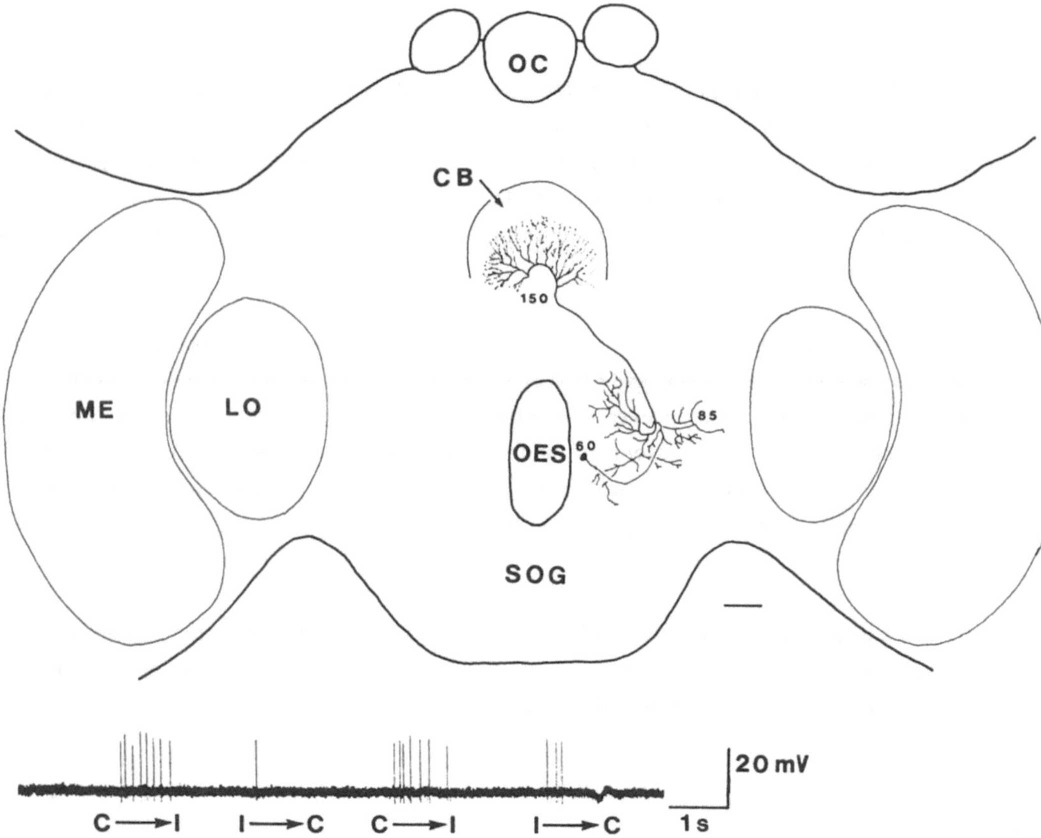

Fig. 10 - Fan-shaped neuron of the central body, in this case with a very blebby dendritic arborization, and a smooth second branching in the lateral protocerebrum. Scale = 100 µm. The neuron shows a directional preference for moving gratings: in the frontal visual field the movement from the contralateral side relative to the cell soma (C) to ipsilateral (I) elicits a much stronger response than movement in the opposite direction.

CONCLUDING REMARKS

Most of the mechanisms underlying the bee's analysis of the visual world remain unresolved, and there are many gaps in our functional map of the brain. Nevertheless, knowledge of basic properties of information processing continues to emerge with ongoing research, and the data now available enable us to put forward a concept of visual signal flux in the bee brain.

Light quanta are absorbed by photoreceptors of the compound eye, which produce an electrical signal proportional to the log quantal flux. This signal is transferred to the lamina monopolar cells. Their function in signal processing in the bee is still, however, not yet clear. In the lamina, amacrine cells provide the visual system with lateral integration. These cells either collect identical information from neighbouring ommatidia (e.g. to feed the responses of photoreceptors of identical spectral information into specific color channels), or they may function in a lateral inhibitory way to enhance the contrast of intensity borders. Additionally, the sensitivity of visual input may be controlled by centrifugal fibers at this first integration level.

In the medulla there is a segregation of the different qualities of a visual signal into different pathways. The spectral composition of the visual world gets a first interpretation by color coding interneurons, giving wavelength dependent antagonistic responses. Moving objects are detected by small field neurons without analyzing the direction of movement, and wide field cells, mostly gathered in the POC, code the locus of a stationary target by antagonistic responses, regardless of its color.

The separated information of medulla neurons partly converges onto some lobula neurons, and these cells code both the position and color of an object in a double antagonistic manner. The main function of the lobula, however, is the detection of moving objects. Wide field neurons analyze the direction of movement and transfer this information to the lateral protocerebrum. From here, this information is either passed on via local interneurons or is directly transferred onto descending interneurons through the suboesophageal ganglion to the thorax.

Many neurons of the medulla and lobula are connected to higher integration centers in the protocerebrum, where their information converges with that coming from other sensory inputs to the brain. These multimodalities are discussed in detail by Erber and Homberg in this volume.

REFERENCES

(1) DeVoe, R.; Kaiser, W.; Ohm, J.; and Stone, L. 1982. Horizontal movement detectors of honeybees: directionally-selective visual neurones in the lobula and brain. J. comp. Physiol. 147: 155-170.

(2) Gronenberg, W. 1984. Das Protocerebrum der Honigbiene im Bereich des Pilzkörpers - eine neurophysiologisch-anatomische Charakterisierung. Ph.D. Dissertation, Freie Universität Berlin.

(3) Hertel, H. 1980. Chromatic properties of identified interneurons in the optic lobes of the bee. J. comp. Physiol. 137: 215-231.

(4) Homberg, U. 1982. Das mediane Protocerebrum der Honigbiene (Apis mellifica) im Bereich des Zentralkorpers: Physiologische und morphologische Charakterisierung. Ph.D. Dissertation, Freie Universität Berlin.

(5) Kaiser, W. 1974. The spectral sensitivity of the honey bee's optomotor walking response. J. comp. Physiol. 90: 405-408.

(6) Kien, J., and Menzel, R. 1977. Chromatic properties of interneurons in the optic lobes of the bee. II. Narrow band and colour opponent neurons. J. comp. Physiol. 113: 35-53.

(7) Laughlin, S. 1984. The roles of parallel channels in early visual processing by the arthropod compound eye. In Photoreception and Vision in Invertebrates, ed. M.A. Ali. New York: Plenum Press.

(8) Menzel, R. 1974. Spectral sensitivity of monopolar cells in the bee lamina. J. comp. Physiol. 93: 337-346.

(9) Menzel, R., Ventura, D.F., Hertel, H., de Souza, J.M., Greggers, U. 1986. Spectral sensitivity of photoreceptors in insect compound eyes: comparison of species and methods. J. comp. Physiol. 158: 165-177.

(10) Meyer, E.P., Matute, C., Streit, P., and Nässel, D.R. 1986. Insect optic lobe neurons identifiable with monoclonal antibodies to GABA. Histochemistry 84: 207-216.

(11) Michael, C.R. 1978. Color vision mechanisms in monkey striate cortex: Dual-opponent cells with concentric receptive fields. J. Neurophysiol. 41(3): 572-588.

(12) Mobbs, P.G. 1984. Neural networks in the mushroom bodies of the honeybee. J. Insect Physiol. 30(1): 43-58.

(13) Ribi, W.A. 1974. Neurons in the first synaptic region of the bee, Apis mellifera. Cell Tissue Res. 148: 277-286.

(14) Ribi, W.A. 1981. The first optic ganglion of the bee. IV. Synaptic fine structure and connectivity patterns of receptor cell axons and first order interneurones. Cell Tiss. Res. 215: 443-464.

(15) Ribi, W.A., and Scheel, M. 1981. The second and third optic ganglia of the worker bee. Cell Tissue Res. 221: 17-43.

(16) Riehle, A. 1981. Color opponent neurons of the honeybee in a heterochromatic flicker test. J. comp. Physiol. 142: 81-88.

(17) Schäfer, S. 1984. Charakterisierung extrinsischer Großfeldneuronen aus der Medulla der Honigbiene (Apis mellifera). Diplomarbeit, Freie Universität Berlin. FB23.

(18) Schäfer, S., and Bicker, G. 1986. Distribution of GABA-like immunoreactivity in the brain of the honeybee. J. Comp. Neurol. 246: 287-300.

(19) Witthöft, W. 1967. Absolute Anzahl und Verteilung der Zellen im Hirn der Honigbiene. Z. Morph. Tiere 61: 160-184.

Motion Sensitive Descending Interneurons, Ocellar L_D Neurons and Neck Motoneurons in the Bee: A Neural Substrate for Visual Course Control in Apis mellifera

Lesley J. Goodman, William A. Fletcher, Richard G. Guy, Peter G. Mobbs and Christopher D. J. Pomfrett

School of Biological Sciences, Queen Mary College, University of London, Mile End Road, London E14 NS, U K

Abstract. The response characteristics of 12, identified, motion-sensitive descending interneurons in the brain of Apis mellifera suggests that they form a significant part of the neural substrate for visual course control. The neurons are sensitive to wide field-motion of the visual surround, non-habituating, non-adapting, velocity sensitive and unresponsive to small target movement. Ten of them show broad band directional sensitivity. Analysis of the preferred directions of the cells shows a polarization towards either the vertical or the horizontal with an asymmetrical distribution of units within one connective. Differences in sensitivity to pitch and to roll simulations is found in some of the vertically sensitive cells. At least one ocellar L_D neuron also carries information about vertical movement over the compound eye. Suboesophageal neck motoneurons are also found to display directional sensitivity to wide field motion.

INTRODUCTION

The honeybee, Apis mellifera, has been studied perhaps more extensively than any other insect in the world yet curiously the neural mechanisms underlying its rich repetoire of behaviors have been neglected by neurophysiologists. We know virtually nothing, for example, about the neural control of flight, fanning behavior, walking, respiration, feeding and trophallaxis and the complex movements underlying the dance. Attention has been focussed upon the response characteristics and processing mechanisms of the visual and olfactory pathways and on the mushroom bodies within the brain (see revs. by Erber and Homberg, and Hertel and Maronde in this volume). Very little is known about interactions between the brain and body ganglia and of control of the motor activity at ganglion level. Recent studies on a number of insects are beginning to reveal the way in which information about whole field displacement of the visual surround of insects is signalled to the motor systems responsible for the appropriate adjustments of head, body and legs in visual course control, (4, 5, 9, 10, 19, 21, 22, 23). This paper attempts both to describe some elements of the neural substrate for visual course stabilization in the bee and, if only for its omissions, to encourage more neurophysiologists to venture down its ventral nerve cord and into the thoracic ganglia.

MOTION SENSITIVE DESCENDING INTERNEURONS RESPONDING TO WIDE FIELD MOVEMENT OF THE VISUAL SURROUND

Twelve unique descending interneurons (DNs) showing tonic or phaso-tonic responses to wide field-movement have been encountered in the cervical connectives (4, 5). All of these cells have their major arborisations in what is now considered to be deutocerebral neuropil (24) immediately posterior to the deutocerebral lobes or in areas at the base of the lobula. Nine of the cell bodies are located in the deutocerebral rind, one in the protocerebrum and two on the boundary of the tritocerebral and suboesophageal ganglion (Fig. 1a). The cells have been classified according to their morphology, anatomically similar cells have been placed together resulting in six groups of descending neurons designated DN I - DN VI. This seems to be the simplest and most useful way of describing the cells at present since it remains possible to add cells to the groups if necessary and does not imply that the cells are purely visual in their response or that they are associated with a particular behavioral response. The anatomy of individual cells is briefly described in the legends to Figs. 1a and 2. The inputs to these DNs are not known. One possible source of input may be the 12 large wide-field neurons in the posterior region of the lobula (Mobbs, pers. obs) which project to the deutocerebrum in posterior optic tract I terminating ipsilaterally in a manner very similar in location and appearance to the VS and HS cells of the fly (rev. 11). Two large fibres project from the lobula into the contralateral posterior deutocerebral/tritocerebral neuropil. The physiological properties of these cells are unknown although wide-field cells sensitive to horizontal motion are known to conjoin the lobulae (2). The bee has several optic foci in the lateral deutocerebrum some of which are visited by individual DNs and many of the DNs visit a common ocellar/compound eye focus at the base of the ocellar tract where the ocellar neurons begin to arborise. An extensive tract of fine fibres leaves the posterior lobula in posterior optic tract II and extends into this region (17). Most of the cells also have arborisations within some part of the dorsolateral posterior slope or perioesophageal region occupied by the arborisations of ocellar neurons, while some send small collaterals up into the ocellar tracts. All of the DNs have been traced as far as the prothoracic ganglion and 5 as far as the meso- and metathoracic ganglion (5).

Response characteristics of the twelve DNs

In our studies intracellar recordings are made from the cervical connectives while stimulating the bee with movement of a large, square-wave grating of vertical black and white stipes in the frontal visual field or by 2 gratings placed lateral, one on either side of the head, and moved either singly or simultaneously. The gratings are moved at 20° or 7 $1/2^{o}$ intervals throughout 360°, for a period of 3s in one direction with an interstimulus of 3s. Spatial wavelength and grating velocity can be adjusted to give a range of contrast frequencies. The response of a cell to movement is obtained by substracting its response during the previous interstimulus interval from its response to the stimulus. To obtain the mean direction of cells whose response appears to be polarized in one overall direction, it is appropriate to calculate the mean vector angle (MVA) (1). Cells are normally marked with cobalt chloride

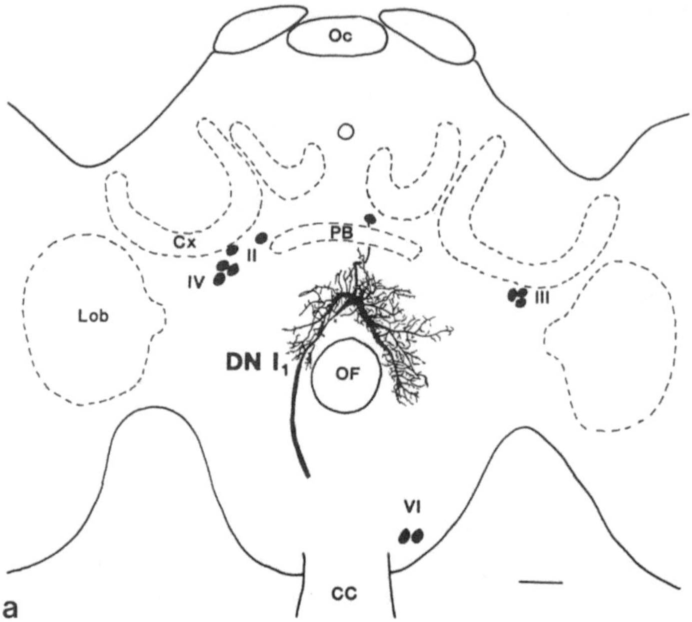

Fig. 1 - (a) A posterior view of the brain to show the postion of the DNs. The unique cell DN I is shown here arching over the gut with arborisations in each half of the brain although the major branching lies in the half contralateral to the axon in the cervical connective, cc. The cell bodies of the remaining cell groups are indicated. Cx, calyx of the mushroom bodies; Oc, ocellus; PB, protocerebral bridge; Lob, lobula. Scale bar 200 um.

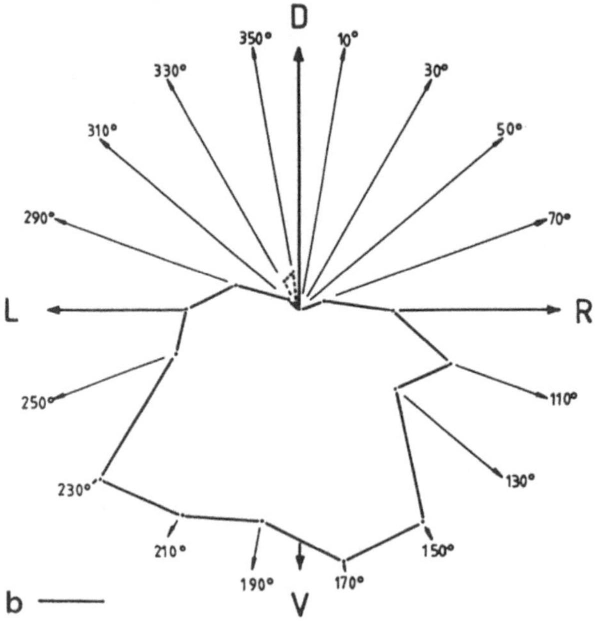

Fig. 1 - (b) - The response of this cell to grating movement in 18 different directions plotted on polar coordinates. The vertical axis DV is aligned with the dorsoventral axis of the bee, 90° is on the bee's right, 270° on the left. Scale bar 25 Hz. From Fletcher et. al. (5).

or Lucifer yellow. Extracellular recordings are made from a preparation in which the bee itself can be rotated in the pitching, rolling and yawing planes. Further details of experimental methods are given elsewhere (5).

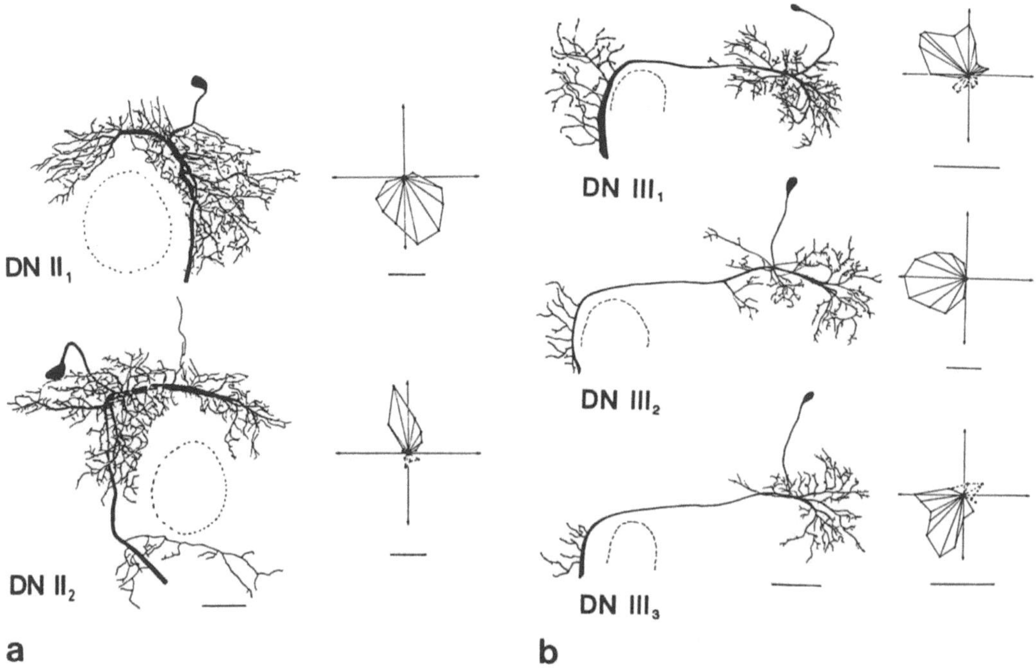

Fig. 2 a, b - Five groups of wide field-motion sensitive DNs together with a polar plot of each cell's response. Dotted lines show inhibition of spontaneous frequency. (a) Cells DN II_1 and II_2 have extensive arborisations medially and lateral to the gut in the posterior deutocerebral neuropil in the contralateral half of the brain. Note that these and other vertically sensitive cells send long trailing collaterals up into the ocellar tracts. Bar 200 um and 10 Hz. (b) Cells DN III_1, III_2 and III_3 have their major, spined arborisations near the base of the lobula contralateral to their axons in the VNC. Their more restricted ipsilateral arborisations in the posterior superficial neuropil beside the gut are blebbed. Bars 200 um and 25 Hz.

The response characteristics of these 12 DNs suggest that they form part of the neural substrate for course control in the bee. The cells show little or no sign of habituation to repeated stimulation when tested with up to 100 stimuli of 1s duration. With the exception of DN IV_1, they show little sign of adaptation, maintaining their response to sustained grating movement over periods of at least 20s and usually for considerably longer (4). They are all velocity sensitive. The cells give little or no response to the movement of small black targets within the visual field. Ten of the cells show directional sensitivity in their response to grating movement although they are not sharply tuned, typically giving some excitatory response to movement throughout at least 150°, usually with 50% response levels around 90° (Figs. 1b and 2). Rarely are the responses so narrowly tuned as the example shown for cell DN II_2 in Fig. 2a.

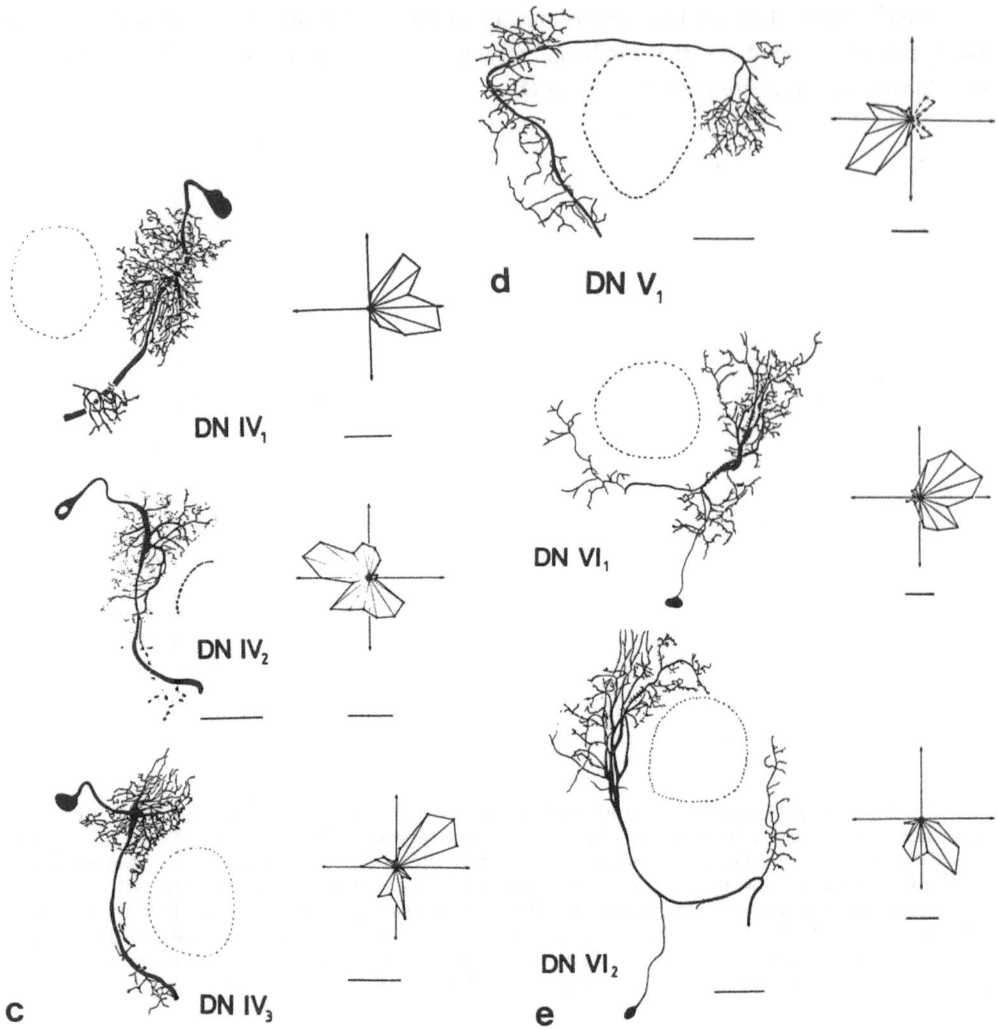

Fig. 2 c, d - (c) Cells DN IV_1, IV_2 and IV_3 have a relatively restricted area of branching in the ipsilateral deutocerebrum. Each of the cells gives off collaterals in the tritocerebrum and suboesophageal ganglion. Bars 200 um and 15 Hz. (d) DNV has a fine-spined arborisation contralateral to its axon and a more extensive network of blebbed arborisations in the ipsilateral half of the brain. The cell body has not been located. Bars 200 um and 25 Hz. (e) The cells of group VI, DN VI_1 and VI_2 have their cell bodies located on the border of the tritocerebral/suboesophageal rind. Both have densely spined arborisations in the posterior deuterocerebrum contralateral to their axons in the VNC. They also show restricted branching ipsilaterally around the oesophageal foramen. Bars 200 um and 25 Hz. From Fletcher et. al. (5).

However, the overall preferred direction of movement for each cell in response to frontal stimulation remains remarkably constant from preparation to preparation and within the same preparation over a period of time, although levels of background discharge, bandwidth of the 50% response level and level of inhibition in the null direction may vary.

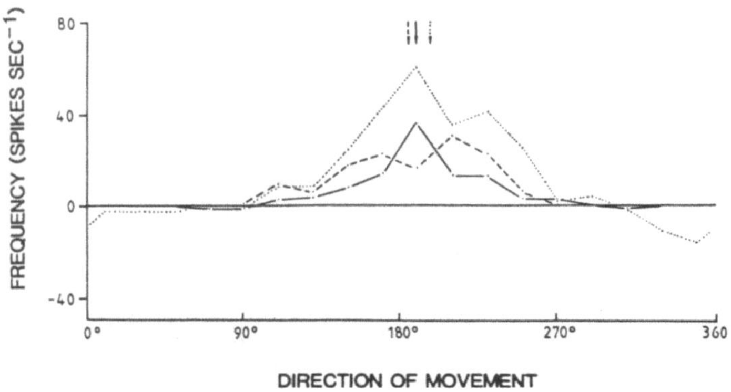

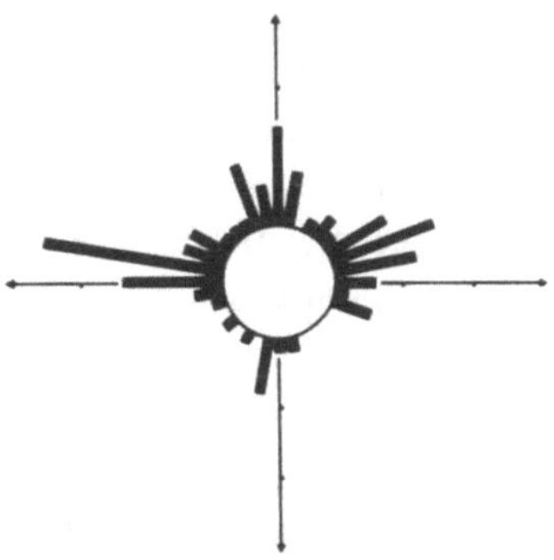

Fig. 3 - The response of three DN VI_2 cells to a moving square-wave grating presented in 18 different directions, contrast frequency 3.7 Hz. At 0° a horizontal grating is moved upwards, at 90° a vertical grating is moved from left to right, at 360° a horizontal grating is moved down and at 270° a vertical grating is moved from right to left across the front of the head. Arrows show the mean vector angle or PD of each cell at 187°, 190° and 180°.

Fig. 4 - The mean vector angles (MVAs) of 89 directionally selective descending cells summarized as a polar histogram. The responses of all the cells are shown as if they were recorded in the left cervical connective. The MVA of most of the vertical DNs lies to one side of the vertical axis. More horizontal DNs are excited by right to left motion in the left connective than by left to right motion. Scale, 5 cells per division. After Fletcher et al. (5).

Figure 3 shows the response of cell DN VI_2 recorded in the left connective in three individuals. Although the shape of the response curve varies somewhat between these cells, the MVAs are very similar, 189°, 190° and 198° respectively. This constancy of overall directional sensitivity is a feature of all the cells comprising groups DN I, II, III, V and VI (5). The cells comprising group DN IV have some features which distinguish them from the other wide field-motion sensitive cells. DN IV_1, is more phasic in its response than the other 11 cells and its level of excitation in response to movement is much more variable. The overall directional sensitivity of the cell is horizontal (see Fig. 6a) but there is often a characteristic notch in the polar plot around the horizontal axis so that two distinct peaks are seen, one above and one below the 90°-270° axis. The most extreme example of this type of response encountered is shown in Fig. 2c. Cells DN IV_2 and IV_3 give some response in all four quadrants at contrast frequencies between 2 and 4Hz.

The distribution of the MVAs of the directionally selective cells encountered (excluding cells with the response characteristics of DN IV_1, for which it is not appropriate to calculate an MVA) shows a polarization towards either the horizontal or vertical, although individual cells can be encountered with preferred directions at most orientations. There is an asymmetrical distribution of the preferred directions of cells encountered in one connective (Fig. 4). In the left connective more cells are encountered with a sensitivity for right to left movement than for left to right movement and, indeed, only one cell type responsive to left to right movement has been identified in the left connective, cell DN VI_1 (Fig. 2e). The MVA of most vertically sensitive cells lies off axis with a bias to the left of the bee's dorso-ventral axis in the left connective and to the right in the right connective (cf. the distribution of directional sensitivity of units in the dragonfly VNC (19)). More cells are sensitive to downward vertical motion than upward vertical motion and this presumably reflects the fact that 4 cell types, DN I, DN II_1, DN III_3 and DN VI_2, sensitive to downward ventral movement have been identified, whilst only two cell types sensitive to upward vertical movement, DN III_1 and DN II_2, have been found. It is not clear why there should be a preponderance of vertically downward sensitive units. Possibly it is associated with an asymmetrical distribution of of flow field stimuli in forward flight since ground and horizon features passing beneath the insect will provide most of the input.

What are the roles of individual DNs?

It is premature to attempt to assign a role to individual DNs without further information on the response characteristics of optomotor torque responses and other wide field-driven behaviors, such as exists for the fly, together with a more detailed knowledge of the neural organization of locomotory systems in the bee. However, initial observations show that there are subtle differences between the response characteristics of individual vertically sensitive cell types and between each of the horizontally sensitive cell types, which suggests that they have distinct roles in visually guided behavior. For example, they are all velocity sensitive, but the shape of the response curves and the peak response differs quiet considerably between cell types although changes in velocity do not alter the overall preferred direction of a cell, Fig. 5. DN II_2 is maximally excited at a lower velocity, equivalent to a constant frequency of 4.3 Hz. Two other vertically sensitive neurons, DN I and DN VI_2, show a peak velocity response between 1.5 and 3 Hz in the slow image velocity range normally shown by optomotor systems, while other vertically sensitive cells are not saturated at 10 Hz (Ibbotson and Goodman, unpublished obs.). Some vertically sensitive units appear to show two distinct peaks when recorded extracellularly, depending on whether the bee is rolling or pitching.

Flies show a good correspondence between the optomotor torque responses and the response characteristics of the tangential cells in the lobula plate (7). In the bee there is a wide discrepancy between the one unidentified horizontally sensitive optic lobe unit measured, which peaks around 2-3 Hz (8), and the optomotor torque response which peaks at 10 Hz (11). The horizontal DNs again show a range of peak sensitivities between 2 Hz and 9-10 Hz. The motion-sensitive units of the bee thus collectively appear to operate over a wide range of velocities with differing peak sensitivities. Behavioral studies of temporal acuity and of visual scanning mechanisms (13) suggest that an active forager such as the bee may employ optomotor-type stabilizing responses in a variety of visual orientation behaviors. Possibly the parameters of the optomotor systems may turn out to be rather different from those of the fly.

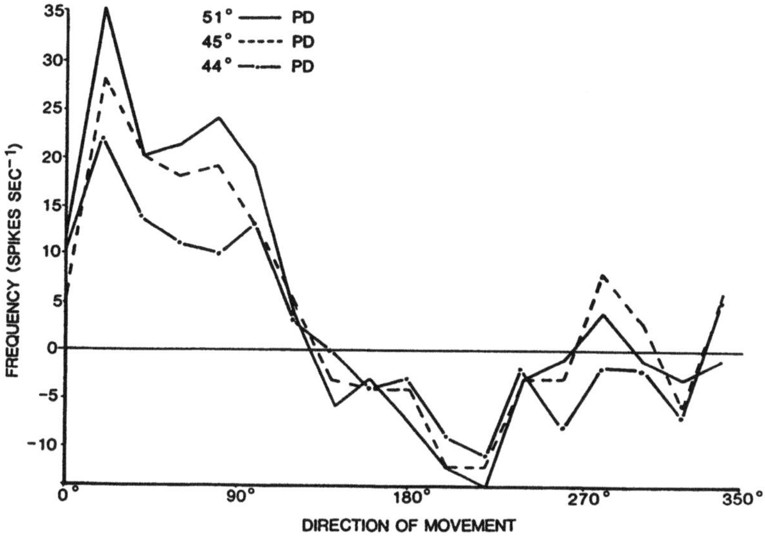

Fig. 5 - The response of one DN II_2 cell recorded in the right connective to grating presentations in 18 different directions at three velocities. Continuous line, 64° sec^{-1} (= 4.3 Hz); dotted line, 129° sec^{-1} (= 8.6 Hz); dot/dashed line 190° sec^{-1} (= 12.7 Hz). Increasing the velocity of grating movement reduces the response of the cell but does not significantly change its MVA.

Analysis of the contribution of each eye and of different regions of the eye can help to suggest a function for individual DNs. Extracellular studies tell us that most vertically sensitive units recorded in the VNC are stimulated to some extent when the insect rolls as well as when it pitches either up or down although some units do seem to be particularly sensitive to either roll or pitch. Intracellular studies suggest that at least two of the DNs are especially sensitive to movement around the longitudinal axis. DN VI_2 is a binocularly driven unit which is sensitive to motion in opposite directions over each eye . It responds strongly to downward movement over the eye ipsilateral to its cell body and weakly to upward movement over the opposite eye (Fig. 6a). Its response to binocular stimulation reflects the dominant downward sensitivity of the ipsilateral eye. Simulation of a left hand roll with grating movements in opposite directions over the lateral regions of the eye results in an enhanced response of this cell in the left connective. DN II_1 shows almost identical responses to DN VI_2, although since this unit is ipsilateral, a left hand roll produces an enhanced response in the neuron in the right connective. DN II_2 differs from these units in being sensitive to motion in the same direction over both eyes and in being preferentially sensitive to movement over the frontal region of the eye, Fig. 6c. The properties of this neuron would seem to suit it for detection of downward pitch of body or head or loss of height in flight.

Studies of head turning movements in the yawing plane have suggested regional specialization within the horizontal motion detecting system of each eye in the bee with the lateral region of one eye and the anterior median region of the opposite eye responding to motion in the same direction (18). So far our examination of horizontally descending sensitive units has revealed no sign of this with most units showing little difference between frontal and lateral stimulation (Fig. 6b), but this may be because the areas of the eye stimulated have been too large to reveal any regional specialization.

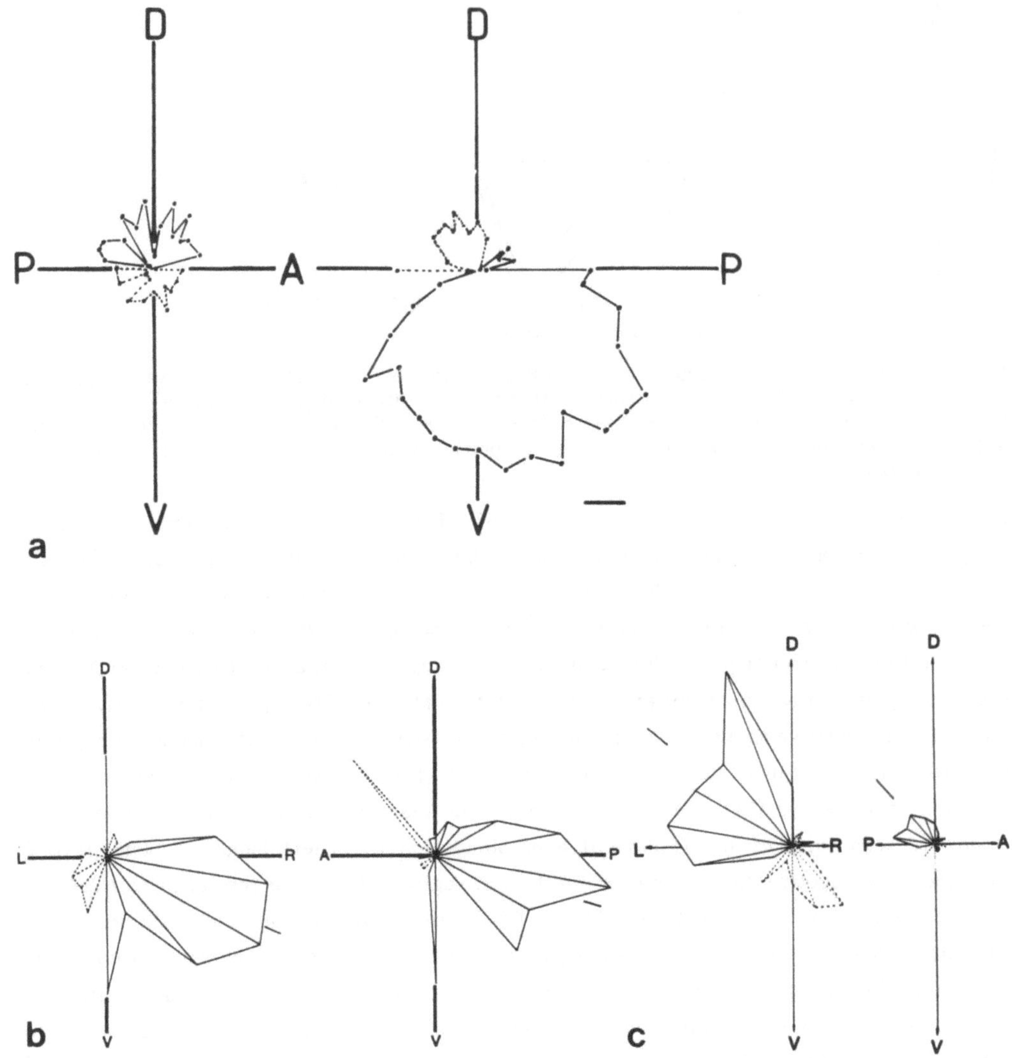

Fig. 6 - (a) The response of cell VN VI_2 to grating motion over the lateral region of each eye recorded in the left connective. The cell responds strongly to downward movement over the right eye ipsilateral to its cell body. A, anterior; P, posterior; D, dorsal; V, ventral. (b) The ipsilateral cell, DN IV_1, stimulated frontally (left polar plot) and laterally (right polar plot) over the right eye. The cell's response does not change markedly when stimulation is confined to the lateral region of the ipsilateral eye. Bar = 1 spike sec^{-1}. (c) Cell DN II_2 stimulated frontally (left polar plot) and laterally over the left eye (right polar plot). A much reduced response is given to lateral stimulation. Bar = 5 spikes sec^{-1}. D, dorsal; V, ventral; L, left; R, right; A, anterior; P, posterior region of the compound eye.

DIRECTIONALLY SELECTIVE RESPONSES IN OCELLAR L_D NEURONS

In the dragonfly "self-movement" detectors recorded in the VNC combine visual and mechanosensory information in such a way as to detect rotation of the insect or of its head within the same plane in space (19). Descending interneurons in the locust can carry both compound eye and ocellar information as well as wind information in some cases. The different inputs are spatially compatible with each other requiring a precise stimulus configuration to effectively excite individual units, but yielding very specific information about the insects course deviations (21, 23). Units formerly regarded as driven only by ocellar and wind stimulation apparently respond to compound eye input if the stimulus configuration is right. The bee possesses pairs of 5 first-order ocellar interneurons which run directly from the ocellar retina to the thoracic ganglia (15, 20). One of these neurons, $Locth_1$, has been shown to respond to other inputs including light on the compound eye and to a variety of mechanosensory stimuli (15). We have found that the ocellar L_D unit $Locth_2$ and its homolog in the wasp, Paravespula vulgaris, is directionally sensitive to wide field motion over the frontal and, in particular, the lateral compound eye. Fig. 7b shows that this unit, which aborises in the left ocellus, is quite sharply tuned to vertical upward movement over the left lateral compound eye, being inhibited in the null direction. Little or no response is given to movement over the right compound eye. This may be a further example of the very precise stimulus configurations required to reveal all of the inputs to some of the descending fibres concerned with course stabilization. The contralateral units shown in Fig. 7a and c could well contribute to the detection and/or correction of downward pitch and more particularly of roll. The latency of response is around 100 msec in the bee and 100-110 msec in the wasp compared with values of 20-30 msec for ocellar 'off' responses in L_D units at the level of the cervical connectives reflecting the additional processing in the compound eye pathway. The interplay between ocellar and compound eye input to this cell is currently the subject of investigation. $Locth_2$ could take its compound eye input from collaterals of the motion sensitive DNs (the upward vertically sensitive cell DN III_1, for example, gives off blebbed branches in an appropriate area of the posterior slope neuropil) or there is the possibility of a direct input from lobula units which terminate in the contralateral posterior deutocerebrum (Mobbs, pers. obs.).

DIRECTIONALLY SELECTIVE RESPONSES IN NECK MOTONEURONS

Head turning movements form part of the visual stabilization mechanism of insects. Compensatory head movements to stabilize the retinal image lead to a mismatch between head and body position which is detected by proprioceptors and may be used to assist in driving steering behavior (6, 9, 10, 12, 16, 25). Such head movements can be readily elicited in flying bees in response to wide field stimuli together with rudder-like movements of the abdomen and hind legs. In view of these observations at least some of the motoneurons should be sensitive to movement of the visual surround, and this has proved to be the case. We have shown that the cervical nerve, IC1 (14), carries at least 8 suboesophageal motoneurons which innervate one muscle from each of the two main groups involved in moving the head, muscles 44 and 51.

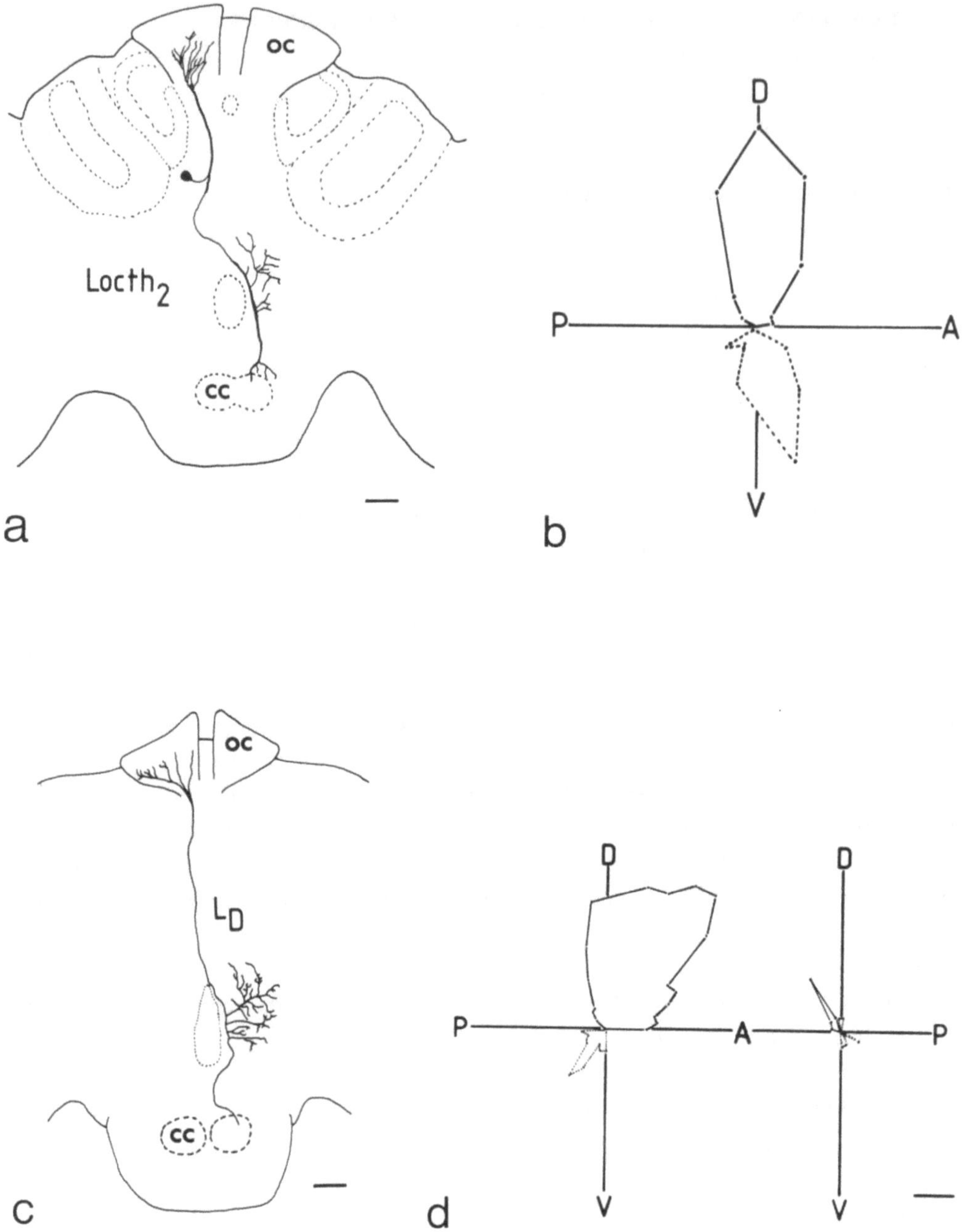

Fig. 7 - A posterior view of the brain of (a) Apis mellifera and (c) Paravespula vulgaris, showing the ocellar L_D neuron Locth2 and an anatomically similar ocellar neuron in the wasp recorded in the right connective and stained with cobalt chloride; OC, ocellus; CC, cervical connectives; Bars 100 um. (b) The response of Locth2 to stimulation of the left lateral eye with a moving grating at 20° intervals. Dotted line shows inhibition. A, anterior; P, posterior. (d) The response of the wasp L_D neuron to lateral stimulation over the left and right eyes. Bars 20 Hz.

All of these neurons are responsive to wide field movement over the compound eyes. Seven of them show a broad band directional sensitivity to movement of a grating, six of them to horizontal movement (Fig. 8b) and one to vertically downward movement. Inhibition of spontaneous activity is often shown to movement in the null direction. Two of the cells are excited by right to left movement across the eye and four by left to right movement when the cells are recorded in the left ICl nerve. They appear to be involved in controlling the antagonistic activity of the pair of large ventral muscles, M 44, which participate in the rotating head in the yawing plane.

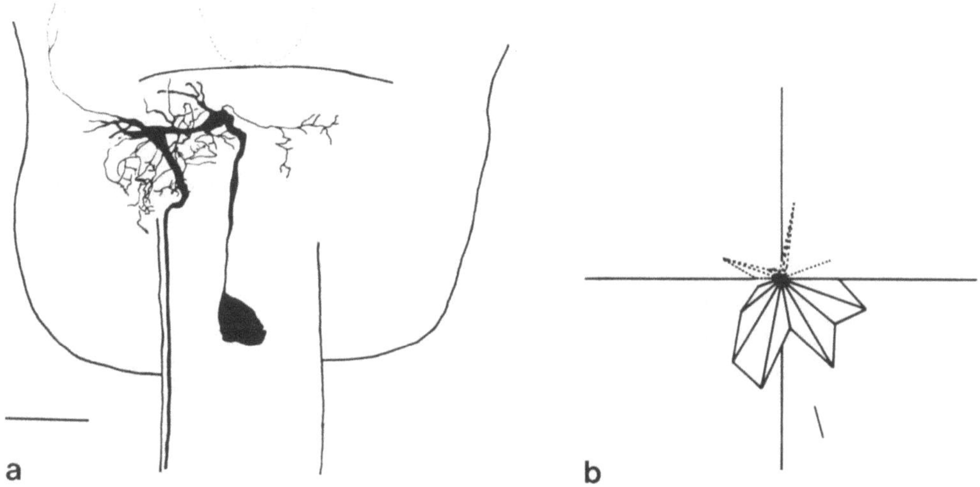

Fig. 8 - (a) Posterior view of the suboesophageal ganglion and cervical connectives showing one of the 4 motoneurons with very large, medial cell bodies recorded in the left hand nerve IC_1. Bar 100 um. (b) The cell gives a broad band response to oblique and horizontal movement from the left to right across the frontal visual field when stimulated with movement in 18 different directions. Dotted lines show inhibition of spontaneous frequency. Bar 5 Hz.

Recordings from motor units in four pairs of peripheral nerves that innervate 19 pairs of neck muscles in the fly, Calliphora erythrocephala, have demonstrated the presence of some motoneurons excited by wide field visual stimuli (16). They are directionally sensitive, responding to either horizontal movement or vertically downward movement, tending to be inhibited by movement in the null direction. A direct pathway has been demonstrated between lobula units and specific motoneurons. Two cervical nerve motoneurons in the brain of the fly have been shown to be cobalt coupled to the terminals of the two frontal VS_2 and VS_3 lobula neurons in the contralateral half of the brain, sharing their receptive fields and directional sensitivity. Other motoneurons have been shown to be cobalt coupled to descending interneurons that in turn are cobalt coupled to wide field lobula units. $DNOVS_1$, for example, is cobalt coupled to VS_{4-9} and also to ipsilateral frontal nerve motoneurons. The frontal nerve motoneurons share the receptive fields and directional sensitivity of the VS_{4-9} cells. Only a few motoneurons are reported to be excited by visual stimuli in the fly. Neuroanatomical studies suggest that many of the neck motoneurons receive sensory input from other modalities including mechanosensory input from the prosternal organ and halteres.

The cell bodies of the eight suboesophageal motoneurons of the cervical nerve ICl of the bee lie in two groups, one containing four cells with extremely large cell bodies situated close to the midline (e. g. Fig. 8a) and one containing four cells with smaller pear-shaped cell bodies lying in the ventrolateral rind. All of the cells arborise extensively in the ipsilaterally dorsal suboesophageal neuropil with some additional contralateral branching. Some of the cells have fine branches extending into the trito and deutocerebrum. They all have part of their arborisations overlapping with those made by descending directionally sensitive DNs and three of the L_D ocellar neurons in the dorsal suboesophageal neuropil. This is one possible site at which these motoneurons could receive directionally selective visual input. The response characteristics of the horizontally sensitive motoneurons differs, for example, they are velocity sensitive and they have rather different operational ranges and peak responses. It is possible to match the response characteristics of individual DNs and motoneurons (Pomfrett and Goodman, in prep.). The mechanoreceptive hairs on the episternal cone also send a few projections into this area of the suboesophageal ganglion (3) as do the hairs on the vertex. Some of the motoneurons are sensitive to wind stimuli, but not all of them. Responses to other mechanosensory stimuli have yet to be tested. Although to understand the complex combination of muscle movements required to turn the head in various ways is challenging, the neck muscle system does afford one accessible approach to the examination of the output end of the visual stabilization mechanism in the bee in the absence of any information about the thoracic neural systems governing steering in flight and walking.

Acknowledgements. This work was supported by the Science and Engineering Research Council and the British Bee Keepers Association.

REFERENCES

(1) Batschelet, E. 1981. Circular Statistics in Biology. London and New York: Academic Press.

(2) De Voe, R.D.; Kaiser, W.; Ohm, J.; and Stone, L.S. 1982. Horizontal movement detectors of honeybees. Directionally-selective visual neurons in the lobula and brain. J. comp. Physiol. 147: 155-170.

(3) Fletcher, W.A., and Goodman, L.J. 1982. The central projections of the hairplate receptors of the episternal cone, petiole and mesocoxa of the honeybee. In The Biology of Social Insects, eds. M.D. Breed, C.D. Michener and H.E. Evans. Boulder, Colorado: Westview Press.

(4) Fletcher, W.A.; Goodman, L.J.; Guy, R.G.; and Mobbs, P.G. 1984. Horizontal and vertical motion detectors in the ventral nerve cord of the honeybee, Apis mellifera. J. Physiol. 351: 15.

(5) Fletcher, W.A.; Guy, R.G.; Mobbs, P.G.; and Goodman, L.G. Directionally selective motion sensitive descending interneurons in the brain of the honeybee, Apis mellifera. J. comp. Physiol., in prep.

(6) Goodman, L.J. 1965. The role of certain optomotor reactions in regulating stability in the rolling plane during flight in the desert locust, Schistocerca gregaria. J. Exp. Biol. 42: 385-407.

(7) Hausen, K. 1981. Monocular and binocular computation of motion in the lobula plate of the fly. Verh. Dtsch. Zool. Ges. pp. 49-70. Stuttgart: Gustav Fischer Verlag.

(8) Kaiser, W., and Bishop, L.G. 1970. Directionally selective motion detecting units in the optic lobe of the honeybee. Z. Vergl. Physiol. 67: 403-413.

(9) Kien, J. 1975. Neuronal mechanisms subserving directional selectivity in the locust optomotor system. J. comp. Physiol. 102: 337-355.

(10) Kien, J. 1977. Comparison of sensory input with motor output in the locust optomotor system. J. comp. Physiol. 113: 161-179.

(11) Kunze, P. 1961. Untersuchung des Bewegungsehens fixiert fliegender Bienen. Z. Vergl. Physiol. 44: 656-684.

(12) Land, M.F. 1975. Head movements and fly vision. In The Compound Eye and Vision of Insects, ed. G.A. Horridge, pp. 469-489. Oxford University Press.

(13) Lehrer, M.; Wehner, R.; and Srinivasin, M. 1985. Visual scanning behaviour in honeybees. J. comp. Physiol. 157: 405-415.

(14) Markl, H. 1966. Peripheres Nervensystem und Muskulatur im Thorax der Arbeiterin von Apis mellifera L., Formica polyctena Foerster und Vespa vulgaris L. unter der Grundplan der Innervierung des Insektenthorax. Zool. Jb. Anat. Bd. 83.S: 107-184.

(15) Milde, J. 1984. Ocellar interneurons in the honeybee. Structure and signals of L-neurons. J. comp. Physiol. 154: 683-693.

(16) Milde, J. J., and Strausfeld, N. J. 1986. Visuo-motor pathways in arthropods. Giant motion-sensitive neurons connect compound eyes directly to neck muscles in blowflies (Calliphora erythrocephala). Naturwiss. 73: 151-154.

(17) Mobbs, P.G. 1984. Neural networks in the mushroom bodies of the honeybee. J. Insect Physiol. 30(1): 43-58.

(18) Moore, D., and Rankin, M.A. 1982. Direction-sensitive partitioning of the honeybee optomotor system. Physiol Entomol. 7: 25-36.

(19) Olberg, R.M. 1981a. Parallel encoding of direction of wind, head, abdomen and visual pattern movement by single interneurons in the dragonfly. J. comp. Physiol. 142: 27-41.

(20) Pan, K.C., and Goodman, L.J. 1977. Ocellar projections within the central nervous system of the worker honey bee, Apis mellifera. Cell & Tissue Res. 176: 505-527.

(21) Reichert, H.; Rowell, C.H.F.; and Gris, C. 1985. Course correction circuitry translates feature detection into behavioural action in locusts. Nature 31(5): 142-144.

(22) Rind, F.C. 1983c. The role of an identified brain neuron in mediating optomotor movements in a moth. J. Exp. Biol. 201: 273-284.

(23) Rowell, C.H.F.; Reichert, H.; and Bacon, J.P. 1985. How locusts fly straight. In Feedback and Motor Control in Invertebrates and Vertebrates, eds. W.J.P. Barnes and M.H. Gladden. London: Croom Helm.

(24) Strausfeld, N.J.; Bassemir, U.; Singh, R.N.; and Bacon, J.P. 1984. Organizational principles of outputs to dipteran brains. J. Insect Phýsiol. 30: 73-93.

(25) Taylor, C.P. 1981a. Contribution of compound eyes and ocelli to steering of locusts in flight. I. Behavioural analysis. J. Exp. Biol. 93: 1-18.

(26) Wehner, R. 1981. Spatial vision in arthropods. In Handbook of Sensory Physiology: Vision in Invertebrates: C Invertebrate Visual Centres and Behaviour, ed. H. Autrum, VII/6C pp. 288-616. Berlin, Heidelberg, New York: Springer Verlag.

Color Vision in Honeybees: Metric, Dimensions, Constancy, and Ecological Aspects

Werner Backhaus, Annette Werner, and Randolf Menzel

Institut für Tierphysiologie, Neurobiologie, Freie Universität Berlin, Königin-Luise-Str. 28–30, D-1000 Berlin 33, FRG

Abstract. The color space of honeybees can be modeled with great precision since we know the spectral sensitivities of the three receptor types very accurately. The predictions of the model are met by color matching experiments (lower colorimetry), and by the judgment of the dissimilarity of colors (higher colorimetry) if we take the receptor noise as the limiting factor for perceptual distance judgment. The behavioral analysis with multifactorial (multidimensional) analysis reveals two perceptual dimensions; the total color distance is the sum of the absolute differences on the two perceptual scales (city-block metric). Color brightness is ignored by the bee in our training experiments. The dissimilarity between color pairs correlates well with the added differences of excitations of a UV/blue-green and a blue/UV-green color opponent system. The corresponding spectrally opponent neurons were found already several years ago. Color constancy is tested in a simultaneous, multi-color arrangement similar to that of Land's (21) "Mondrian" experiment. It is concluded that color constancy in bees is a consequence of antagonistic color coding, and that ratio-making operations are an essential part of this function. It can be quantified with the algorithm developed for human color constancy. Higher order color phenomena of color vision like asymmetric color discrimination between pairs of signals, color specific differences in learning acquisition, context specific discrimination of color signals are described. The phenomena indicate a central nervous representation of color and not just a neural coding of the inputs from the three spectral receptor types.

INTRODUCTION

The study of color vision in honeybees began with a historical controversy. V. Hess (13), an influencial physiologist early this century claimed that bees are color blind because in his experiments their choice preference for colored lights or pigment paints resembled that of color blind people. He came to the conclusion: "At the present time there is not one single fact that would make the assumption even probable, that the bee has a color sense that is comparable to our own sense of color. In fact, my earlier experiments with spectral and glass lights, as well as my new experiments with colored paper, have finally shown this assumption to be unfounded. Considering also the results of previous experiments , all of which are easily reproducable, it is no longer possible to defend Sprengel's spiritual doctrine (Sprengel 1795)(see 45) which is concerned with the meaning of flower color with regards to insect visitation."

As so often in science, v. Hess was not completely wrong. Indeed his early experiments were actually correct and bees are color blind in the behavioral context in which he tested them. However, he made the important mistake to conclude that bees are, therefore, also color blind in other behavioral contexts e.g. at the feeding place. In addition, he made serious experimental mistakes when he tried to repeat v. Frisch's experiments. Hess tested the bees in their phototactic response when they tried to escape from an enclosure spontaneously to the light. We repeated these experiments under better controlled conditions and also found that bees direct their escape runs towards a light source only with respect to the effective photon flux without any indication of color effects (32). For example, mixtures of UV and green (or UV and blue or UV and violet) lights were chosen relative to monochromatic green light with a frequency which can be predicted by simple addition of the effective photon flux of each of the two mixed wavelenghts. Apart from phototaxis, bees are also color blind in their optomotor response (16) and in the orientation of their flights along vertical contrast borders (scanning behavior) (25). Both these behaviors are dominated by the green receptors, whereas in phototaxis all three photoreceptors contribute about equally. Furthermore, bees are color blind in training experiments at low light intensities. For example, bees were trained to walk to one side (e. g. left) in a T-maze when a spectral light was presented from below at the decision point, and to walk to the other side (e. g. right) when the presented light was achromatic white. At low intensities of the spectral light the bees walked to the left, whereas at higher intensities they chose the right side. The spectral light thus appeared achromatic to the bees at lower intensities, and colored at higher intensities (28). This result is supported by the finding that free flying bees loose color vision at low ambient light before they are unable to visually control their flight behavior (27, 41).

Bees see color contrast at the feeding place and at the hive entrance. Since Frisch's (6) first experiments, color training experiments have been repeated many times with varying experimental arrangements. The result of these efforts is that their tri-chromatic color vision system, which partly consists of UV, blue and green receptors, is well documented with behavioral and electrophysiological experiments. Recently, quantitative models have been developed which try to explain the color matching and the color discrimination behavior on the basis of the properties of the photoreceptors and the visual interneurons. (30, 2, 3). We shall first outline the major arguments of these quantitative studies. Further aspects of the color vision system have been described particularly with respect to color constancy, and these shall be presented in the second part of this article. The perceptual dimensions of color vision in bees derived from multiple choice experiments and the interpretation of color opponent systems are presented in the following two chapters. Finally, the question of a connection between color memory and color categories (basic colors) is discussed. We shall demonstrate that color opponency, color constancy and categorial color coding are the basic features of the color vision system in bees.

Chromaticity Diagrams and Photoreceptor Properties

Daumer (5) showed in color mixture experiments with free flying bees, that the Graßmannian mixture laws formulated for human color vision (7) also apply to the color vision system of the bee. As an analogy to human color vision, he presented color mixtures in a chromaticity diagram for bees, i.e. the edges of a symmetric triangle represent three basic lights (primaries); the loci of light mixtures are constructed by dividing the straight line between the loci of two lights of the mixture into the same but inverse ratios of the light intensities used (center-of-gravity construction, see Fig. 1b). In particular, Daumer proved the continuity of a series of mixtures of UV and yellow ("bee-purple"), which have no correlating spectral light. Furthermore, he measured the proportions of complementary spectral lights that are necessary to produce metameric light mixtures (physical different but undistinguishable) to "bee-white".

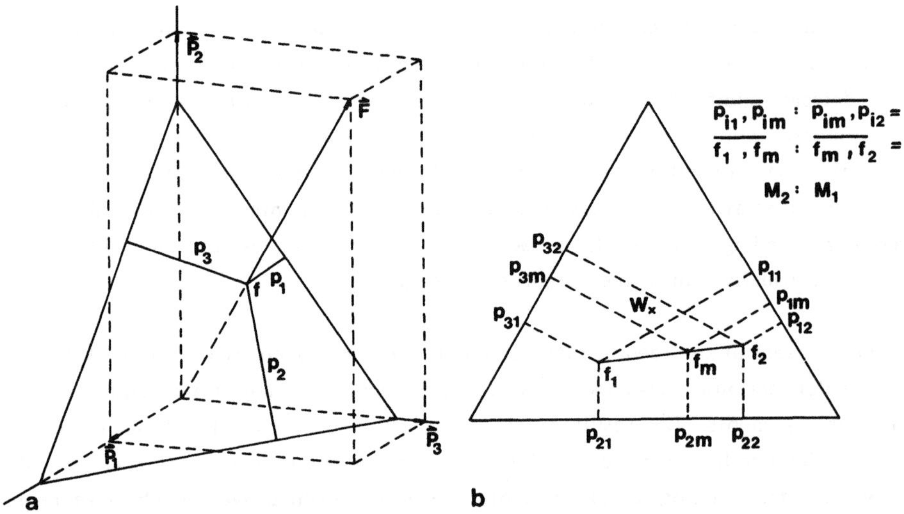

Fig. 1 - a. The receptor plane as a section through the receptor space. The geometrical connection of the chromaticity coordinates p of the color stimulus f and the components P constituting the corresponding color stimulus vector **F**. b. Center-of-gravity construction of the mixture locus f_m from the amounts M of the mixed color stimuli f_1 and f_2. The proportional relations hold for the chromaticity coordinates p as well. Geometrical distances are indicated by a line.

Equivalent to the chromaticity diagram, is the concept of a three dimensional color space where the three primaries are denoted as orthonormal basis vectors. The Graßmannian mixture rules are realized by vector addition. Fig. 1a shows the interpretation of the chromaticity diagram as a section through the color space. Brightness can be included in a color luminance space by multiplying the basis vectors by their luminance coefficients (43, 44). The brightness of a color is calculated as sum of the absolute values of the components of the color brightness vector (Abney's law).

The primaries can be changed to other lights, in general to all linear functionals of light intensity, e.g. absorbed photon fluxes; the loci of the lights change in different color spaces but the Graßmannian mixture laws (and Abney's law) hold (18). This allows the construction of a physiological color stimulus space (tristimulus space) (4, 42, 40) The primaries correspond to the photon fluxes P (tristimulus values) absorbed by each of the three receptors:

$$P_i = \int_{-\infty}^{+\infty} s_i(\lambda) I(\lambda) d \qquad (1)$$

I denotes the spectral photon flux density (spectral intensity) as emitted or reflected from color signals; s are the spectral sensitivities of the three receptor typs. "Bee-luminance" is assumed to be proportional to the sum of the tristimulus values; i.e. the "bee-brightness" only depends on the spectral sensitivities. The color stimulus space corresponds to the color luminance space. The corresponding physiological chromaticity diagram represents a plane of constant "bee-brightness" (constant totally absorbed photon flux). The chromaticity coordinates p are defined as:

$$p_i = P_i / \sum_{j=1}^{3} P_j, \text{ thus} \qquad (2)$$

$$\sum_{i=1}^{3} p_i = 1 \qquad (3)$$

Changes of photon fluxes absorbed by the three receptors cause perceptual changes in chromaticness and brightness. If the lights are changed in such a way that the total absorbed photon flux is kept constant, changes occur only in chromaticness. Variations of the total absorbed photon flux change the brightness of the color. Lights which are indistinguishable for the receptors cause matching colors. On the other hand, it is not obvious whether two lights, which are distinguishable for one or more of the receptors, will be judged as different colors. One may ask, therefore, what is the relationship between color difference and receptor properties?

The resolution of the color vision system in bees has been measured in behavioral experiments with respect to wavelength discrimination (11), brightness discrimination (20) and first saturation threshold that surrounds the white point (24). Since the concept of chromaticity diagram and color space is based on color matching judgments (metameric colors), the results of color difference judgments cannot be predicted in a simple way from the differences of tristimulus values or chromaticity coordinates. In the case of "small field color vision" (one ommatidium, three receptor types 3 UV, 2 blue, 4 green receptors, 31, 34), the color vision system can not resolve better than the photoreceptors. The resolution of the photoreceptors is limited by the fluctuations of the receptor potential. Each photon absorbed by the receptors is transduced into a unit of transmembrane currents, the sum of which is coded as the relative magnitude of the graded receptor potential:

$$V/V_{max} = (RI)^n / ((RI)^n + 1) \qquad (4)$$

The photon absorption process and the transduction process cause fluctuations of the receptor potential (shot noise and transducer noise) (23). These fluctuations were found to be independent of the magnitude of the potential (23) as we also observed in our intracellular recordings (34, Fig. 6). The fluctuation amplitude of the receptor potential never exceeds a boundary of 1.2% of the maximal potential, and this is identical with the 3s interval when assuming (proofed by eye), that the fluctuation is Gaussian distributed. One standard deviation s turns out to be 0.4% of the maximal response.

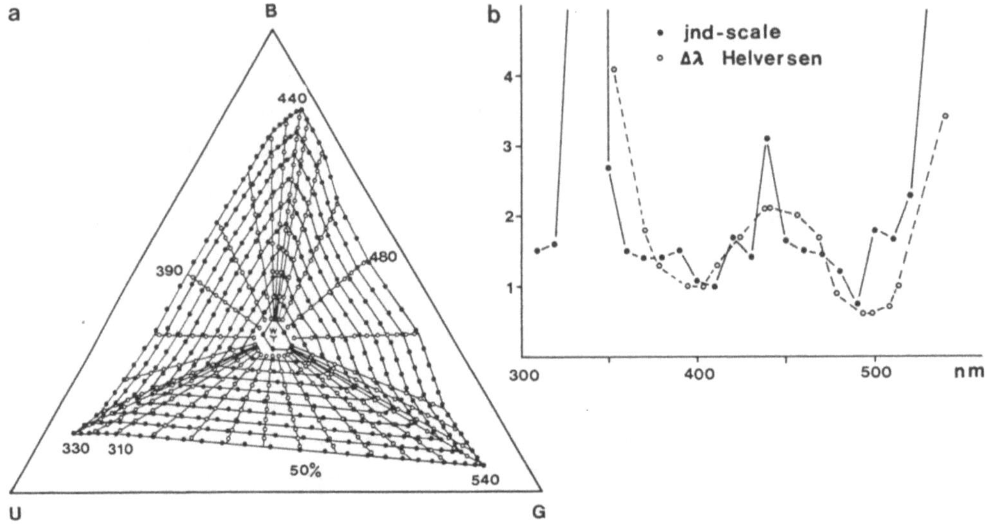

Fig. 2 - a. pjnd-scales calculated for variations in wavelengths (black dots) and variations of the white-spectral light mixtures (circles). The distance between the marked loci represents 10 pjnd steps. The closed curves (black dots) are calculated for white-spectral light mixtures that differ by 10% in the mixture coefficient. The radial curves (circles) are calculated for spectral and purple lights that differ by 10nm and 10% in the green-UV mixture coefficient. b. Comparison of normalized wavelength discrimination functions of the bee derived from the pjnd-scales of the receptor model (black dots) and of that measured in behavioral experiments by Helversen (11) (circles). The two functions are normalized at their minima at about 410nm. The unit of the ordinate corresponds to 8nm of Helversen's function and to the reciprocal value of 38 pjnd steps per 10nm in the model calculation.

What are the consequences of this limitation in accuracy of the light intensity coding in the receptor potentials with respect to the resolution of the bees color vision? To analyze the limitation of the perceptual just noticeable difference steps (pjnd) by the just noticeable difference steps in the receptors (rjnd), we simulated stimulation of the receptors by changing mixtures of spectral light and white light which cause a constant total absorbed photon flux i.e. which only cause differences in chromaticness (see above). In the first series the mixture varied continuously in the wavelength of the spectral light changing the white-light proportion in 10% steps. In a second series, the mixture varied continuously in the white-light proportion whilst the spectral light changed in 10nm steps (Fig. 2a). One rjnd step is reached if the variations of the mixtures cause a significant (50% threshold: 0.3% of V_{max}) change in at least one of the three receptor types (a dot denotes ten rjnd steps). As seen in

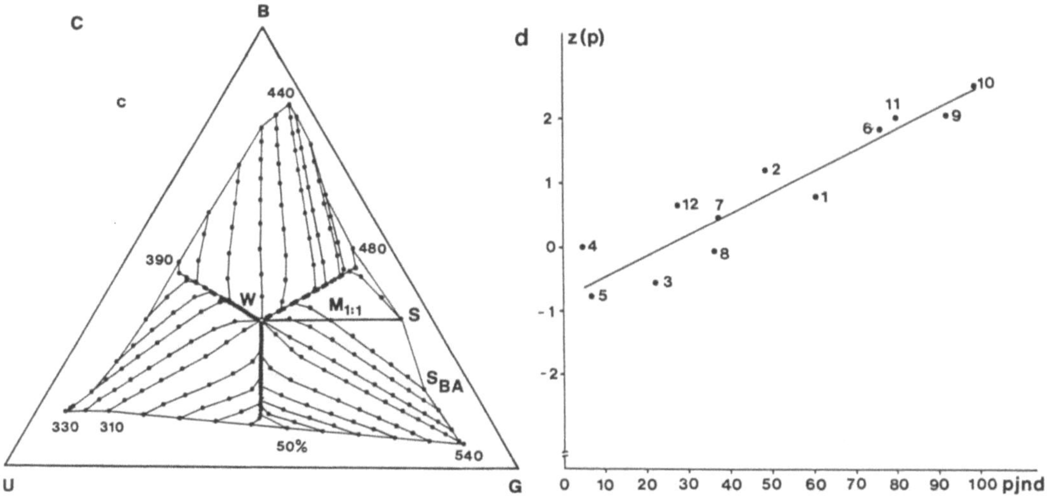

Fig. 2 - c. Mixture lines corresponding to the most similar colors caused by the mixture of spectral light and white light. The distance between the marked loci represents 10 pjnd steps. The lines are calculated with the aid of the step-by-step procedure explained in (2). The curved lines differ in the spectral and purple lights used for the mixture by 10nm and 10% in the green-UV mixture coefficient. The value of the Bezold-Abney hue shift can be derived graphically as explained in the text. d. Comparison of the probability transformed choice frequencies z(p) with the pjnd scales derived from the receptor model. Each number gives a pair of color stimuli which have been tested in a dual forced choice discrimination test after training bees to one or the other color stimulus. 1: BG12 (U=.519, B=.744, G=.181) vs. BG28 (U=.189, B=.670, G=.288) (n=476), 2: BG18 (U=.270, B=.743, G=.834) vs. BG28 (n=1084), 3: BG28 + B4 (U= .146, B=.807, G=.322) vs. BG28 (n=504), 4: BG28/2 (U=.066, B=.279, G=.107) vs. BG28 (n=219), 5: BG28 + V3 (U=.200, B=.874, G=.324) vs. BG28 (n=227), 6: VG6 (U=.038, B=.341, G=.514) vs. BG28 (n=842), 7: BG25 + B5 (U=.317, B=.751, G=.186) vs. BG28 (n=179), 8: BG25 + B3 (U=.286, B=.710, G=.179) vs. BG28 (n=281), 9: BG28 vs. UG3 (U=.768, B=.525, G=.164) (n=99), 10: BG28 vs. BG3 (U=1.132, B=.729, G=.223) (n=286), 11: BG28 vs. BG25 (U=.511, B=.503, G=.123) (n=77), 12: BG28 v.s. BG23 (U=.499, B=1.029, G=.808) (n=348). n gives the total number of choices in the two series of experiments of each pair of color stimuli. The notations indicate broad band color filters (1mm thick, besides BG28/2 which is 2mm thick) of Schott, Mainz, which are lying on top of a sanded aluminium disc or on a cardboard (e.g. + B4 a blue cardbord, + V3 a violet cardbord). The tristimulus values U,B,G are calculated for a grey background (U=1, B=1, G=1).

Fig. 2a, areas with high (many dots between the lines) or low resolution (few dots between the lines) do not correspond to areas where the lines are more or less dense. It is obvious from this calculation that there exists no simple relationship between color resolution and the geometrical distance of the loci of the stimuli in the chromaticity diagram. We found a very good agreement between the calculated resolution of the color vision system for spectral lights, as the number of pjnd's, and the spectral discrimination function as determined by Helversen (11) by training experiments (see (2), Fig. 2b).

The dissimilarity of colors can be measured as the minimal number of pjnd steps (10, 44). The paths of most similar colors follows (in general) curved lines in the chromaticity diagram. We derived an approximation procedure to find the shortest (minimal number of pjnd steps) mixture line between two colors (2). In Fig. 2c, the shortest mixture lines are drawn for a starting point at pure spectral lights in 10nm intervals and increasing proportions of white light. The model predicts that bees trained to a 1:1 mixture M of white and spectral light should judge a spectral light of longer wavelengths S_{BA} more similar than the spectral lights used for the mixture (Bezold-Abney hue shift). The hue shift occurs more or less to longer and shorter wavelengths respectively, and is caused by the nonlinearity of the transduction function of the receptors. The Bezold-Abney shift has still to be demonstrated for bees.

The application of the receptor model to natural objects, which reflect light varying in all physical parameters, makes a further assumption necessary. Natural objects do not adjust the lights so that only chromaticness changes. A change from one light to another causes changes in the potentials of the three receptors. The color vision system has to derive a measure of color distance from the differences in the potentials. We investigated two different possibilities for the color vision system to compute a neuronal representation of a color distance measure. 1) The maximum information about changes in absorbed photon fluxes is obtained when the system determines the rjnd steps separately in each receptor as a difference in receptor potential weighted by a factor for converting rjnd to pjnd, and then simply adding the weighted differences as a dissimilarity measure. 2) Since the tranduction function (with n = 1) is approximately a logarithmic function (V/V_{max} .576 log(7.38 RI)) the receptor channels can be subtractively connected to make the resulting excitation independent of changes in intensity. The dissimilarity measure can simply be represented as the difference in excitation of a cell. The non-linearity of the transduction process causes the linear dissimilarity measure to appear from the measurements as complicated functions of the chromaticity coordinates (curved similarity lines in the chromaticity diagram), since color measurements can only be performed in terms of light intensities or absorbed photon fluxes respectively.

The first possibility predicts that the bee weights brightness differences equal to differences in hue and saturation. The second possibility predicts that the bee weights differences in chromaticness higher, and that differences in brightness do not contribute to the dissimilarity of colors. We found a much better correlation of the choice behavior with the second measure (two dimensional) than with the first measure (three dimensional). Fig. 2d shows the correlation of the z-values of the measured choice proportions of Apis with the second jnd measure (two dimensional) for color distance. The scatter is homogeneous arround the regression line. The same was found for the stingless bee Melipona (35).

Thus bees ingnore differences in brightness when trained to colors (not specially trained to brightness differences). Color distance is dominated by the receptor properties spectral sensitivity, phototransduction, and noise. The independency of intensity differences is taken into account in the model by the simple assumption that the receptor potentials are linearly subtracted. This model predicts that the nonlinear transduction process makes the linear (neuronal) dissimilarity measure appear very complex in psychophysical experiments. The resulting curved similarity lines in the chromaticity diagram should be directly measurable as Bezold-Abney hue shift.

Color Contrast and Color Constancy

Color contrast effects can be demonstrated by training bees to one of several color signals on a grey background and presenting the same color signals on different backgrounds during a test situation (36, 37). The colors used by Neumeyer differed in hue along a blue-yellow axis, and the backgrounds surrounding the colormarks were either grey, yellow or blue. If the background color was changed from grey to blue, the bees shifted their choice behavior to more blue colors, whereas if it was changed to yellow they chose more yellow colors. The hue shift was also induced by a small colored ring surrounding the color mark, even if the colored ring was separated from the color mark by a thin black annulus.

A particular kind of color contrast effect has been found in pattern discrimination experiments (33). A vertically arranged circular pattern consisting of two half circles with two different colors is readily discriminated from a similar but differently oriented pattern. The sensitivity to the change in orientation of the pattern depends on the color of the half-circles. For example, there is a change in the upper field of view if the area is UV light reflecting. The spatial dependence is reversed for a bluish-green appearing area; a similar antagonism was observed for blue and yellow. Although this orientation specific color effect is not yet well understood, it demonstrates clearly a combined spatial-chromatic antagonism along the vertical axis.

Connected with color contrast is the ability of a color vision system to see the color of objects unchanged while the illuminating light changes both in intensity and/or spectral composition, a phenomenon called "color constancy" (10) or "color transformation" (15). In humans, the effect of color constancy is particularly impressive in an experimental arrangement which Land (21) calls the "Mondrian-experiment"; the "Mondrian" arrangement is composed of many rectangular colored plates with different reflectance coefficients. The arrangement is equally illuminated by three adjustable light beams containing light of long, middle, and short wavelengths respectively. When the intensities of the illuminating light beams are changed, the colors of the Mondrian areas remain the same or change very slightly. Slow receptor adaptation is unlikely to be involved because the colors appear to be the same even when the arrangement is illuminated for 100 msec (22). It is concluded, therefore, that color constancy results from neural processes in the retina and cortex (retinex-theory). The color of an area in such an arrangement is determined not only by the photon flux coming from this area but also depends on the relative photon fluxes of the whole arrangement. An adequate way to describe color in this context is the representation as points in a retinex three-space composed of three (short-, middle-, and longwave) designators on orthogonal axes. The contributions of the photon fluxes of all areas to the three designators corresponding to the color of an area are computed independendently from each other according to the retinex algorithm: Starting at random positions in the arrangement, all logarithms of the relative photon fluxes (above a threshold) of one waveband of every two neighbouring areas are summed on the way to the area in question. The designators of the area are the average of these sums. The procedure converges quickly; only a few paths have to be considered. Overall changes in illumination do not change the designators and, therefore, do not change the color appearence of the arrangement.

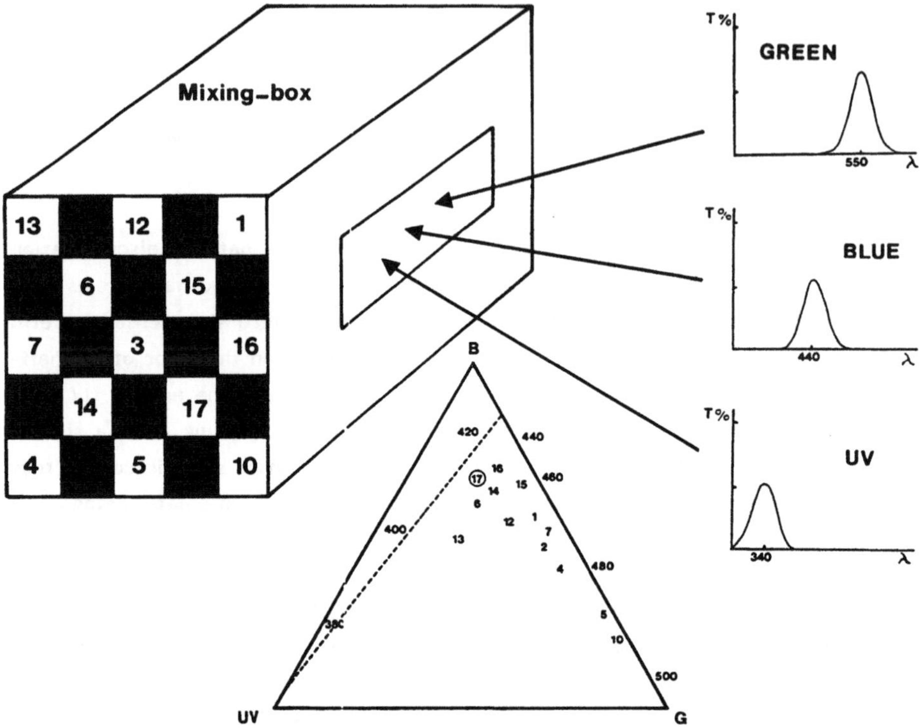

Fig. 3 - A multicolored checkerboard arrangement ("Mondrian") is illuminated from behind by a mixture of the three wavelength bands (UV max=340nm, blue max=440nm, green = 550nm). The numbers of the "Mondrian"-areas indicate the types of glassfilters.

A similar experiment was carried out in order to study the color constancy of bees (47, 48). Freely flying bees were trained to collect a sucrose solution from one of 13 colored filters, which were arranged like a checker-board (Fig. 4). This arrangement was illuminated from behind by three broadband light beams (UV, blue, green), whose spectral composition was matched to the spectral properties of the three color receptors in the bee eye. After training the bee to discriminate one color from all the others, the three light beams were changed in such a way that one of the unrewarded filters transmitted the same amounts of the photon fluxes of the three light beams as did the rewarded filter during training. If the color of a filter would be determined by the photon flux passing through it, the bee should choose this filter. As Fig. 3 shows, the bee still preferred the trained filter despite the fact that the

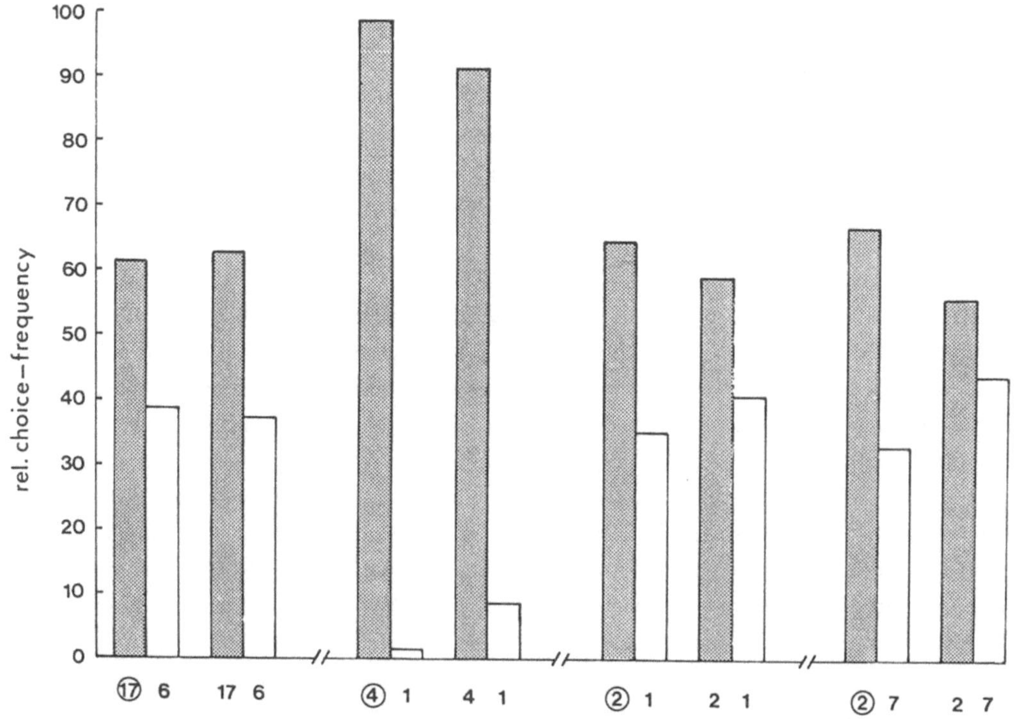

Fig. 4 - Performance of color constancy, tested for four color matches between violet and blue-green colors. In all cases, the distribution of choices between training (**O**) and matching color remained almost constant during training illumination (first double block of every experiment) and during matching illumination (second double block of every experiment).

spectral composition of the transmitted photon flux changed considerably, and that the actual signals in the photoreceptors changed accordingly.

A convenient way to explain the independency of color appearence from the actual photon flux of the three light beams is to assume a ratio making principle which adjusts the neural representation of a color such that each color representation is expressed in relative terms of the photon fluxes from all other areas in the visual field. A neuronal correlate for such a process may be seen in (double) opponent cells which combine spatial and chromatic opponency in their response properties (22, 49). Simple color opponent cells with overlapping receptive fields of their antagonistic responses ($U^-B^+G^+$; $B^+U^-G^-$) have been recorded in the visual system of the bee many times (see below; Hertel and Maronde, this vol.); recent investigations have also been carried out on double opponent cells with a UV-green antagonism combined with spatial antagonism. Centre-surround double opponency is not known from any insect visual interneuron, but more complex combinations of spatial and chromatic contrast have been found (17). Such neurons are equally suitable for the proposed mechanism of ratio making if they exist in many positions of their receptive fields. It might well be that only a limited number of such neurons exist with particular positions of their receptive fields, in which case one should expect color constancy to be limited to certain arrangements of color areas in the visual field. An indication for preferred combinations of chromatic and spatial contrast comes from the color pattern experiments described above. More experiments with the "Mondrian" are required to investigate whether or not color constancy is limited to certain spatial and chromatic combinations, and to determine the range of variations in illumination where color constancy holds.

Dimensions of color perception

Multiple color choice experiments as in the "Mondrian arrangement" are also suitable for analyzing the perceptual dimensions of color vision. In these experiments the color marks are presented as small (50 or 70 mm ⌀) discs on a grey background and are so far apart (more than 20cm) that the individual test bee views each test color signal independently. Twelve different signals are presented simultaneously. Each of the twelve signals was trained in turn using a new bee for each new signal and the choice behavior to all twelve colors determined in many tests. Metric (46) and nonmetric (19) multidimensional scaling procedures can be applied to the dissimilarities derived from the choice frequencies (8, 46). The dissimilarities are easily reproduceable from only two subjective scales by the city-block metric (sum of the absolute differences on the scales) (3).

Although the light reflected by the color signals differed in intensity over a wide range, brightness did not correlate with any of the two scales (nor with a third scale). The bee ignores differences in brightness in this color choice situation, and this is in good agreement with the findings of Daumer (5) and Helversen (11). Fig. 5b shows the twelve color stimuli used in the experiment. The subjective color loci with the two scales as components are presented in Fig. 5a. The two configurations are topographically equal to each other.

The subjective color scales can be interpreted in two ways: 1) The scales correlate with a UV/blue-greenness and blue/greeness dimension. The similarity measure can be represented neuronally as the sum of the differences in the excitations of two opponent color systems. 2) The scales correlate with a hue and saturation dimension. The similarity measure has to be calculated by the nervous system in a complicated way from the receptor potentials as absolute sum of the differences in saturation S and hue H derived as $\Delta S=\sqrt{(\Delta(U^-B^+G^+))^2+(\Delta(B^+U^-G^-))^2}$ and $\Delta H=\Delta \mathrm{arctg}(U^-B^+G^+/B^+U^-G^-)$ from the excitations of the respective color opponent system UBG (14).

Color Opponency

We tested the first hypothesis which is supported by our receptor model and which assumes linear subtraction of the receptor potentials (see above). We calculated the coefficients as the least square solution of the general linear equation (without assuming anything about opponency) of the two scale values A and B (Fig. 5a) obtained for twelve colors of the multiple choice experiment (see above) and the corresponding three receptor excitations E

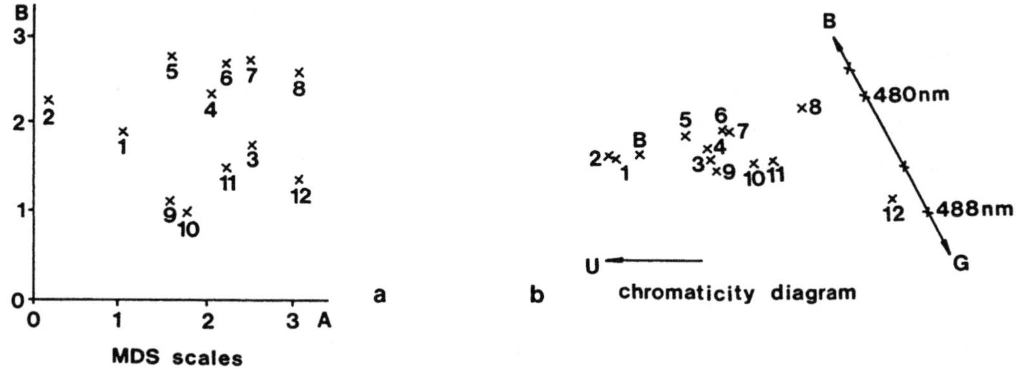

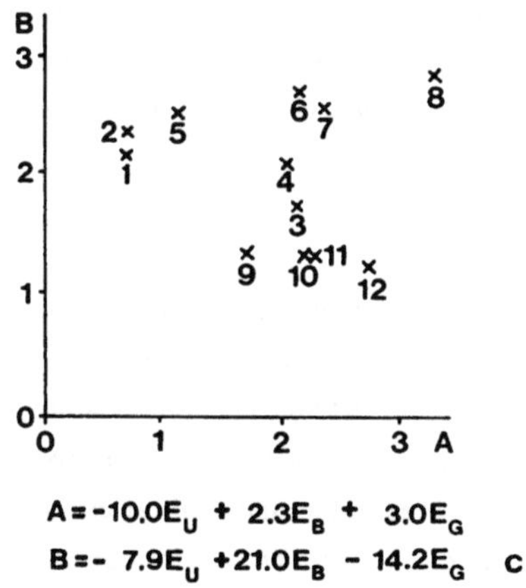

Fig. 5 - a. Result of non-metric multidimensional scaling: The two color similarity scales A and B for the case d=2 and city-block metric (p=1). The scales are a measure for color dissimilarity between the twelve colors as they appear to the bee. This subjective arrangement of colors is topologically similar to the arrangement of color stimuli in the chromaticity diagram (see Fig. 2b). b. Chromaticity diagram of the bee. The numbers denote the color stimuli which are defined by the relative numbers of photons absorbed by each of the receptors per unit time. The corresponding color signals illuminated by daylight used in our experiment were:

1: Alu+F 2: Gray 3: BV1 4: BV2 5: BV3 6: BV3+F 7: BV3+2F 8: BG18 9: GR4 10: GR4+F 11: GR4+2F 12: VG6. F denotes a gray foil which decreases in general total reflection. The color signals were covered with UV transparent plexiglas except the two glass filters (8, 12). c. Scale values for blue/purpleness and UV/blue-greenness derived from our color opponent model (linear connection of the receptor excitations) with the coefficients which give the best fit (least square solution) to the scale values derived by multidimensional scaling.

caused by the twelve color stimuli (Fig. 5b).

$$A = -10.0\, E^U + 2.3\, E^B + 3.0\, E^G \quad (5)$$

$$B = -7.9\, E^U + 21.0\, E^B - 14.2\, E^G \quad (6)$$

The result is that scale A corresponds to a UV/blue-green opponent system, and that scale B corresponds to a blue/purple opponent system. The reproduced subjective color loci from the receptor excitations are shown in Fig. 5c. We found that the derived subjective scales A' and B' are very sensitive to changes of the coefficients (e.g. rank changes occur because of the nonlinearity of the transduction function). On the other hand the coefficients change very little if the sample is reduced by two of the color stimuli. Thus the nervous system can obtain the color dissimilarity measure as the sum of the absolute differences in the exitations in the two opponent systems when two color stimuli are presented after each other, or simultaneously, at different areas in the visual fields. Since the sum of the coefficients is not equal to zero, our opponent color model predicts the dependence of color on the light intensity (Bezold-Brücke effect). Both the light intensity dependent and the wavelength dependent (Bezold-Abney) hue shift are a consequence of color opponency. Both dependencies have yet to be measured.

The model calculations explain the results of the color choice experiments and support strongly opponent color coding mechanisms. Neuronal correlates of the predicted opponent mechanisms have been recorded from the second and third visual neuropile (medulla, lobula) in the bee brain (17, 12, 39, see also Hertel and Maronde this volume). As Fig. 6 shows, two main classes of chromatic opponency are found: an antagonism between UV / blue and green, and one between blue / UV and green ("purple").

Memories for Colors and Color Categories

There is some evidence that the choice behavior depends on the behavioral context, i.e. that the information represented by the color vision system is used selectively by the bees like in human color vision, where color naming uses different color attributes (hue names, saturation, red/greenness, blue/yellowness, brightness) depending on the kind of experiment and the instructions given by the experimenter (14, 38, 9). Besides color discrimination and color distance experiments, in which the judgment of the bee is based on the dimensions UV/blue-greenness and blue/purpleness, there exist other behavioral aspects which are better explained by hue and saturation as perceptual dimensions.

Colors are meaningful signals to the bee. They mark a food source or the entrance to the hive. The meaning of the color signal is derived from the information gathered by the species through the evolutionary process and by the learning processes of an individual animal. The choice behavior towards a color signal is not only determined by perceptual aspects but also by the meaning of it. In honeybees, the individual learning process is so strong that the choice behavior can be manipulated by training procedures. In such a situation, most of the information available to the nervous system to discriminate colors is actually used and this permits the kind of psychophysical analysis as described above. However, under certain conditions the bias of the evolutionary predispositions shines through the individual learning process. For example, the acquisition of spectral colors as food markers is faster for violet and slower for bluish-green (Fig. 7a) (26). This is independent of the photon flux and of the

Fig. 6 - A summary of all kinds of spectrally opponent neurons recorded in the visual system of the honeybee. Except for the very lowest trace (UV-off, B-on, G-off) all neurons display tonic spectral opponency. The lowest trace gives an example for a phasic opponent neuron. The neuron $U^-B^+G^+$ in the middle of the figure has been marked intracellularly (courtesy by S. Schäfer). It receives input from the proximal medulla and projects to the distal dorsal lobula. (From 12, 17 and unpublished data).

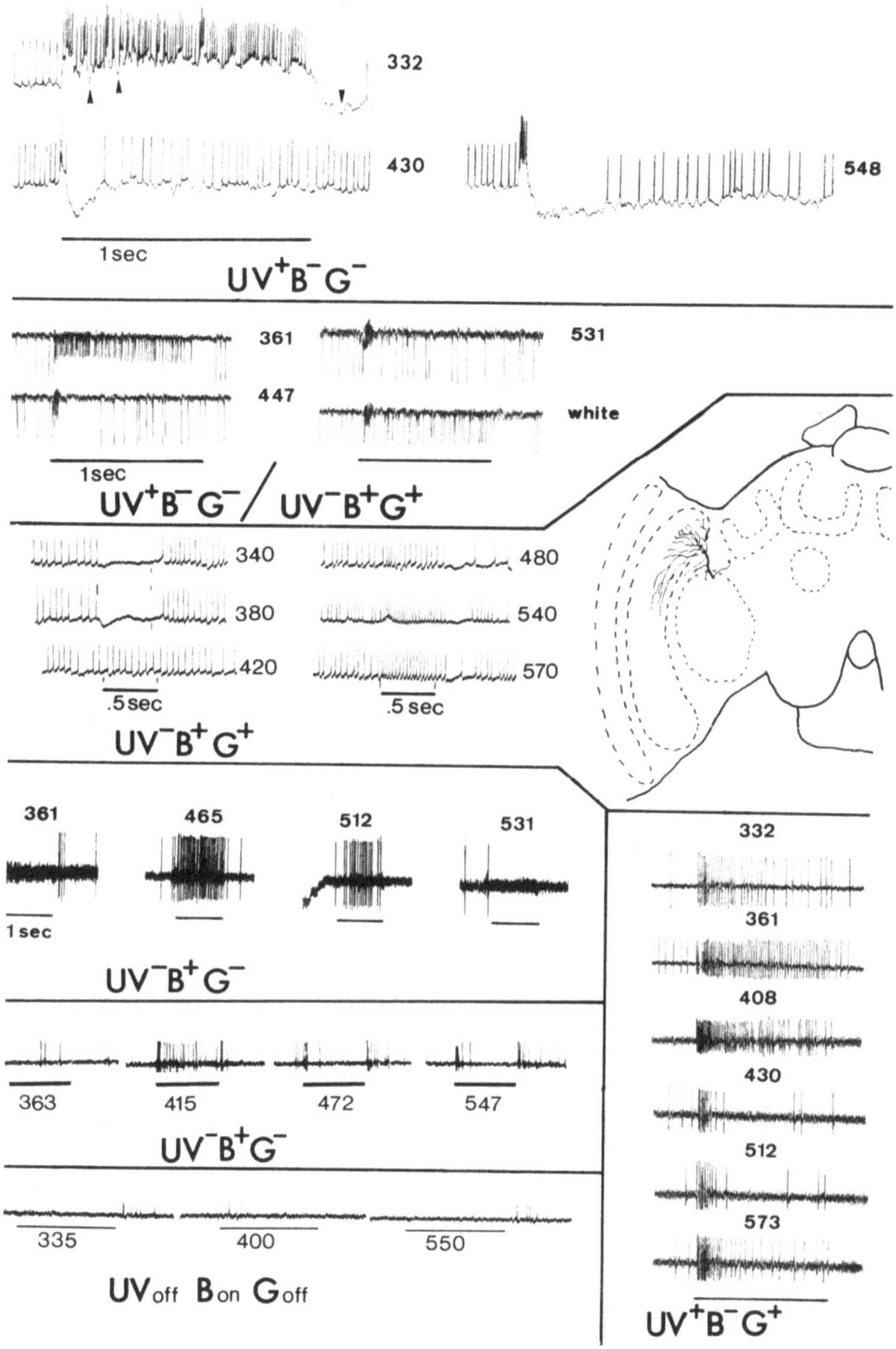
332
430
548
1sec
UV⁺B⁻G⁻
361
447
531
white
1sec
UV⁺B⁻G⁻/ UV⁻B⁺G⁺
340
380
420
.5sec
480
540
570
.5sec
UV⁻B⁺G⁺
361
465
512
531
1sec
UV⁻B⁺G⁻
363
415
472
547
UV⁻B⁺G⁻
335
400
550
UVoff Bon Goff
332
361
408
430
512
573
UV⁺B⁻G⁺

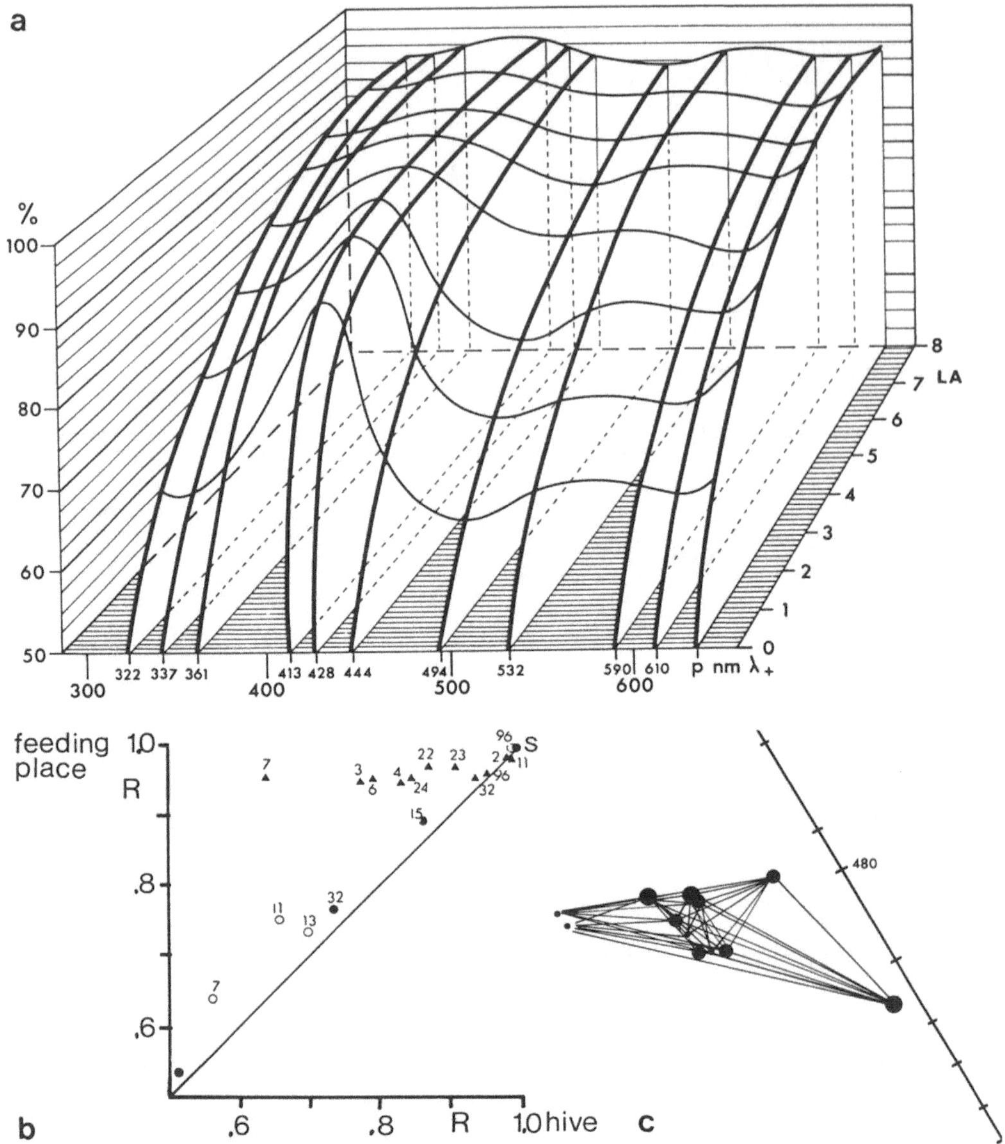

Fig. 7 - a. Learning curves for the spectral colors. The bees are trained to monochromatic light with a wavelength indicated at the abscissa, and the choice behavior is tested after each learning trial (z-axis). The respective alternative color in the dual forced choice test is the complementary color to the trained color. Response R (ordinate) is the percentage of correct choices. b. Twelve pigment colors in the bluish-green region are trained and tested in all possible combinations (full matrix). Four categories of asymmetric choice behavior are indicated by the diameter of the black spot at the respective color locus. Thick dots indicate those colors which were chosen more frequently if they were trained, whereas small dots refer to lower choice behavior for the respective trained color. (see text). c. Color discrimination depends on the behavioral context. This graph gives the percentage of correct choices of the stingless bee, Melipona quadrifasciata, after training to the same blue color at the feeding place and at the hive entrance. The alternative colors in the dual forced choice test were various colors (indicated by numbers) in the violet to bluish-green region. The dots indicate identical test situations at the two behavioral contexts (see text).

wavelength used as an alternative color in the dual choice test. Colors of low saturation are learned slower than those of high saturation (5, 24), although they are very well discriminated (24). Achromatic white is very hard to train at all (5, 24, 26).

Asymmetries in the choice behavior are an additional indicator for color biased behavior. Fig. 6 gives an example of a matrix of twelve color signals which were all trained individually and tested against the other 11 signals. If only the perceptual distance between the colors A and B would determine the choice behavior it should not matter whether A or B was trained. It is obvious from Fig. 7b that significant asymmetries exist, and that they indicate an improved choice for the more saturated colors.

Color discrimination may also depend on the behavioral context. We found a particular interesting example in the stingless bee, Melipona quadrifasciata (Fig. 7c), which distinguishes bluish-green colors much better at the hive entrance than at the feeding station (35). No such large differences were found in Apis mellifera (30). The preferred choice of color signals which is not overcome by learning is of much greater influence in Melipona than in Apis. For example, the asymmetries mentioned above are more pronounced in Melipona, and the response/jnd-functions depend much more on the color signals tested than in Apis (35).

A bias towards certain colors may indicate a neural process which categorizes the color signals into a small number of unique or basic colors. We have not yet collected enough data throughout the whole color space of the bee to determine these basic colors, but we believe that the analysis of asymmetries, as in Fig. 7, will give us the answer.

CONCLUSION

Seventy years of active research on color vision in bees has revealed a large body of knowledge at various levels of neural integration and behavioral analysis. The accurate determination of the spectral sensitivity functions of the three receptor types enables us to construct a receptor model of color vision. This in turn allows to make predictions about color mixing (lower colorimetry) and the dissimilarities of colors (higher colorimetry), if we take the receptor noise as the limiting factor for perceptual difference judgment. The behavioral analysis with multifactorial (multidimensional) analysis has revealed the perceptual dimensions of color vision in bees. The perceptual dimensions UV/blue-greenness and blue/purpleness are not separately affectable by single variations of the physical parameters of wavelength or white proportion as performed in conventional color discrimination experiments. The dissimilarity between two colors correlates well with the added differences of excitations of a UV/blue-green and a blue/purple color opponent system. The corresponding spectrally opponent neurons were already described ten years ago. The properties of these neurons are interpreted to underlie also the observed phenomena of color contrast and color constancy.

However, there exist parameters measured in the bee's color choice behavior which are not explainable in relation to the one dimensional dissimilarity measure. White is learned very slowly, whilst spectral colors are learned much faster depending on the color range. It is possible that the speed and acquisition niveau of color learning depends on the saturation and hue of colors, which are other color attributes than UV/blue-greenness and blue/purpleness. Asymmetries in color discrimination, seem to correspond to distinct areas in the color plane (basic colors). The memory of colors induces distortions in the perceptual representation of remembered colors, which in turn leads to generalization processes biased to certain colors. This bias is not very pronounced in the honeybee and its influence on color perception experiments can be overcome by a symmetrical arrangement of all the color discrimination tests. Although of relatively small effect, the color bias may be interpreted to indicate the existence of unique or basic colors in bees. These colors have still yet to be determined.

The knowledge of the opponent system in the color coding of bees offers a convenient way of describing the color of natural objects, which are important for the orientation of the bee (flowers, natural background etc.). The application of such a system would facilitate the elucidation of co-evolutionary relationships between flowers and bees, and the ecological constraints of the chromatic light climate in which bees live. In contrast to v. Hess, whom we cited at the beginning of this paper, we can conclude that the results presented here not only give further support to Sprengel's spiritual doctrine, but that we now also have the possibility to present this doctrine in the form of a quantitative investigation.

REFERENCES

(1) Backhaus, W.; and Menzel, R. 1984. Bestimmung der Farbwahrnehmungskomponenten bei Bienen durch multidimensionale Skalierung. Verh Dtsch Zool Ges 77: 230, Stuttgart: Fischer.

(2) Backhaus, W.; and Menzel, R. in press. Color distance derived from a receptor model of color vision in the honeybee. Biol Cybern.

(3) Backhaus, W.; Menzel, R.; and Kreißl, S. in press. Multidimensional scaling of color similarity in bees. Biol Cybern.

(4) Cornsweet, T. N. 1970. Visual perception. New York: Academic Press.

(5) Daumer, K. 1956. Reizmetrische Untersuchungen des Farbensehens der Bienen. Zeitschr vergl Physiol 38: 413-478.

(6) Frisch, K. v. 1914. Der Farbensinn und Formensinn der Biene. Zool J Physiol 37: 1-238.

(7) Graßmann, H. 1853. Zur Theorie der Farbenmischung. Ann Phys Chem 89: 69-84.

(8) Guilford, J. P. 1937. Scale values derived from the method of choices. Psychometrika 2: 139-150.

(9) Helm, C. E. 1964. Multidimensional ratio scaling analysis of perceived color relations. J opt Soc Am. 54: 256-262.

(10) Helmholtz, H. v. 1896. Handbuch der physiologischen Optik, edn. 2., Hamburg: Voß.

(11) Helversen, O. v. 1972. Zur spektralen Unterschiedsempfindlichkeit der Honigbiene. J Comp Physiol 80: 439-472.

(12) Hertel, H. 1980. Chromatic properties of identified interneurons in the optic lobes of the bee. J Comp Physiol 137: 215-231.

(13) Hess, C. v. 1913. Experimentelle Untersuchungen über den angeblichen Farbensinn der Bienen. Zool Jahrb Abt allg Zool Physiol 34: 81-106.

(14) Indow, T. 1974. Applications of multidimensional scaling in perception. In Handbook of perception Vol.II, ed. E. C. Carterette, M. P. Friedman, pp 493-530, New York: Academic Press.

(15) Jaensch, R. E.; and Müller, E. A. 1919. Über die Wahrnehmung farbloser Helligkeiten und den Helligkeitskontrast. Z Psychol 83: 266-341.

(16) Kaiser, W.; and Liske, E. 1974. Die optomotorischen Reaktionen von fixiert fliegenden Bienen bei Reizung mit Spektrallichtern. J Comp Physiol 89: 391-408.

(17) Kien, J.; and Menzel, R. 1977. Chromatic properties of interneurons in the optic lobes of the bee. II. Narrow band and colour opponent neurons. J Comp Physiol 113: 35-53.

(18) Krantz, D. H. 1975. Color measurement and color theory: I. Representation theorem for Graßmann Structures. J math Psychol 12: 283-303.

(19) Kruskal, J. B. 1964. Multidimensional scaling by optimizing goodness of fit to a nonmetric hypothesis. Psychometrika 29: 1-29.

(20) Labhart, T. 1974. Behavioral analysis of light intensity discrimination and spectral sensitivity in the honey bee, Apis mellifera. J Comp Physiol 95: 203-216.

(21) Land, E. H. 1983. Recent advances in retinex theory and some implications for cortical computations: Color vision and the natural image. Proc Natl Acad Acad Sci. 80: 5163-5169.

(22) Land, E. H. 1986. Recent advances in retinex theory. Vis Res 26: 7-21.

(23) Laughlin, S. 1981. Neural principles in the peripheral visual systems of invertebrates. In Handbook of Sensory physiology. Vol. VII/6B, ed. H. Autrum, pp 133-280, Berlin: Springer.

(24) Lieke, E. E. in press. Honeybees have a perceptual dimension of color saturation. J Comp Physiol.

(25) Lehrer, M.; Wehner, R.; and Srinivasan, M. 1985. Visual scanning behaviour in honeybees. J Comp Physiol A 157: 405-415.

(26) Menzel, R. 1967. Untersuchungen zum Erlernen von Spektralfarben durch die Honigbiene (Apis mellifica). Z vergl Pysiol 56: 22-62.

(27) Menzel, R. 1980. Verhaltensuntersuchungen zum Farbensehen der Biene nahe der Perzeptionsschwelle. Verh Dtsch Zool Ges, pp 26-40.

(28) Menzel, R. 1981. Achromatic vision in the honeybee at low light intensities. J Comp Physiol 141: 389-393.

(29) Menzel, R. 1985. Learning in honey bees in an ecological and behavioral context. In Experimental behavioral ecology, eds. B. Hölldobler, M. Lindauer, pp 55 74, Stuttgart: G. Fischer.

(30) Menzel, R. 1985. Colour pathways and color vision in the honeybee. In Central and peripheral mechanisms of colour vision, eds. D. Ottoson, S. Zeki, pp. 211-233, London: MacMillan Press.

(31) Menzel, R.; and Blakers, M. 1976. Colour receptors in the bee eye morphology and spectral sensitivity. J Comp Physiol 108: 11-33.

(32) Menzel, R.; and Greggers, U. 1985. Natural phototaxis and its relationship to colour vision in honeybees. J Comp Physiol 157: 311-321.

(33) Menzel, R.; and Lieke, E. 1983. Antagonistic color effects in spatial vision of the honey bees. J Comp Physiol 151: 441-448.

(34) Menzel, R.; Ventura, D.; Hertel, H.; de Souza. J.; and Greggers, U. 1986. Spectral sensitivity of photoreceptors in the insect compound eyes: Comparison of species and methods. J Comp Physiol 158: 165- 177.

(35) Menzel, R.; Ventura, D. F.; Werner, A.; and Backhaus, W. Submitted. Spectral sensitivities of single photoreceptors and color vision in the stingless bee, Mellipona quadrifasciata. J Comp Physiol.

(36) Neumeyer, C. 1980. Simultaneous color contrast in the honeybee. J Comp Pysiol 139: 165-176.

(37) Neumeyer, C. 1981. Chromatic adaptation in the honeybee: Successive color contrast and color constancy. J Comp Physiol 144: 543-553.

(38) Ramsey, J. O. 1968. Economical method of analyzing perceived color differences. J opt Soc Am 58: 19-22.

(39) Riehle, A. 1981. Color opponent neurons of the honey bee in a hetero-chromatic flicker test. J Comp Physiol. 142: 81-88.

(40) Rodieck, R. W. 1973. The vertebrate retina. San Francisco: Freeman.

(41) Rose, R.; and Menzel 1981. Luminance dependence of pigment color discrimination in bees. J Comp Physiol 141:379-388.

(42) Rushton, W. A. H. 1972. Pigments and signals in colour vision. J Physiol 220: 1-31.

(43) Schrödinger, E. 1920. Grundlinien einer Theorie der Farbenmetrik im Tagessehen. Ann Physik 63: 397-426; 427-456.

(44) Schrödinger, E. 1920. Grundlinien einer Theorie der Farbenmetrik im Tagessehen: Der Farbenmetrik II. Teil: Höhere Farbenmetrik (eigentliche Metrik der Farbe). Ann Physik 63: 481-520.

(45) Sprengel, C. K. 1793. Das entdeckte Geheimnis der Natur im Bau und in der Befruchtung der Blumen. Berlin.

(46) Torgerson, W. S. 1958. Theory and methods of scaling. New York: Wiley.

(47) Werner, A. in press. Farbkonstanz der Honigbiene - ist die Biene ein Retinex-Tier? Verh Dtsch Zool Ges.

(48) Werner, A. in press. Die Biene in einem "Mondrian-Experiment" - Farbkostanzleistung und Retinex-Theorie. Neurobiologentagung-Abstract.

(49) Zeki, S. 1984. Colour pathways and hierarchies in the cerebral cortex. In Central and peripheral mechanisms of colour vision, eds. D. Ottoson, S. Zeki, pp. 19-44, London: MacMillan Press.

The Ocellar System of the Honeybee

Jürgen J. Milde

European Molecular Biology Laboratory, Meyerhofstraße 1, D-6900 Heidelberg, FRG

Abstract. Intracellular recording and staining has revealed new aspects of the anatomy and physiology of ocellar interneurons in the honeybee (Apis mellifera). Homologous large first-order interneurons (L-neurons) from different individuals vary in their responses to light, which present a continuum from graded to spiking responses. The response depends on the state of the L-neuron and cannot be correlated with particular morphological types. Graded responses can be elicited exclusively by stationary illumination of the ocelli, whereas spiking L-neurons can also respond to stimuli of other sensory modalities. The existence of two response patterns in the same cell that can encode different information may be important with respect to the processing of information in the brain. There appears to be a variety of different pathways enabling interaction of ocelli and compound eyes either by direct contact between ocellar and optic lobe neurons or by convergence to a common descending or local interneuron. The results presented here provide insight into the complexity of the ocellar system and may help to clarify its function.

INTRODUCTION

The compound eyes of the honeybee have been the subject of numerous investigations leading to a detailed knowledge of signal processing and function. The single-lensed eyes, the ocelli, as a second visual system, are often neglected and, indeed, it is not easy to perceive their necessity. However, when all the available anatomical, physiological, and behavioral data are considered (4), the ocelli comprise a well-developed sensory system which offers a small number of identifiable first-order interneurons with large axon diameters (L-neurons). L-neurons are the largest interneurons in the honeybee brain and are easily accessible for intracellular recording and iontophoretic staining. Such studies should help to elucidate the role of the ocelli in controlling behavior, a fundamental question that still cannot be answered sufficiently.

Structural organization of the ocellar system

In worker bees (Apis mellifera), each of the three ocelli contains about 800 photoreceptors (20), which are linked to the brain by 30 L-neurons and approximately 80 (small-axon-diameter) S-neurons (17). The axons of the interneurons form a nerve bundle, which arises from the ocellar plexus (receptor/interneuron synaptic neuropil) and enters the caudal part of the brain medially (Fig. 1). The L-neurons exist as 15 homologous pairs. Their morphology and nomenclature has been worked out extensively on the basis of cobalt fills (4).

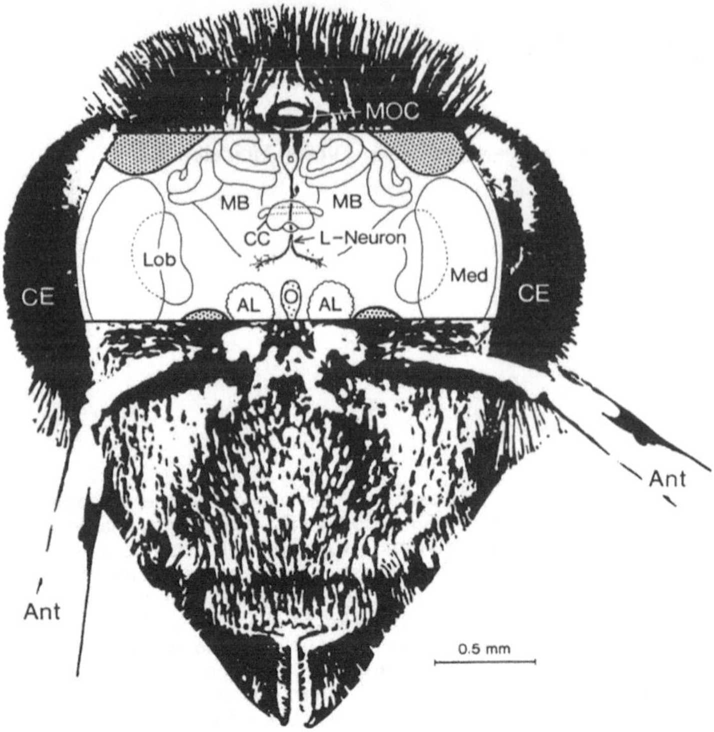

Fig. 1 - Frontal view of a bee's head with a window cut into the head capsule. Outlines of prominent brain structures are indicated. A single L-neuron from the median ocellus can be seen behind the central complex (CC). AL = antennal lobe; Ant = antenna; CE = compound eye; Lob = lobula; MB = mushroom body; Med = medulla; MOC = median ocellus; O = oesophagus.

Two L-neuron subclasses can be distinguished: (a) 20 L-neurons leading from the ocellar plexus terminate in the posterior slope of the brain. This group includes all 12 neurons of the median ocellus (one representative is shown in Figs. 1 and 3) as well as 4 neurons from each of the lateral ocelli (Fig. 3). (b) 10 descending L-neurons (termed L_D-neurons), which finally terminate in the thoracic ganglia (Fig. 3). Each lateral ocellus has 5 L_D-neurons. Figure 1 illustrates the relative size of L-neurons with respect to the head of a worker bee and the general outline of the brain.

Light responses in L-neurons

The intracellularly recorded L-neuron responses to stationary wide-field light of high intensity range from non-spiking to spiking patterns with all intermediate forms (Fig. 2). The graded responses characterize L-neurons in accordance with other intracellular studies as "non-spiking", e.g. locust (21); dragonfly (2); honeybee (6). However, responses with one or a few spikes can also be observed as well as inhibition of spontaneous spiking activity by light with or without a graded response (Fig. 2).

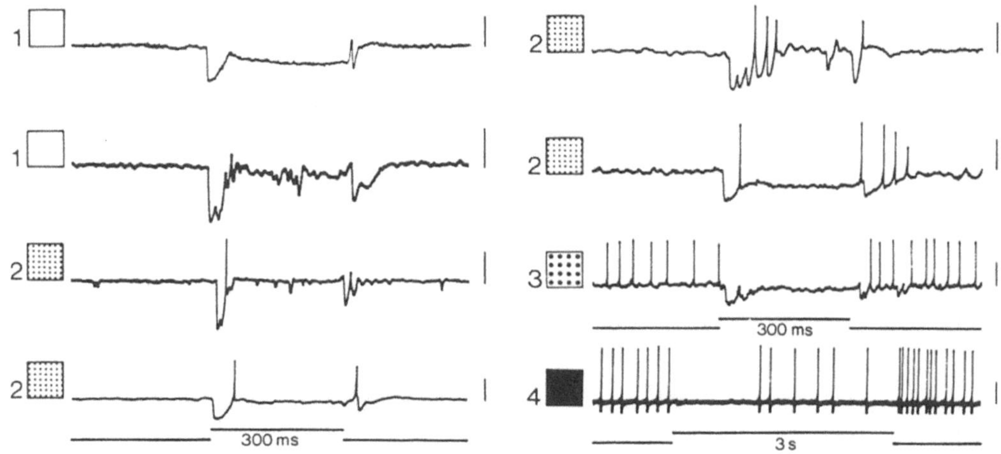

Fig. 2 - L-neuron light responses. Numbers and squares indicate four response classes: 1, graded responses only; 2, graded responses with one or a few additional spikes; 3, graded responses and spontaneous discharge of action potentials; 4, spiking responses only. Vertical bar = 20 mV.

Do particular L-neurons exhibit particular light responses?

To answer this question the response patterns were subdivided arbitrarily into four classes (Fig. 2) and correlated with anatomical groups. Figure 3 shows the response distribution for all recorded L-neurons and for the subsets of median, lateral and descending L-neurons. The distribution of response patterns differs in the three subsets. Although lateral L-neurons with a pure spiking discarge cannot be observed, regenerative potentials appear in all subsets. L_D-neurons always exhibit at least one on- and off-spike and should therefore be considered to be spiking neurons. The median L-neurons show all four response classes. Due to the low number of recordings (74) compared with the 15 morphological L-neuron pairs, it is difficult to describe the distribution of the particular response patterns for single L-neurons. However, at least one L-neuron of the median ocellus exhibits all four response classes (13) and its individual anatomical variability is not related to the variety of responses (12). Hence, it does not appear to be an anatomical correlate for a particular signal pattern. This is supported by the observation of changes in light responses during recording from a single L-neuron.

Are there graded and regenerative signals in the same L-neuron?

The response pattern of an L-neuron can be changed with successive light stimulations (Fig. 4). Every light flash hyperpolarizes the membrane potential and induces spontaneous activity, which finally results in a steady discharge of action potentials. This can also be achieved by injection of hyperpolarizing current into the cell. Moreover, L-neurons which are able to change their response pattern by shifting the membrane potential to more negative or positive values even without any light stimulations can be observed. This clearly indicates that both spiking and non-spiking responses can be present in a single cell. L-neurons in the

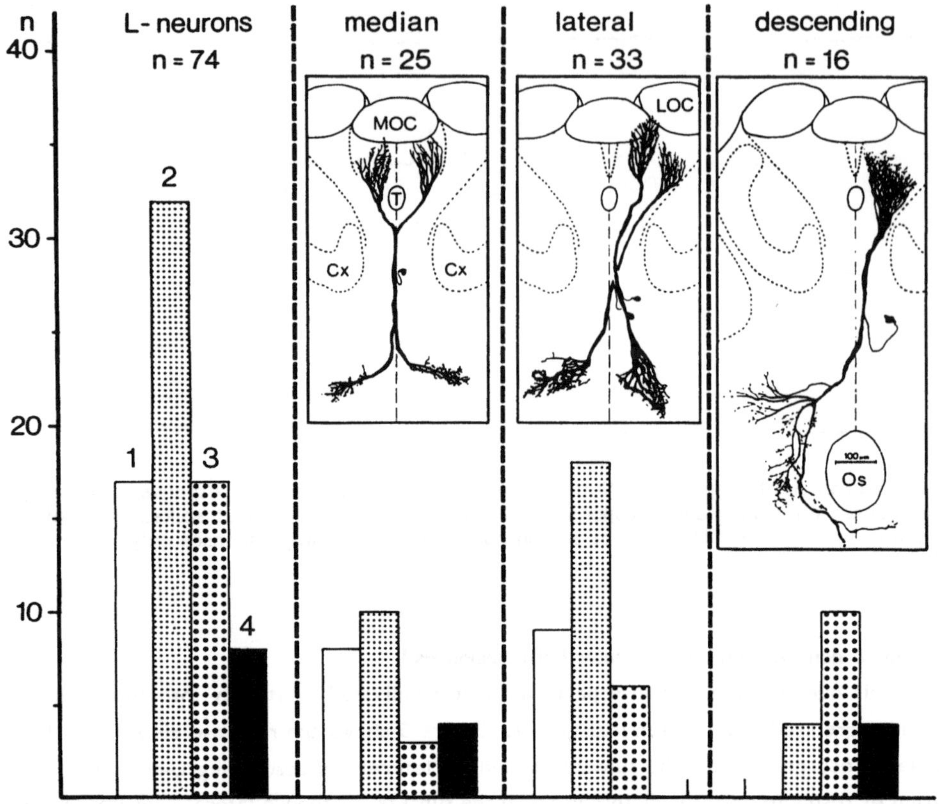

Fig. 3 - Frequency distribution of the classified response pattens (see Fig. 2) in all recorded large ocellar interneurons (n = 74) and in the subsets median (n = 25), lateral (n = 33) and descending (n = 16) L-neurons. The insets illustrate representative anatomical types, but omit the L_D-neuron terminals in the thorax. Cx = Calyx; LOC = left ocellus; MOC = median ocellus; OS = oesophagus.

non-spiking state appear to be refractory due to a maintained depolarisation that blocks their regenerative capabilities (11), as is the case for lobula plate giant neurons of the fly (7). The mechanism generating the depolarization is unknown and honeybee L-neuron membrane properties have not yet been subject to detailed investigation. However, the rigid distinction between spiking and non-spiking neurons, as for example in the case of thoracic interneurons of locusts (1), cannot be applied to L-neurons.

Do L-neurons in the non-spiking and spiking state encode the same light information?

Stimulating a non-spiking L-neuron with white light, a short-latency, fast-adapting response can be obtained over an intensity range of 5 log units (Fig. 5). The amplitude of the on-transient gives a steep response/intensity (R/I) function that saturates one log unit above the threshold. Such a function is well suited for the detection of small changes in illumination

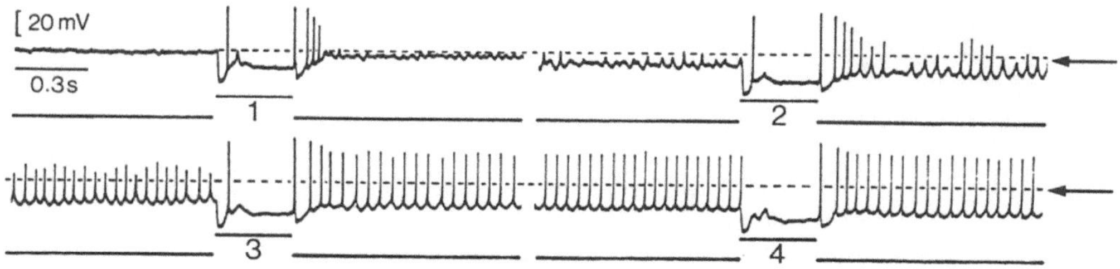

Fig. 4 - Subsequent and identical light stimulation results in hyperpolarization of the cell, inducing spontaneous background activity which finally leads to discharge of action potentials. The arrows at the end of each row and the broken line indicate the initial membrane potential.

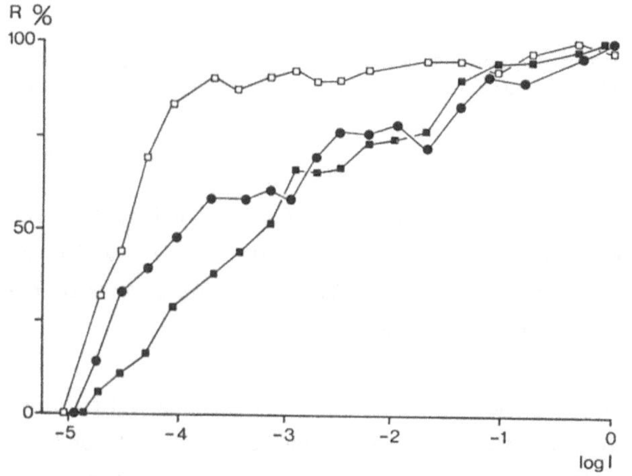

Fig. 5 - Response/intensity (R/I) functions of two L-neurons in the non-spiking state. Different parameters were evaluated: amplitude of the hyperpolarizing on-transient ( ), area of the on-transient (same neuron) ( ), area of the on-transient (O).

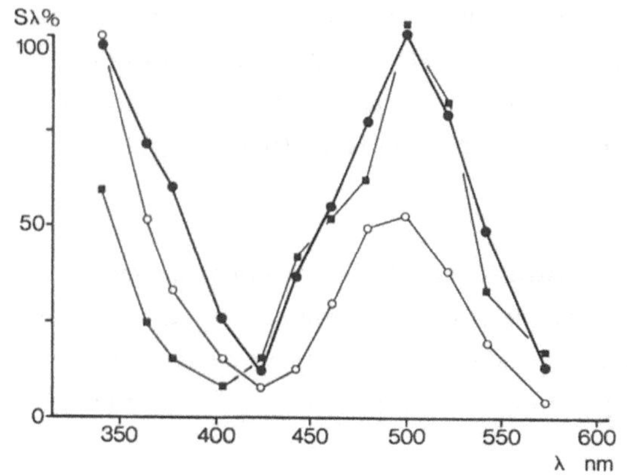

Fig. 6 - Relative spectral sensitivity. Average of 11 L-neurons (O). The peaks are at about 350 and 500 nm with a nearly 1:1 ratio. The two curves with the most extreme difference between UV and Green peak are also shown.

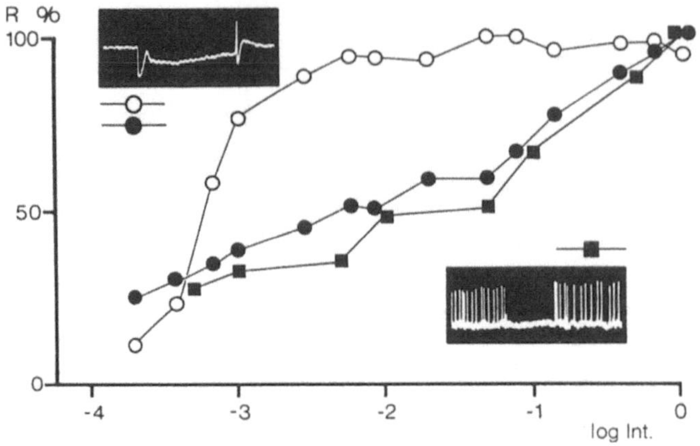

Fig. 7 - L-neuron showing alternating graded (upper inset) and spiking responses (lower inset) during recording. R/I functions for: O amplitude of the on-transient; O area of the on-transient and inhibition of spike discharge.

over a narrow intensity range. In contrast, the response magnitude defined by the area between the baseline and the on-transient increases continuously with intensity and could thus encode both the appearance of light and its intensity. Thus different aspects of the graded response could serve to encode different stimulus parameters.

All tested L-neurons in the graded state respond to stimulation with spectral light flashes from 340 to 600nm. The relative spectral sensitivity (Fig. 6) has peaks at about 350 and 500 nm, which correspond with the peak sensitivity of the ocellar photoreceptors (3). The two L-neuron peaks are almost equal, which indicates an equal input from the receptor populations to the interneuron, imparting a spectral broad-band character (10).

L-neurons that switch from graded to spiking mode during a recording make it possible to compare spiking and non-spiking light responses in a single cell (Fig. 7). The R/I function for the area of the graded on-transient and for spike inhibition appear to be similar. This suggests that the same ocellar light information is encoded in the two different signals.

Multimodality in L-neurons

Tests with multimodal stimulation clearly demonstrate that the information relayed by L-neurons can be different depending on whether they are in the graded or spiking state. Moving gratings, stationary light flashes given to the compound eyes as well as air puffs to the head and body, which are ineffective in non-spiking L-neurons, can elicit responses in spiking L-neurons (13).

The result of eight recordings from the same spiking L_D-neuron in different individuals is presented in Figure 8. The spectrum of stimulus responses varies from recording to recording

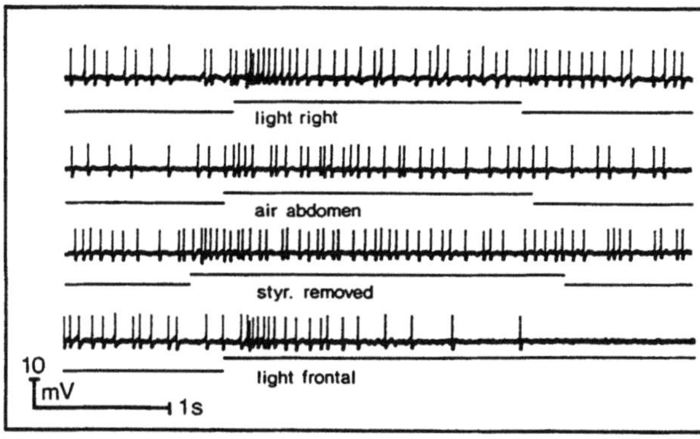

n	Light	Styr. rem.	Air Head	Air Abd.	Sugar	Odour
1	●		○	○	○	○
2	●		○	○	○	○
3	●		○	○	○	○
4	●		○	○	●	○
5	●	●	●	○	●	○
6	●	●	○	●	○	○
7	●	●	●	●	●	○
8	●	●	●	●	○	○

Fig. 8 - Response spectrum of the same L_D-neuron recorded from 8 individuals. Stimuli were: light, removal of styrofoam substrate from the bee's tarsi, airpuffs onto the head and abdomen, a drop of sugarwater applied to the antennae and the proboscis and an airstream containing odour. Closed circles indicate response; open circles, no response; blank, not tested. Four original responses are shown to the left.

and the same cell can change its response if the same stimulus is repeated (13). This demonstrates a considerable degree of plasticity in L-neurons, which excludes a classification on the basis of effective stimuli.

What is the meaning of a mechanism that enables a nerve cell to carry different information depending on whether it is spiking or non-spiking? If, for example, some of the terminals of an L-neuron are selective for action potentials, then these terminals would be active in the spiking mode and might transmit exclusively multimodal information. Consequently, the cell may be able, depending on the kind of signal, to distribute different information (uni- or multimodal) to different sets of postsynaptic targets. Such a mechanism would greatly increase the capacity of a single interneuron to carry and process information, a useful design for the densely packed, size-limited insect brains.

Interaction of ocelli and compound eyes

It seems reasonable to suggest that the ocelli and the compound eyes should combine their information on the visual surround and interact at distinct neuronal levels. As already mentioned, spiking L-neurons receive input from the compound eye though the anatomical basis remains obscure.

A second level of interaction might be provided by a few S-neurons connecting the ocellar retina to the medulla and lobula (4, 17). A cobalt fill of such an S-neuron reveals bleb-like structures (indicating presynaptic specializations) in the extensive arborisation in the lobula output region as well as in the inner plexiform layer of the medulla (15). Such cells may

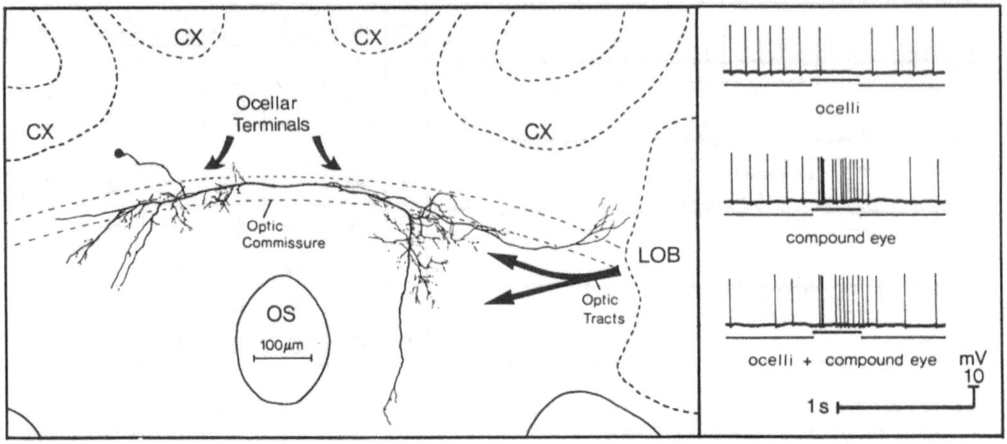

Fig. 9 - A local interneuron in the posterior slope of the midbrain arborising amongst L-neuron terminals and within the posterior optic tracts and the psoterior optic commissure connecting both lobulae. Illumination of the ocelli inhibits the cell, whereas illumination of the right compound eye excites it (right). The result of simultaneous stimulation of ocelli and compound eye does not differ from a compound eye stimulation alone. CX = calyx; LOB = lobula; OS = oesophagus.

represent a short-latency pathway from the ocellus to modulate the information processing in the compound eye.

The architecture of the posterior midbrain favors a role as a location for interactions between both visual systems. It contains optic commissures connecting the visual neuropils of both compound eyes as well as optic tracts leaving the lobula (16). The L-neurons arborize in the posterior midbrain where the dendrites of descending neurons originate. Since all these are in close proximity, it is likely that synaptic contact can be mediated directly or via local interneurons. Figure 9 presents an example of a local interneuron, demonstrating its position relative to the optic neuropils. This cell exhibits responses to ocellar and compound eye stimulation. A variety of such local interneurons have been recorded (15). Interaction of ocellar and compound eye signals at a common descending neuron has been postulated by Guy et al. (6). Because of latency differences simultaneous stimulation of both visual pathways would first result in an ocellar signal, which could modulate the compound eye input.

CONCLUDING REMARKS

In the honeybee, the multiple ocellar connections to specific brain targets as well as the variety of responses within a single species of interneuron demonstrate the high complexity and support the idea of ocellar multifunctionality (21). The optical characteristics of the ocelli (underfocussed lens, large area of view) together with the high neuronal convergence confer a high absolute sensitivity and rule out the perception of sharp images. The fast and sensitive light responses are best suited for a role in visual flight control as shown for locusts (18). However, a comprehensive functional characterization is not yet available, though a variety of different functions have been discussed. Ocelli, for instance, can alter the long-term sensitivity of the compound eyes during phototactic and foraging behavior (19) or the waggle dance (5). Recently, ocellar participation in turning behavior during phototactic runs (9) and flight (8) have been reported. A recent physiological analysis demonstrates that the modulations of the compound eye sensitivity via the ocelli are not present in the retina and are thus likely to occur at more central levels (14). The ocellar system of the honeybee certainly reflects a compromise between numerous functions especially adapted to the different requirements. Our understanding of the ocellar system is still at the beginning.

Acknowledgements. I wish to thank Harjit Seyan for critically reading the manuscript, Renate Weisskirchen for photographic assistance and Wendy Moses for typing the manuscript. I am especially grateful to Prof. Randolf Menzel. Supported by a grant from the Deutsche Forschungsgemeinschaft.

REFERENCES

(1) Burrows, M., and Siegler, M.V.S. 1982. Spiking local interneurons mediate local reflexes. Science 217: 650-652.

(2) Chappell, R.L., and Dowling, J.E. 1972. Neural organization of the median ocellus of the dragonfly. I. Intracellular electrical activity. J. Gen. Physiol. 60: 121-147.

(3) Geiser F.X., and Labhart, T. 1982. Elektrophysiologische Untersuchungen an der Ocellen-Retina der Honigbiene (Apis mellifera). Verh. Dtsch. Zool. Ges. 75: 307.

(4) Goodman, L.J. 1981. Organization and physiology of the insect dorsal ocellar system. In Handbook of Sensory Physiology, Vol. VII 6C, ed. H. Autrum, pp. 201-286. Berlin, Heidelberg, New York: Springer-Verlag.

(5) Gould, J.L. 1975. Communication of distance information by honeybees. J. Comp. Physiol. 104: 161-173.

(6) Guy, R.G.; Goodman, L.J.; and Mobbs, P.G. 1979. Visual interneurons in the bee brain: Synaptic organization and transmission by graded potential. J. Comp. Physiol. 134: 253-264.

(7) Hengstenberg, R. 1977. Spike responses of 'nonspiking' visual interneurons. Nature 270: 338-340.

(8) Kastberger, G., and Kral, K. 1985. Flugsteuerung bei Hymenoptera: Die Rolle von Komplexaugen und Ocellen bei photoaktischen und photokinetischen Reaktionen. Verh. Dtsch. Zool. Ges. 78: 230.

(9) Kral, K., and Heran, H. 1983. Phototaktische Wendreaktionen der Honigbiene (Apis mellifera carnica POLLM) nach Eingriffen in das Ocellensystem. Zool. J. Physiol. 87: 127-140.

(10) Menzel, R. 1979. Spectral sensitivity and colour vision in invertebrates. In Handbook of Sensory Physiology, Vol. VII 6A, ed. H. Autrum., pp. 503-580. Berlin, Heidelberg, New York: Springer-Verlag.

(11) Milde, J.J. 1981. Graded potentials and action potentials in the large ocellar interneurons of the bee. J. Comp. Physiol. 143: 427-434.

(12) Milde, J.J. 1984. Ocellar interneurons in the honeybee. Structure and signals of L-neurons. J. Comp. Physiol. A 154: 683-693.

(13) Milde, J.J., and Homberg, U. 1984. Ocellar interneurons in the honeybee. Characteristics of spiking L-neurons. J. Comp. Physiol. 155: 151-160.

(14) Milde, J.J. 1985. Circadian change of compound eye sensitivity is not governed by the ocelli in honeybees. Exp. Biol. 44: 241-145.

(15) Milde, J.J. 1986. Characteristics of interneurons in the ocellar system of the honeybee. Exp. Biol. (in press).

(16) Mobbs, P.G. 1984. Neural networks in the mushroom bodies of the honeybee. J. Insect Physiol. 30: 43-58.

(17) Pan, K.C. 1981. The neural organization of the ocellar system and associated pathways in the central nervous system of the worker honeybee, Apis mellifera. Ph.D. thesis, University of London.

(18) Rowell, C.H.F.; Reichert, H.; and Bacon, J.P. 1985. How locusts fly straight. In Feedback and Motor Control, eds. W.J.P. Barnes and N.H. Gladden, pp. 337-354. London: Croom Helm Ltd.

(19) Schricker, B. 1965. Die Orientierung der Honigbiene in der Dämmerung. Zugleich ein Beitrag zur Frage der Ocellenfunktion bei Bienen. Z. Vergl. Physiol. 49: 420-458.

(20) Toh, Y., and Kubawara, M. 1974. Fine structure of the dorsal ocellus of the worker honeybee. J. Morphol. 143: 285-306.

(21) Wilson, M. 1978. The functional organization of locust ocelli. J. Comp. Physiol. 124: 297-316.

Neuroanatomy and Signal Processing in the Brain

Chemical Neuroanatomy of the Honeybee Brain

G. Bicker, S. Schäfer, and V. Rehder

Institut für Tierphysiologie, Neurobiologie, Königin-Luise-Str. 28–30, D-1000 Berlin 33, FRG

Abstract. This review provides a brief survey of the major neuropiles in the brain of the worker honeybee. The distribution of putative neurotransmitters was investigated in these neuropiles with antisera raised against GABA- and serotonin-protein conjugates. Immunocytochemistry revealed new cell types, pathways, and homologies to neurons of other insect species. The pattern of GABA-immunoreactivity suggests that GABA is more important in mediating local interactions rather than more distant neural ones. Serotonin-immunoreactive neurons interconnect and cover large areas within and between neuropiles. Release of serotonin from these neurons may thus help to coordinate neural activity between several neuropiles.

INTRODUCTION

The nervous system of the worker honeybee provides the substrate for some remarkable information processing tasks. For example, visual information about the location and distance of a food source can be memorized and transformed into a motor program which results in the recruitment of other workers from the hive (12). The elegance of the bee's behavior may have helped to stimulate the many anatomical investigations of its brain since the beginning of the century (21, 22, 23, 54). These classical studies have already been compiled by Bullock and Horridge (4). The purpose of our review is to survey recent progress made in the anatomy of the bee brain with emphasis on new developments in chemical neuroanatomy. This term was borrowed from the title of Björklund and Hökfelt's "Handbook of Chemical Neuroanatomy"(3) which reviews the analysis of transmitter related substances in the vertebrate nervous system. Chemical neuroanatomy bridges the gap between anatomy and biochemistry by providing information about the distribution of possible neurotransmitters and their receptors within specific pathways.

This approach encompasses several histochemical techniques. Monoamines can be visualized with the histofluorescence technique (10) which, in favorable circumstances, allows one to distinguish among the various amines (25). Mercer et al. (29) applied a refined histofluorecence method, based on glyoxylic acid, to locate biogenic amines in the brain of the bee. These studies are presently complemented by autoradiographic localizations of the biogenic amine receptors with labelled ligands (9, 45). Recently, it has become possible to visualize several classical transmitters and transmitter enzymes directly with antibodies (see review in (3)). So far, only the distribution of serotonin- and GABA-immunoreactivity has been studied in the bee brain (2, 31, 34, 39, 44, 48). GABA is thought to be a classical neurotransmitter, whereas serotonin may function as a classical neurotransmitter, but may also be nonsynaptically released as a neuromodulator or neurohormone. For information about the immunocytochemical localization of a peptide transmitter candidate, or the ultrastructural localizations of other transmitter substances we refer to the articles of Noble and Goodman (36) and Schürman and Elekes (43).

INTRODUCTION TO THE BEE BRAIN

The nervous system of the bee includes a cerebral ganglion (brain) (Fig. 1), a suboesophageal ganglion (SOG), and a ventral nerve chord. According to Witthöft (55) the worker's brain contains approximately 850,000 cells, about half of which belong to the optic lobes. The insect brain has been traditionally divided into the proto-, deuto-, and tritocerebral parts which are comprised of several neuropilar masses interconnected by nerve cell processes. It is not known how many segmental ganglia are actually incorporated into the brain. The suboesophageal ganglion of the bee arises from the fusion of three ganglia and is attached to the deuto- and tritocerebral parts of the brain. The protocerebrum incorporates the largest part of the insect brain and contains ocellar tract neuropile, mushroom bodies, central complex, pars intercerebralis, and lateral protocerebrum. There is some debate in the literature about whether the optic ganglia should be incorporated into the protocerebrum, as conventional wisdom holds, or into the deutocerebrum as suggested by Strausfeld and Bacon (50). The deutocerebrum consists of antennal- and dorsal-lobe neuropiles and some projection areas of antennal lobe relay fibers. The tritocerebrum is a neuropile without obvious landmarks. It lies in the ventral part of the brain bordering on the deutocerebrum and the SOG and connects the brain to the stomatogastric nervous system. The exact borderlines between proto-, deuto-, and tritocerebrum are somewhat arbitrary because detailed observations about their embryological origin are lacking. Furthermore, it should be stressed that the arborisations of intersegmental interneurons, projection fibers, serially repeated interneurons, and even motorneurons are not limited by the boundaries but interconnect the various segmental parts of brain and SOG. The projection fibers of many neurons bundle together in commissures and tracts linking the neuropilar areas. It should, however, be mentioned that many neurons do not follow these main fiber tracts. In addition, fibers of one tract may eventually separate and project to different neuropilar areas.

Ocellar tract neuropile

The protocerebrum is topped by three dorsal ocelli (Fig.5a) whose photoreceptor cells synapse within the ocellar plexus onto interneurons of large diameter. These large ocellar fibers (L-

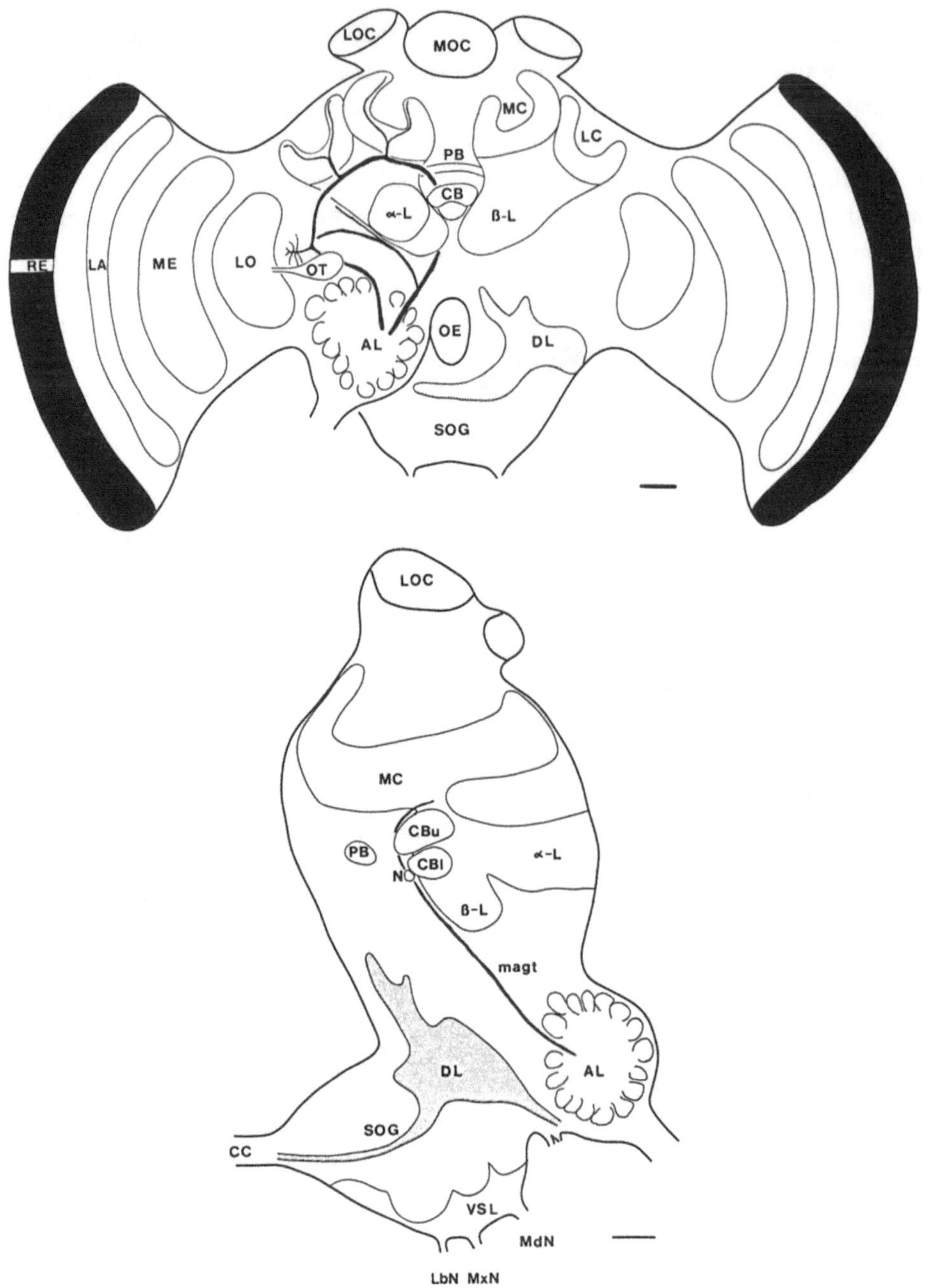

Fig. 1 - Frontal a) and side view b) of the bee brain focussing on sensory projections from the antennal lobe. RE: retina, LA: lamina, ME: medulla, LO: lobula, OT: optic tubercle, AL: antennal lobe, OE: oesophagus, SOG: suboesophageal ganglion, DL: dorsal lobe, CB: central body, CBu: upper division of central body, CBl: lower division of central body, a-l: a-lobe, ß-L: ß-lobe, PB: protocerebral bridge, LOC: lateral ocellus, MOC: median ocellus, CC: cervical connective, magt: median antennoglomerular tract, LbN: labial nerve, MxN: maxillary nerve, MdN: mandibular nerve. Stippled area indicates primary sensory projections from the antennae. Scale bar 100 um.

neurons) project behind the protocerebral bridge into the posterior slope neuropile; some terminate there. However, five pairs are known to descend through the ventral nerve chord to the thoracic ganglia (15).

Mushroom bodies

The mushroom bodies or corpora pedunculata are paired neuropilar structures in the dorsal protocerebrum (Fig. 5a) which are extensively developed in social hymenopterans. Each mushroom body consists of a lateral and a medial calyx connected to the a- and ß-lobes via the pedunculus. The calyces are packed with the somata of the ca. 170,000 intrinsic Kenyon cells whose dendrites ramify within the cup-shaped neuropile of the calyces. Based on the morphology of their dendritic arborisations, Kenyon cells can be divided into five groups (32). The long projection fibers of the Kenyon cells pass through the pedunculus, branch at its base from where they send one process into the a- and one into the ß-lobe (23). Since their discovery by Dujardin (7), the mushroom bodies have been considered to be neuropiles of multimodal sensory convergence representing an association center in the insect brain. Visual, olfactory, and possibly mechanosensory information reaches the calyces that are predominantly described as sensory input regions, while the a- and ß-lobes are, on the other hand, thought to be output regions of the mushroom bodies (32, 33, 46). The antennoglomerular tracts (a.g.t.) provide the main sensory input from the antennae, whereas the visual input from the medulla and lobula enters via the anterior-superior-optic tract (a.s.o.t.). The calycal neuropile can be subdivided into lip, collar, and basal ring regions. These calycal zones differ with respect to afferent sensory modalities. Antennal sensory input is restricted to the lip (Fig. 4a), whereas the collar receives mainly visual input. Input to the basal ring is thought to derive from the tritocerebrum and suboesophageal ganglion. The closed contour of the calycal neuropile opens up in the pedunculus to form curved horseshoe-shaped bands which finally flatten into sheets in the lobes. Thus fibers preserve their relative position suggesting that a map-like arrangement of the calycal neuropile is conserved in the lobes. Arborisations of extrinsic neurons form layers oriented perpendicularly to the Kenyon cell projections, particularly in the a-lobe. The neuroanatomical organization of the mushroom bodies thus resembles the cerebellum (23), where hundred thousands of parallel fibers synapse onto the perpendicularly oriented planes formed by the dendrites of Purkinje cells. Many protocerebral fibers form an unstructured neuropile that surrounds the mushroom bodies and the central complex.

Central complex

The central complex in the midbrain (Fig. 5) consists of the central body, the two glomerular noduli, and the protocerebral bridge (pons) (22, 23). The central body has been divided into an upper and a lower division. Both divisions are accessed by fibers running through the isthmus tracts and the anterior bundle (9, 19). The projections into the central body arborise in a dorsally directed, fan-shaped pattern in eight segments. The protocerebral bridge is an elongated medial neuropile posterior to the upper division of the central body, that crosses

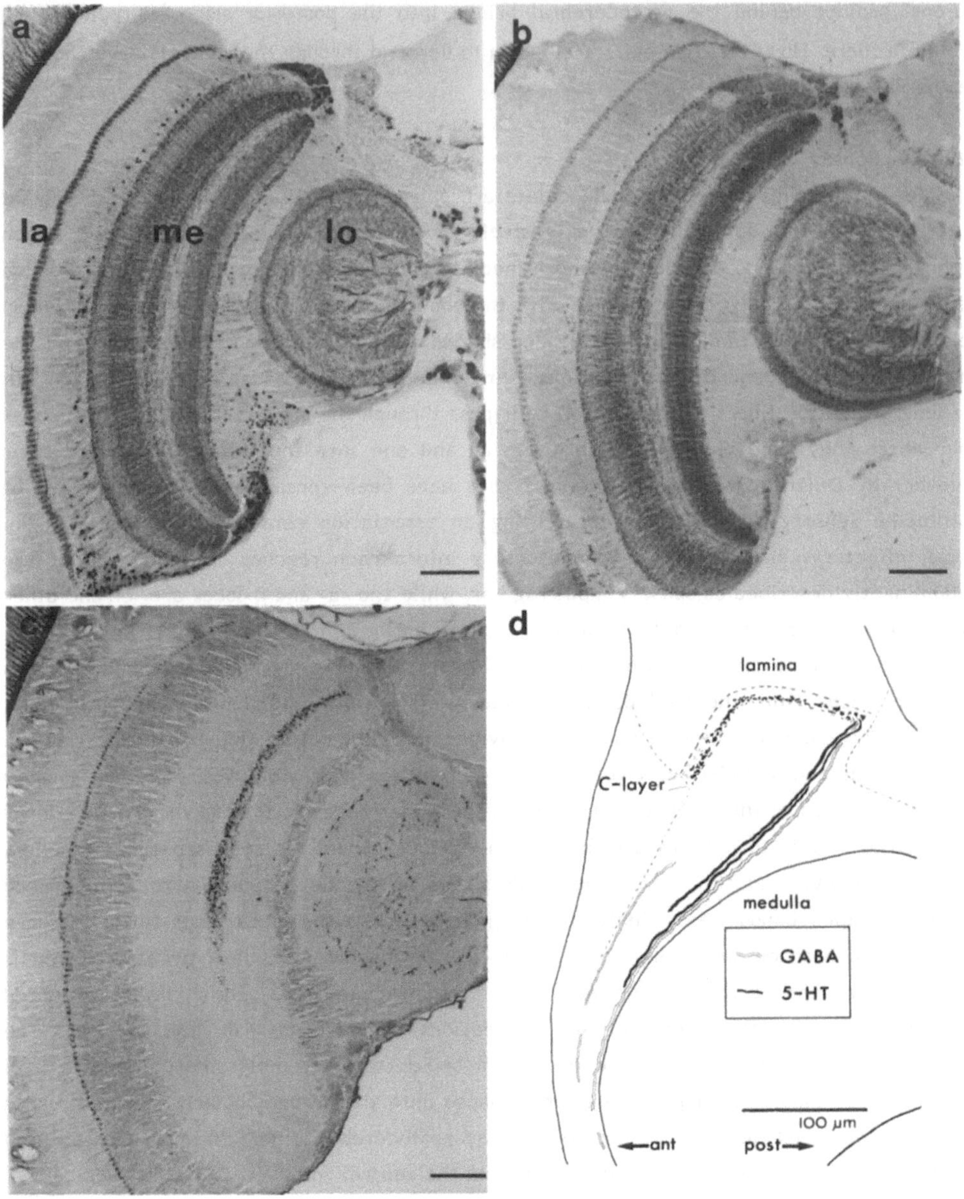

Fig. 2 -a) Frontal section through the visual ganglia showing the stratification of the GABA-immunoreactivity and labelled somata in and around the outer and inner chiasma. la: lamina, me: medulla, lo: lobula. b) Frontal section showing GAD-immunoreactivity. c) Frontal section showing serotonin-immunoreactivity. d) Compound drawing of horizontal sections showing tracings of GABA-and serotonin-immunoreactivity. GABA and 5-HT-(serotonin) immunoreactivity was detected on the same section by rhodamine and fluorescein isothiocyanate labelled secondary antibodies. All scale bars 100 um.

between the two brain hemispheres. Segmentally arranged neurons link the protocerebral bridge and central body.

Pars intercerebralis

The pars intercerebralis is dorsomedially situated above the central body and is flanked laterally by the mushroom body neuropile. It contains different cell populations with an aggregation of about 116 neurosecretory cells (55), many of which send projections through a nerve leading to the the corpora cardiaca at the posterior side of the brain.

Lateral protocerebrum

This area summarizes the remaining, mainly lateral, portions of the protocerebrum that lack obvious structured neuropiles, groups of large cell bodies or other prominent structures. The neurons in this area run their individual courses apart from the main tracts forming an unstructured neuropile. Again there is some disagreement in the literature about which part of this neuropile really belongs to the protocerebrum, or whether some parts of it may be attributed to the deutocerebrum. Neurons projecting their axons through the antennoglomerular tracts form a plexus in its lateral portion. Mobbs incorporated this terminal projection area of the a.g.t. as lateral deutocerebral neuropile area (Fig. 4a) into the deutocerebrum (33).

Optic lobes

The optic lobes of the honeybee contain three distinct neuropilar masses: the lamina, medulla, and lobula (Fig. 1 and 2). Most anatomical studies on this part of the brain have concentrated on the structure and ultrastructure of the outermost ganglion, the lamina, which receives input from the photoreceptors of the compound eye. The lamina can be subdivided into a cell body layer that contains the somata of monopolar cells and a fiber layer that has been further subdivided into an external plexiform A, B, and C layer (40, 41). The outer chiasma connects the lamina and the second optic ganglion, the medulla. In the chiasma, bundles of fibers cross in the horizontal plane before they enter the medulla, which shows a pronounced layering reflecting the distribution of diverse cell types and their branching pattern (42). The third optic ganglion, the lobula, is connected to the medulla through the inner chiasma where fiber bundles also cross in the horizontal plane. The lobula shows distinct layers, which in contrast to the lamina and the medulla, are almost parallel to the frontal plane. A columnar organization perpendicular to the layers is a general feature of all three optic ganglia. This results from the preservation of the retinotopic array of fiber bundles from one processing stage to the next. Several fiber pathways connect the medulla and the lobula to the optic foci within the deutocerebrum and into the protocerebrum. There are several commissures that interconnect the optic ganglia of the two brain hemispheres (17). The optic tubercle is a glomerulus lying above the antennal lobe which is associated with the visual system near the anterior base of the optic lobes.

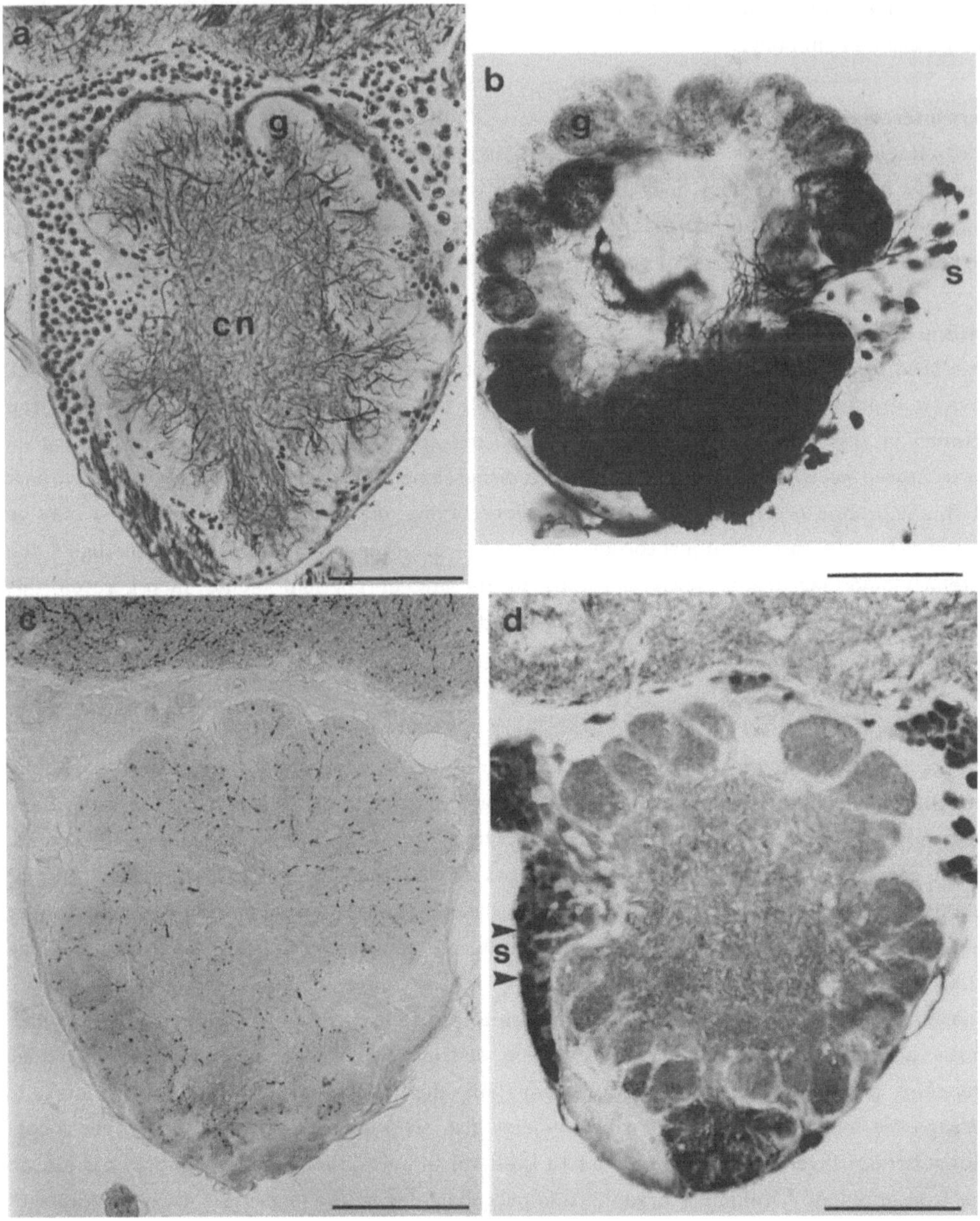

Fig. 3 - Frontal section through the antennal lobe. a) Bodian staining showing the central neuropile (cn) and glomeruli (g). b) Cobalt-backfill of the antennal nerve stains the spherical glomeruli (g) which are invaded by arborisations of interneurons. (s): somata of interneurons. c) Serotonin-immunoreactive arborisations of varicose appearance in the antennal lobe. d) GABA-immunoreactivity in the antennal lobe. The glomeruli, central neuropile, lateral soma group to the left, and somata lying mediodorsally are labelled. All scale bars 100 um.

Posterior slope area

The posterior slope is an integrating neuropile where proto- and deutocerebral brain areas are confluent. In this area, on the posterior surface of the brain, (which includes the perioesophageal neuropile) visual, ocellar, and antennal information converge. The information is then transmitted to the ventral nerve chord by descending interneurons. The physiology of motion-sensitive interneurons with dendritic arborisations in the posterior slope is described by Goodmann (16).

Antennal and dorsal lobes

Antennal and dorsal lobes are glomerular neuropile areas in the deutocerebral part of the brain. The antennal lobes receive their principal sensory inputs from olfactory receptors on the antennae (Fig. 3a,b), whereas antennal mechanosensory fibers mainly project to the dorsal lobes (38, 52). In the antennal lobe, the sites of synaptic contacts between receptor cells, local interneurons, and output relay neurons are arranged as egg-shaped or spherical glomeruli (Fig. 3) which surround the central neuropile (1, 16, 18). Arnold et al. (1) have proposed that the number, position, and dimensions indicate an univarying organization of approximately 166 identified glomeruli in the worker bee. The output relay neurons of the antennal lobes project via three tracts into the ipsilateral protocerebrum and eventually terminate in or near the calyces of the mushroom bodies and projection areas of lateral neuropilar compartments (Fig. 4a). According to the terminology introduced by Mobbs (32,33), these tracts are called the median, lateral, and mediolateral antennoglomerular tracts (m.a.g.t., l.a.g.t., and m.l.a.g.t.). Some fibers from the dorsal lobe and the SOG join the m.a.g.t.. Arnold et al. (1) observed, in addition, direct fiber projections into the a-lobe and a posterior medio-lateral tract that passes behind the ß-lobe into the lateral protocerebrum. In the bee, there is no evidence for direct projections of the antennal receptors to the contralateral antennal lobe, however, a small tract interconnects the two neuropiles. The dorsal lobe neuropile lies posterior to the antennal lobe (Fig. 1), sends motorneurons into the antennal and inner antennal motor nerve, and receives mechanosensory projections from the antennae. It also contains projections from neurons that descend into the ventral nerve chord.

Tritocerebrum

In the honeybee-larva, the tritocerebral part of the nervous system consists of two separate ganglia which are linked via the preoral connectives to the frontal ganglion and are interconnected by the postoral commissure (51). In the imago, the tritocerebrum is fused to the deutocerebral and the suboesophageal ganglion. The tritocerebrum anteriorly gives rise to the labral nerve and the frontal connective. The labral nerve contains sensory fibers from the labrum and projections of motoneurons. The frontal commissure connects the brain with the frontal ganglion, which serves the stomatogastric system. There are no body appendages that correspond to the tritocerebral segment.

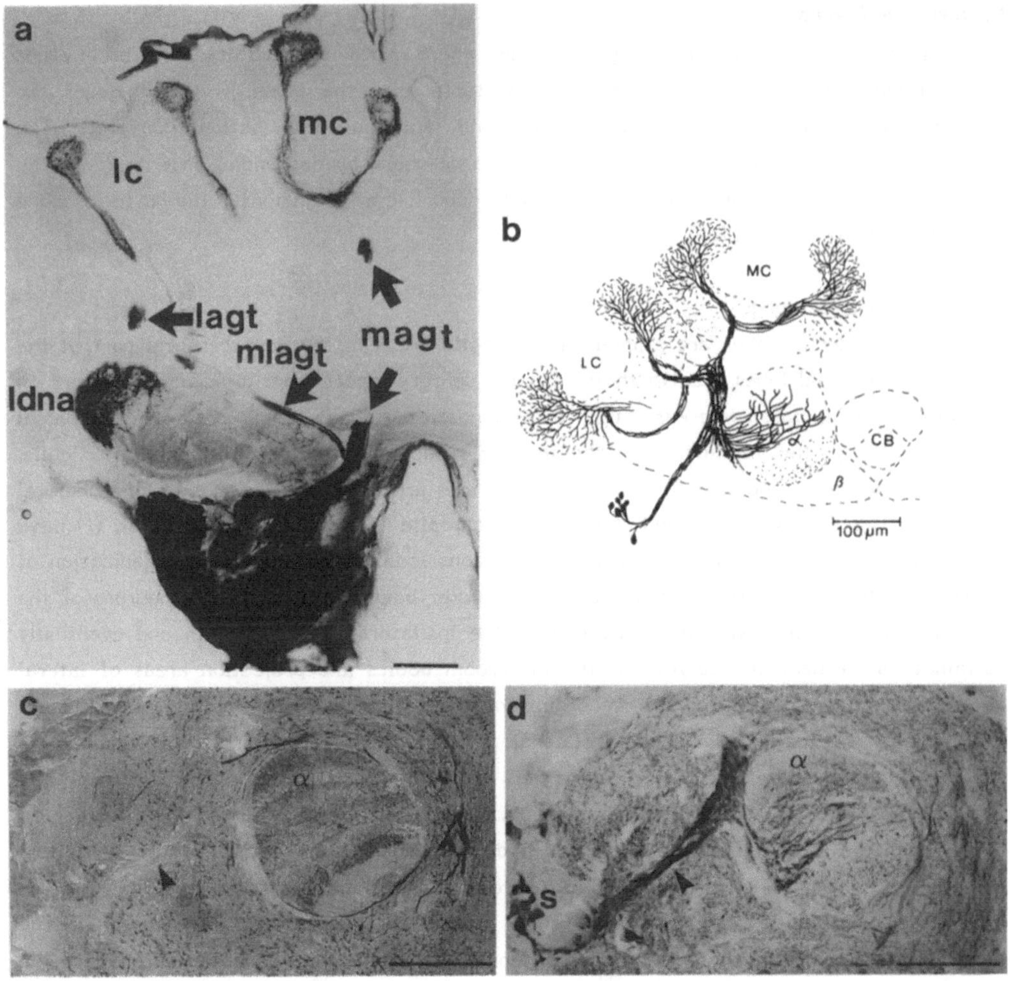

Fig. 4 - Frontal sections through the brain. a) Projection areas and tracts of antennal relay fibers are revealed by a cobalt-backfill of the antennal nerve. lc: lateral calyx, mc: median calyx, magt: median antennoglomerular tract, lagt: lateral antennoglomerular tract, mlagt: mediolateral antennoglomerular tract, ldna: lateral deutocerebral neuropile area. b) Composite drawing of GABA-immunoreactive p.c.t. fibers. a: a-lobe, ß: ß-lobe, CB: central body. c) Serotonin-immunoreactive fibers surround the a-lobe (a). Serotonin-immunoreactivity in the a-lobe shows pronounced layering. Note that the tract (black arrowhead) containing the primary neurites of the GABA-immunoreactive p.c.t. fibers is devoid of serotonin-immunoreactivity. d) GABA-immunoreactive main axonal projections of the p.c.t. fuse with their primary neurites (black arrowhead) coming from the lateral soma cluster. All scale bars 100 um.

Suboesophageal ganglion

The SOG is contiguous with the deuto- and tritocerebral parts of the brain (Fig.1)and arises from the embryonic fusion of three neuromeres: the mandibular, maxillary, and labial neuromeres (Fig. 6a). The neuropilar structure of the SOG is complicated because it serves at least two very general funtions. It innervates the mouthparts and neck muscles, and serves as a relay and transit station for the information flow between brain and the cervical connective (Fig. 6a). The neuromeres contain local and intersegmental interneurons, receive sensory projections from the nerves of the mouthparts and a few from the antennal nerve, and project motorneurons through the corresponding mandibular, maxillary and labial nerves. In addition to the descending interneurons of the brain which branch in the SOG before projecting into the ventral nerve chord, it contains clusters of descending neurons.

CHEMICAL ANATOMY

In the following chapters we will try to outline the flow of information from sensory to central neuropiles and compare some functional aspects of the distribution of serotonin- and GABA-immunoreactivity in selected areas. For our immunocytochemical studies we used a well established commercially obtainable serotonin antiserum, generated against a conjugate of serotonin and bovine serum albumin. The GABA antisera which were raised against GABA conjugates to bovine serum albumin (BSA) and keyhole-limpet hemocyanin (KLH) were prepared according to the method of Storm-Mathisen et al. (83) by T.G.Kingan (Columbia Univ. NY). Although the honeybee brain contains large amounts of GABA, ca.10.9 X 10^{-4}g/g wet weight (13), before the use of antisera there was no information available on its localization. The inhibitory effect of GABA on the crustacean stretch receptor led to its identification as neurotransmitter in invertebrates. Since there is considerable evidence for inhibitory transmitter action of GABA in insect CNS (5,8,24), an antiserum specific for GABA might thus allow us to reveal presumed inhibitory pathways. GABA is synthesized from l-glutamic acid by a decarboxylation step which is catalyzed by l-glutamic acid decarboxylase (GAD). The kinetic parameters of this enzyme have been determined by Fox and Larsen (11) in the honeybee. A constant worry of all immunocytochemical studies is the specificity of the antisera. In order to obtain independent evidence for the localization of GABA we, therefore, used an antiserum against GAD and compared the staining pattern to the one acquired with the GABA antiserum. It appeared that both staining patterns are virtually identical. A comparison is given in Figure 2a,b. Therefore, we hereafter use the term GABA-immunoreactivity instead of GABA-like-immunoreactivity. In contrast to the GABA antiserum, the GAD antiserum does not stain the nuclei, and the cell bodies of GAD-reactive cells appear faint. It should be noted that the GAD antiserum was raised against GAD isolated from rat brain (37). The polyclonal antiserum probably recognizes epitopes common to GAD in the rat and bee brain.

Optic lobes

Immunohistochemical investigations of the distribution of serotonin in the visual system of the worker bee revealed a distinct pattern of labelled layers in the three visual ganglia (34, 41, 48). The layers extend perpendicularly to the columnar organization of the visual system (Fig. 2c) and a common finding of all studies is that the serotonin-immunoreactivity derives from widefield tangential neurons. According to Schürmann and Klemm (48), there are only

20-30 serotonin-immunoreactive somata in each optic lobe. We examined the brain of the honeybee for GABA-like immunoreactivity and found approximately 9000 immunoreactive somata - which is less than five percent of the neurons in the visual system (43). The reactive somata belong to amacrine and other local interneurons and a small number of widefield tangential cells.

Lamina

GABA-immunoreactivity is found neither in the photoreceptor axons nor in the lamina monopolar cells (Fig. 2a). Therefore, it is likely that a transmitter other than GABA directly transforms the depolarizing receptor potential into a hyperpolarizing monopolar cell potential. An overview of the serotonin- and GABA-immunoreactivity in the optic lobes at comparable planes of sectioning is shown in Figure 2. Apparently the neuropiles contain much more GABA- than serotonin-immunoreactivity. In the lamina, we found an overlap of serotonin- and GABA-immunoreactivity in the external plexiform C-layer, which is a narrow stratum closest to the outer chiasma. In both cases the immunoreactivity derives from a set of at least five wide-field tangential interneurons which project through the outer chiasma and invade the lamina at its posterior margin (43, 44, 48). They then spread tangentially across the proximal border of the entire lamina neuropile. The somata of both the serotonin and the GABA-reactive fibers lie at the anterior margin of the medulla. There are, however, differences in the appearance and extension of the stained lamina stratum. In contrast to the GABA-immunoreactivity, which is fairly homogenous and occupies the entire lamina C-layer, the arborisations of the serotonin-immunoreactive fibers have a distinctly varicose appearance and are restricted to the proximal half of the lamina C-layer. Numerous smaller amacrine cell types contribute to the GABA-immunoreactivity in the lamina C-layer (43,44). We could not identify this cell type because its processes are too fine to be resolved by our method in the densely stained lamina stratum. Conceivably, these could be amacrine fibers of the am_{i2} type, which is the only neuronal type restricted to the lamina C-layer whose somata location (40) coincides with the immunoreactive cell bodies around the outer chiasma. From the above comparison, it cannot be definitivly determined whether the GABA- and the serotonin-immunoreactive widefield tangential cells are identical or belong to separate sets of interneurons with different transmitter phenotypes. Double labelling experiments on the same section (44) revealed that the GABA- and serotonin-immunoreactive cells form two subsets of fibers with projections and arborisations in close apposition to each other (Fig. 2d). Nässel et al. (34) performed EM studies in three insect species on similar looking HRP-labelled tangential fiber profiles. In the honeybee, they found these fibers were presynaptic to second order neurons in the lamina and contained large granular and small clear vesicles. Based on fiber morphology they assumed that their HRP-labelled fibers are the serotonergic tangential neurons. However, it should be borne in mind that fibers of similar morphology but different transmitter phenotype exist close to each other. Be this as it may, Nässel et al. (34) provided evidence that tangential fibers may constitute a centrifugal pathway in the visual system because they are presynaptic to lamina elements.

Medulla

The second visual ganglion contains one serotonin-immunoreactive stratum which partly overlaps with the proximal rim of one of the nine GABA-immunoreactive strata (Fig. 2a,c). The serotonin-immunoreactive stratum contains the arborisations of tangential fibers which invade the medulla at its anterior margin where they wrap around the fibers of the anterior commissure, which connects the medulla with the calyces of the mushroom bodies (17). Horizontal sections of the medulla show nine identifiable GABA-immunoreactive strata (31, 43). Only the sixth stratum (counting from the outer chiasma) shows little labelling. The distinctly layered staining in the medulla seems to result from labelling of tangential and amacrine cells that project perpendicular to the retinotopically organized columnar array of centripetal elements. These elements may be involved in lateral inhibition between adjacent columns. In contrast to Meyer et al. (31), we did not find labelled transmedullary cells that run through all layers of the medulla to terminate in the lobula. The stained tangential fiber elements of the outermost stratum cover the medulla surface like a mesh. Together with the labelled wide-field tangential fibers in stratum five that could be traced to the median protocerebrum, they may constitute a pathway centrally controlling the synaptic gain in the periphery of the visual system.

Lobula

Horizontal sections show that the arborisations of serotonin-immunoreactive fibers in the lobula are limited to three separate layers. The fibers, of which there seem to be only two, approach the lobula from the posterior protocerebrum. The stratification of the GABA-immunoreactivity in the lobula is less pronounced than that of the medulla (Fig. 2a). Stained fibers that approach the lobula from the inner chiasma are very thin. Other fibers that depart from the medulla, and follow the course of the chiasma, enter the lobula at its outermost layer. There are only a few thicker wide field fibers labelled which presumably leave the lobula through the anterior bundle. All other stained extrinsic lobula fibers project through the most posterior of the lobula exits to the posterior slope region. These fibers may exert their influence onto the pathways linking the brain and the ventral nerve chord.

Mercer et al. (29) described narrow bands of rapidly fading weak fluorescence in the optic lobes after treatment with glyoxylic acid. The histofluorescence corresponds to the serotonin-immunoreactive strata (28). The large arborisations of the few serotonin immunoreactive tangential fibers that span the strata of the visual system seem to be well suited to influence large portions of the visual field. The common projections of serotonin- and GABA-immunoreactive fibers in the lamina suggest that serotonergic and GABA-ergic pathway may interact in visual information processing. Whether this interaction is limited to the C-layer of the lamina or extends to other parts of the visual system remains to be explored. Release of serotonin may be a molecular signal for a rearrangement of synaptic transmission at various stages of the visual system. The fine varicose extensions that the serotonin-immunoreactive fibers project up to the fenestrated layer indicate that other parts distal to the lamina C-layer could be influenced. Electrophysiological recordings of the electroretinogram show that the plateau which is largely ascribed to the summed response of the photoreceptors is sensitive to serotonin (Bicker unpublished).

Ocellar tract neuropile

There is a certain similarity in the distribution of GABA-immunoreactivity in the protocerebral ocellar system and the optic lobes. In both cases, neither the photoreceptors nor the first order interneurons are labelled. However, thin GABA-immunoreactive fibers wind around the first order L-neurons and arborise in the ocellar plexus. These fibers may belong to efferent small ocellar interneurons. Thus both in the ocellar system and the optic lobes GABA-immunoreactive fibers approach synaptic sites of first order interneurons and may provide a GABA-mediated inhibitory gain control.

Antennal and dorsal lobes

The antennal lobes are chemosensory neuropiles and the first relay station of the olfactory receptors on the antennae (38, 52). This glomerular neuropile receives the terminals of the chemoreceptor axons via the antennal nerve and sends projections into other deuto- and protocerebral areas (Fig. 3a,b; Fig. 4a). The approximately 166 glomeruli are the location for sensory integration and lateral interactions. Intracellular recordings were made from extrinsic relay fibers (18); however, no information is yet available on local interneurons of the lobe neuropile. Cobalt fills of the antennal nerve and injections into the lobe neuropile revealed the multiple connections into deuto- and protocerebral areas of the brain and some minor connections into the tritocerebrum and suboesophageal ganglion (1, 32, 52). Fig. 4a depicts a cobalt fill of the antennal nerve which fortunately showed also secondary fills into other brain areas.

Schürmann and Klemm (48) described blebbed serotonin-immunoreactive fibers that invade antennal and dorsal lobes but could not delineate the position of the corresponding cell somata. The immunoreactivity is found predominantly in the outer parts of the glomeruli. Our serial reconstructions of the serotonin immunoreactivity show that one single, identified interneuron contributes to most, if not all, immunoreactivity in the antennal lobe (39). Due to the position of its soma in the lateral cell body rind of the dorsal deutocerebrum and its extensive projections in the deutocerebral neuropiles, it has been termed the deutocerebral giant. The antennal nerve is devoid of immunoreactivity and no prominent arborisations from other neurons invade the antennal lobe (Fig. 3c). GABA-immunoreactivity is evenly distributed throughout the antennal lobe neuropile (Fig. 3d) but not found in the antennal nerve. The number of ca. 750 immunoreactive somata in the antennal lobes certainly exceeds the number of immunoreactive extrinsic relay fibers. Thus the GABA-immunoreactivity in the antennal lobes seems to predominate in the local interneurons whose somata cluster mainly in the lateral and dorsomedial soma rind (Fig. 3d). Extrinsic GABA-immunoreactive projection fibers were found in the small commissure that interconnects the antennal lobes.

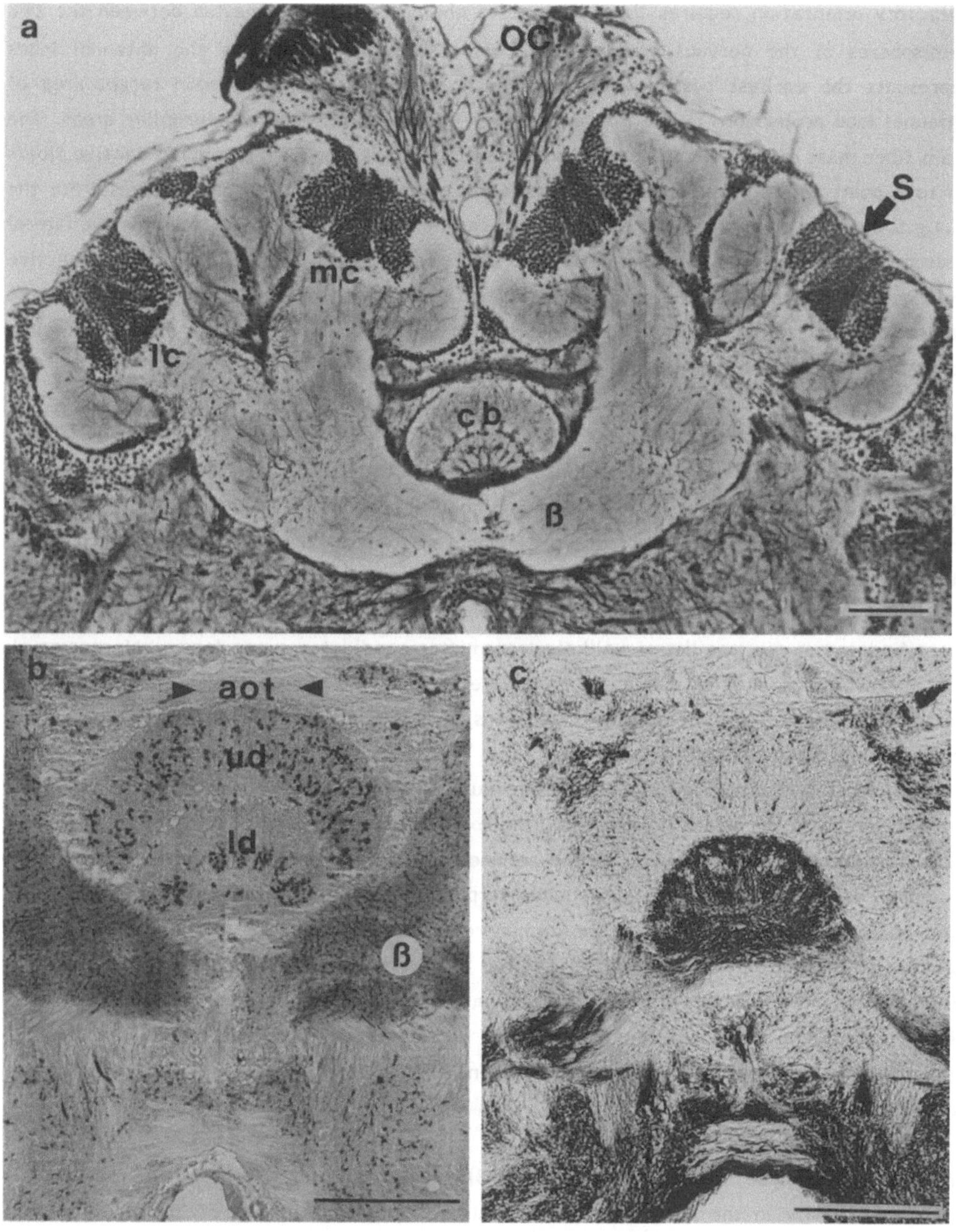

Fig. 5 - Frontal sections through the mushroom bodies and central body. a) Bodian staining shows the ocellar neuropile (oc) central body (cb), ß-lobe (ß), Kenyon cell somata (S) within the lateral and median calyces (lc) (mc),and the anterior optic tract dorsal to the central body. b) Serotonin-immunoreactivity in the upper division (ud), and lower division (ld) of the central body. Note the dense immunoreactivity in the ß-lobe (ß) of the mushroom bodies. Anterior optic tract (aot) is devoid of immunoreactivity. c) Stained GABA-immunoreactive fibers project into the lower division of the central body, which is stronger labelled than the upper division. All scale bars 100 um.

Olfactory orientation requires the exchange of chemosensory information between the two hemispheres of the nervous system. The commissure interconnecting the antennal lobes represents the earliest possible stage for such an integration. One main target area of antennal lobe projections is the mushroom body neuropile and lateral neuropilar areas. The main fiber mass of the m.a.g.t. contains no staining, but is flanked by immunoreactive fibers up to a point where it bypasses the ß-lobe. The m.l.a.g.t. that laterally diverges from the m.a.g.t. contains a few reactive fibers. These can be traced on their way towards the lateral deutocerebral neuropile area, dorsolateral to the antennal lobe (33). Another immunoreactive branch of this fiber bundle runs in close apposition laterally to the pedunculus toward the calyces; then it turns sharply toward the midline of the brain and finally arborises mainly around but also within the pedunculus neuropile.

Mushroom bodies

The histofluorescence and biochemical studies of Mercer at al. (29) demonstrated the presence of biogenic amines in the mushroom body neuropile. Some fluorescent fibers were found in the calyces, but no fluorescent Kenyon cell somata could be detected. Most of the fluorescence is found in the lobes and pedunculus and predominantly originates from extrinsic fibers. The transmitter of the intrinsic mushroom body fibers, the Kenyon cells, remains to be identified, but so far, the list of unlikely transmitter candidates grows longer. Mercer et al. (29) suggested octopamine as a likely candidate because the uptake of neutral red indicates an aminergic nature of these cells (28), and considerable quantities of octopamine were found in the isolated calyces. Schürmann and Klemm (48) described a regular but complex pattern of serotonin-immunoreactivity in the pedunculus and lobes of the mushroom body neuropile. Except for some occasionally observed fine extensions, the calycal neuropile is devoid of serotonin-immunoreactive fibers. In the pedunculus, the a-, and ß-lobe extrinsic serotonin-immunoreactive fibers show fine branches perpendicular to the projections of the intrinsic Kenyon-cells. A general feature of the immunoreactive fiber system is that it spreads mainly radially in the pedunculus and ß-lobe, and has a layered appearance in the a-lobe (Fig. 4c). Even though some fibers have been observed entering the neuropile of pedunculus and lobes, the origin of the serotonin-immunoreactivity is not totally clear. Some immunoreactive somata in the posterior pars intercerebralis send their fibers anteriorly which then ramify around the a-lobe.

Immunocytochemical investigations (2, 48) show neither serotonin- nor GABA-immunoreactivity in the Kenyon cells. This also applies in the case of the main sensory projections into the calyces: the anterior superior optic tract, and the lateral and median antennoglomerular tracts. At least two large extrinsic fibers that leave the a-lobe ventromedially show GABA-immunoreactivity (43). These fibers may represent inhibitory output neurons of the mushroom bodies. Although the main output region of the ß-lobe, the ß-exit, contains no labelled fibers, the commissure linking the two ß-lobes shows dense GABA-immunoreactive labelling. This commissure may conceivably mediate bilateral interactions within the mushroom body system.

Several authors described the anatomy (32, 33) and electrophysiology (9, 20) of a set of fibers which link the a-lobe with the calyces via the protocerebrocalycal tract (p.c.t.). These fibers show a striking varicose appearance in the calyces which is missing in the lobes. The above investigators referred to these fibers as "feedback interneurons" even though they could not provide evidence for the direction of information flow. The p.c.t. fibers are GABA-immunoreactive, allowing a complete anatomical description of this fiber system which displays prominent arborisations in the whole mushroom body neuropile (Fig. 4 b,d). Assuming that these fibers do, indeed, feed information back to the calycal input sites, Bicker et al. (2) suggested that they may function as a negative feed back loop. Cross sections of the p.c.t. bundle showed that it contains ca. 110 GABA-immunoreactive fibers. We found labelled projections of the p.c.t. fibers in the four dorsal bands of the a-lobe and in all calycal regions. The stained fibers seen in the pedunculus, the ß-lobe, or in the remaining two bands of the a-lobe may also be constituents of the p.c.t. fibers (43). The somata are clustered dorsolaterally around the antennal lobe and send their primary neurites in a bundle towards the p.c.t. (Fig. 4d). In order to infer the direction of information flow within this fiber system, a detailed quantitative analysis of input and output synapses in all projection areas is desirable. However, an electronmicroscopical analysis of the p.c.t. fibers in the lobes is complicated because in this region other extrinsic neurons contribute to the GABA-immunoreactivity (43).

Central complex

The function and connectivity of the central complex are largely unknown. Except for the intrinsic neurons of the pons, which process visual stimuli, most neurons in the other parts of the bee's central complex are either multimodal or respond only vaguely to a variety of stimuli (19). Serotonin immunoreactivity of the central body is concentrated in the upper division, the ventral parts of the lower division and the noduli (48). In the lower division, it reflects the segmental structure of the neuropile. Thick serotonin-immunoreactive fibers approach the central body anterioventrally and invade the segments in a dorsally directed manner (Fig. 5b). In frontal sections anterior to the central body these fibers can be traced as they project dorsally around the a-lobe. The GABA-immunoreactivity of the central body is distinct in that the lower division shows an extreme dense staining whereas the upper division contains only few reactive fibers (Fig. 5c). Similar to the serotonin-immunoreactivity in the lower division, the overall pattern of GABA-immunoreactivity in both divisions reflects the segmental structure of the neuropile. Strong immunoreactivity is found in the isthmus tracts and the anteriodorsally projecting anterior bundle. Projections through the isthmus tracts have their corresponding somata dorsomedial to the antennal lobes. No immunoreactivity could be detected within the noduli and the protocerebral bridge.

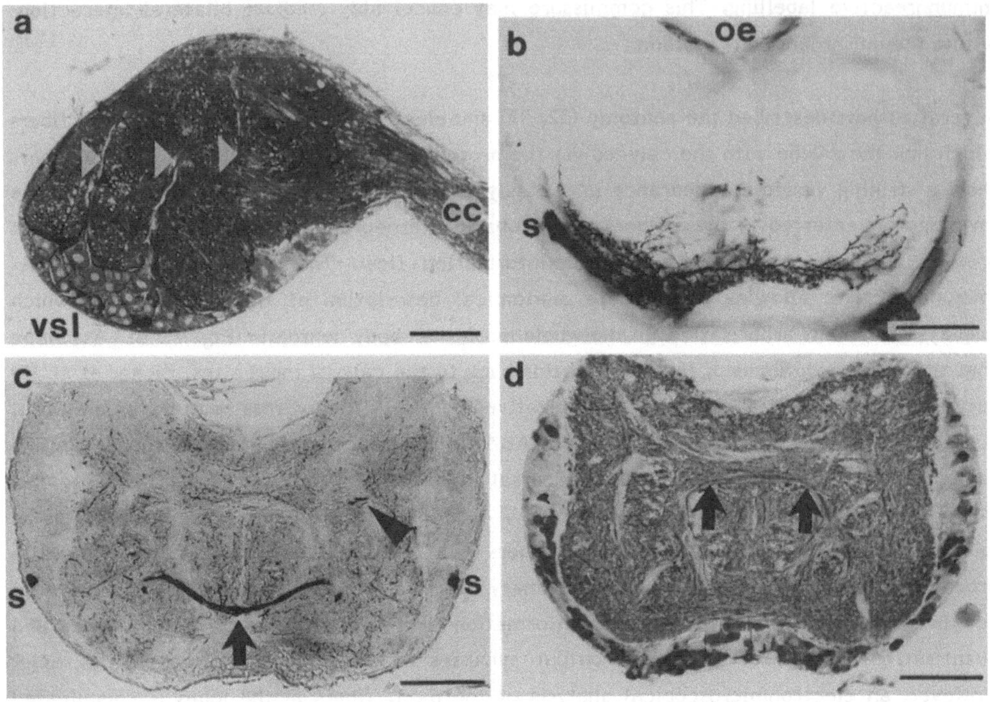

Fig. 6 - Suboesophageal ganglion. a) Sagittal section through the midline of the SOG stained with toluidine blue. White arrows point towards three prominent midline tracts corresponding to the three neuromeres. vsl: ventral soma layer, cc: cervical connective. b) Frontal section through SOG. Cobaltfill of the labial nerve stains retractor glossa motor neuron M 20. oe: oesophagus, s: soma of motorneuron. c) Frontal section through the SOG. Serotonin-immunoreactive serial homologue projects through ventral commissure (arrow) of the maxillary neuromere. The somata (S) lie in the lateral soma rind. Arrowhead points towards projection fibers of two immunoreactive descending neurons. d) Frontal section through the SOG. Most parts of the neuropile show dense GABA-immunoreactivity. Reactive somata are found in lateral and ventral portions of the soma rind. Ventromedially located somata direct their neurites either straight up or through the horseshoe-shaped structure (arrows). All scale bars 100um.

Suboesophageal ganglion and cervical connective

The distribution of serotonin-immunoreactivity reflects the segmental nature of the suboesophageal ganglion in that each neuromere contains the somata and main processes of two bilaterally paired neurons (39). The two somata of each side send their major projections through the same ventral commissure into the contralateral ganglion hemisphere, where they branch extensively and send thinner projections into the adjacent neuromeres (Fig. 6a). Thus, all three neuromeres are linked by serotonin-immunoreactive processes that traverse the boundaries (Fig. 7). We propose that these cells form a set of serial homologues because their patterning in each segment is so similar. However, the only reliable method for establishing serial nomology at the level of the identified neurons is a detailed comparison of their developmental origins. A serotonin-immunoreactive cell type with striking morphological similarities was found in the SOG and ventral nerve chord of the locust (53). Thus transmitter immunohistochemistry may offer the rather unique possibility of establishing homologies at the single cell level between different species even though the phylogenetic distances across which such comparisons can be made have not yet been determined.

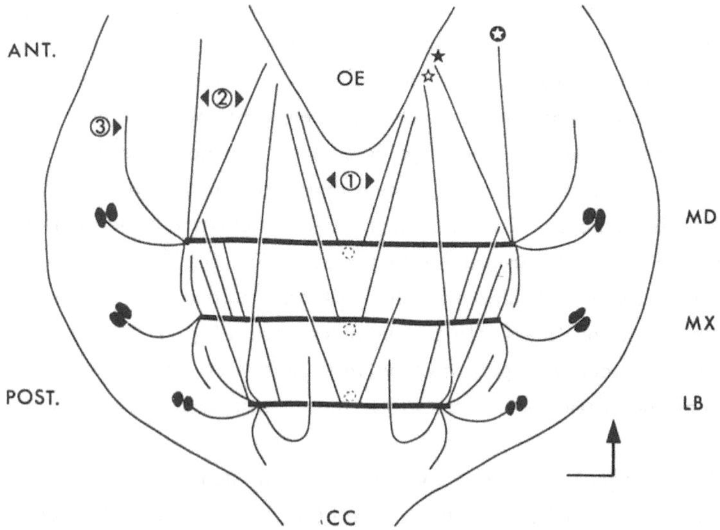

Fig. 7 - Schematic drawing of serotonin-immunoreactive serial homologue neurons in the SOG drawn in the horizontal plane. Medial (1), medio-lateral (2) and lateral projections (3) are labelled only in the mandibular neuromere. black asterisk: ascending projection from the mandibular commissure ending between the a-lobes. white asterisk marks the ascending fiber originating in the labial commissure and ending in the deutocerebrum. white asterisk on black background: fiber of the mandibular commissure leaving the SOG via the frontal connective. Dotted circles mark prominent dorso-ventrally directed midline tracts shown in Fig. 6a. Scale bar 100 um.

While serotonin-immunoreactive profiles form an extensive network in the SOG, all peripheral nerves, except the frontal connective, remain unstained. The frontal connective contains a single fiber originating in the mandibular segment and, additionally, some diffuse varicose arborisations. The origin of a second fiber in the frontal connective remains to be established. We found no fibers in the mandibular nerve, as reported for locusts by Tyrer et al. (53). The lack of serotonin-immunoreactivity in the peripheral mouth nerves is surprising. Nässel and Elekes (35) described an extensive plexus of immunoreactive varicose fibers in the neural sheath of the maxillary-labial and labro-frontal nerves of the blowfly. This difference may suggest that in the bee serotonin is used more as a transmitter in the CNS, and to a lesser extent as neurohormone in peripheral organs.

In the neurobiological analysis of behavior the knowledge of anatomical connectivity is of considerable importance. For instance, antennal and suboesophageal neuropiles mediate the proboscis extension reflex. Cobalt fills of the antennal nerve showed a few direct sensory projections of tract T6-2, leading from the antennal receptors to the dorsal SOG (1, 52). These projections, however, do not overlap with the dendritic arborisations of motor neurons (Fig. 6) responsible for the extension of the proboscis (14; Rehder, in prep.). After complete ablation of the protocerebrum, the proboscis extension reflex can still be elicited. This demonstrates the existence of direct functional pathways between antennal lobes and SOG. The proboscis extension reflex of the honeybee, which is subject to associative learning (27), provides a neural system to study aminergic neurotransmission at a behavioral level. Mercer and Menzel (29) showed that injection of serotonin into the bee brain, before and after single-trial conditioning, reduces the percentage of bees responding to the conditioned stimulus. The use of the immunocytochemical method allowed the mapping of so far unknown, presumably serotonergic, pathways. The deutocerebral giant constitutes a direct connection between the antennal lobe and the SOG. A second serotonin-immunoreactive neuron joins the projection of the deutocerebral giant and links the protocerebrum with the SOG (Fig. 6c). Projections of the mandibular serial homologues could be followed to the ipsilateral a-lobe, and the most posterior labial serial homologues extend fibers into the deutocerebrum (Fig. 7). Our studies mapped identified, presumably serotonergic, pathways between antennal lobes and SOG, which may influence the response properties of neurons within these neuropiles.

The neuropile of the suboesophageal ganglion contains a high density of GABA-immunoreactivity (Fig. 6d). The majority of the labelled somata (ca. 1000) in the SOG belong to interneurons because there are no labelled fibers in the nerves leading to the mouthparts (43). The cervical connective which links the SOG to the thoracic ganglia contains GABA-immunoreactive fibers. Judging by their location in the connective, some of them belong to the descending type. In order to be certain that these neurons descend to the thoracic ganglia, we performed a tandem Lucifer Yellow backfilling of the connective combined with an immunocytochemical staining. This study revealed GABA-immunoreactive descending neurons originating in the SOG. We could not demonstrate GABA-immunoreactivity in the larger, descending neurons of the brain. Insect thoracic and abdominal ganglia are known to contain the essential neural circuits for behavioral subroutines like flight, walking, jumping, stridulation, ventilation, oviposition, etc. (6). In bees, one can commonly observe that the transsection of the ventral nerve chord leads to antenna- and head-cleaning movements of the legs. It is likely that in intact animals the expression of these and other behavioral patterns are under inhibitory control of the brain. This inhibitory control could either be mediated by excitatory descending neurons activating thoracic inhibitory circuits or more directly by inhibitory descending GABA-immunoreactive neurons.

CONCLUSIONS

Classical neuroanatomy has generated a massive amount of data about the organization of the bee brain in its neuropilar compartments. Studies with antibodies to transmitter and transmitter enzymes provide information about possible neurotransmitters within specific anatomical pathways. In addition, immunocytochemistry can reveal the morphology and some biochemical pathways expressed in a single particular neuron. Thus this method is a powerful chemoanatomical approach allowing us to elaborate neuronal circuits and assemblies with known chemical components. Even though immunocytochemistry of the bee's brain is in its infancy, it has already disclosed so far unknown anatomical pathways. It has delineated common projection areas of neurons with different transmitter phenotypes, serial homologies at the single cell level and possible homologies between bee and locust neurons. The localization of a classical transmitter which is thought to open chloride channels (GABA), provided clues for interpreting inhibitory anatomical connections. The distribution of immunoreactivity in an insect brain suggests that GABAergic pathways predominantly mediate local interactions whereas serotonergic pathways may influence synaptic transmission across large neuropilar areas. As with all approaches that try to unravel the brain of the bee, the strength of chemoanatomy lies in its thoughtful application in conjunction with other convergent methods.

Acknowledgments. We thank T.G. Kingan, J.G. Hildebrand, and W. Oertel for generously providing us with antisera prepared and characterized in their laboratories; and S. Schaare for photographic assistance.

REFERENCES

(1) Arnold, G.; Masson, C.; and Budharugsa, S. 1985. Comparative study of the antennal lobes and their afferent pathway in the worker bee and the drone (Apis mellifera). Cell Tissue Res 242: 593-605.

(2) Bicker, G.; Schäfer, S.; and Kingan, T.G. 1985. Mushroom body feedback interneurones in the honeybee show GABA-like immunoreactivity. Brain Res 360: 394-397.

(3) Björklund, A., and Hökfelt, T. (eds.) 1984. Handbook of Chemical Neuroanatomy. Vol.II,III Amsterdam: Elsevier Science Publications.

(4) Bullock, T.H., and Horridge, G.A. 1965. Structure and function in the nervous system of invertebrates, Vol. II. San Francisco: Freeman

(5) Callec, J.J. 1974. Synaptic transmission in the central nervous system of insects. In Insect Neurobiology, ed. J.E. Treherne, pp. 119-185. Amsterdam: Elsevier Science Publishers.

(6) Delcomyn, F. 1980. Neural basis of rhythmic behavior in animals. Science 210: 492-498.

(7) Dujardin, T. 1850. Mémoire sur le système nerveaux des insects. Ann. Sci. Nat B 14: 195-206.

(8) Emson, P.C.; Burrows, M.; and Fonnum, F. 1974. Levels of glutamate decarboxylase, acetyltransferase, and acetylcholine esterase in identified motor neurons of the locust. J. Neurobiol. 5: 33-42.

(9) Erber, J., and Homberg, U. 1986. Neurophysiology of the bee brain. In this volume.

(10) Falck, B.; Hillarp, N.A.; Thieme, G.; and Torp, A. 1962. Fluorescence of catecholamines and related compounds condensed with formaldehyde. J Histochem Cytochem 10: 348-354.

(11) Fox, P.M., and Larsen, J.R. 1972. Glutamic acid decarboxylase and the GABA shunt in the supraesophageal ganglion of the honeybee, Apis mellifera. J Insect Physiol 18: 439-457.

(12) Frisch, K.v. 1967. The Dance Language and Orientation of Bees. Cambridge, Mass: Harvard University Press.

(13) Frontali, N. 1964. Brain glutamic acid decarboxylase and synthesis of GABA in vertebrate and invertebrate species. In Comparative Neurochemistry, ed. D. Richter, pp. 185-192. Oxford: Pergamon Press.

(14) Gaide, M. 1983. Die Projektionen des Labial- und Maxillarnerven im Unterschlundganglion der Biene. Diplomarbeit, Freie Universität, Berlin.

(15) Goodman, L.J. 1981. Organization and physiology of the insect dorsal ocellar system. In Handbook of Sensory Physiology, Vol. VII/6C, ed. H. Autrum, pp. 201-286. Berlin, Heidelberg: Springer-Verlag.

(16) Goodman, L.J. 1986. Motion sensitive descending interneurons, ocellar L_D neurons and neck motoneurons in the bee: A neural substrate for visual course control in Apis mellifera. In this volume.

(17) Hertel, H., and Maronde U. 1986. In this volume.

(18) Homberg, U. 1984. Processing of antennal information in extrinsic mushroom body neurons in the bee brain. J. Comp. Physiol. A. 154: 825-836.

(19) Homberg, U. 1985. Interneurons of the central complex in the bee brain (Apis mellifera, L.). J. Insect Physiol. 31(3): 251-264.

(20) Homberg, U., and Erber, J. 1979. Response characteristics and identification of extrinsic mushroom body neurons in the bee. Z. Naturforsch. 34c: 612-615.

(21) Jawlowski, H. 1957. Nerve tracts in bee (Apis mellifica) running from the light and antennal organs to the brain. Annales Univ. Mariae Curie-Sklodowska Lublin (D). XII/22: 307-323.

(22) Jonescu, C.n. 1909. Vergleichende Untersuchungen über das Gehirn der Honigbiene. Z. Naturwiss. 45: 11-180.

(23) Kenyon, F.G. 1896. The brain of the bee. A preliminary contribution to the nervous system of the Arthropoda. J. Comp. Neurol. 6: 133-210.

(24) Kerkut, G.A.; Pitman, R.M.; and Walker, R.J. 1969. Sensitivity of neurones of the insect central nervous system to iontophorectically applied acetylcholine or GABA. Nature 222: 1075-1076.

(25) Klemm, N. 1976. Histochemistry of putative transmitter substances in the insect brain. Prog. Neurobiol. 7: 99-167.

(26) Masson, C. 1982. Basic mechanisms of sensory antennal information processing in insects, with special reference to social insects. In The Biology of Social Insects, eds. M.D. Breed, C.D. Michener, and H.E. Evans. pp. 380-384 Boulder, Colorado: Westview Press.

(27) Menzel, R. 1983. Neurobiology of learning and memory: the honey bee as a model system. Naturwiss. 70: 504-511.

(28) Mercer, A.R. 1986. Biogenic amines in the bee brain. In this volume.

(29) Mercer, A.R., and Menzel, R. 1982. The effects of biogenic amines on conditioned and unconditioned responses to olfactory stimuli in the honeybee (Apis mellifera). J. Comp. Physiol. 145: 363-368.

(30) Mercer, A.; Mobbs, P.; Davenport, A.P.; and Evans, P.D. 1983. Biogenic amines in the brain of the honeybee (Apis mellifera). Cell Tissue Res 234: 655-677.

(31) Meyer, E.P.; Matute, C.; Streit, P.; and Nässel, D.R. 1986. Insect optic lobe neurons identifiable with monoclonal antibodies to GABA. Histochem 84: 207-216.

(32) Mobbs, P.G. 1982. The brain of the honeybee Apis mellifera. I. The connections and spatial organization of the mushroom bodies. Phil. Trans. R. Soc. (B) 298: 309-354.

(33) Mobbs, P.G. 1984. Neural networks in the mushroom bodies of the honeybee. J. Insect Physiol. 30(1): 43-58.

(34) Nässel, D.R.; Meyer, E.P.; and Klemm, N. 1985. Mapping the ultrastructure of serotonin-immunoreactive neurons in the optic lobes of three insect species. J. Comp. Neurol. 232: 190-204.

(35) Nässel, D.R., and Elekes, K. 1985. Serotonergic terminals in the neural sheath of the blowfly nervous system: electron microscopical immunocytochemistry and 5,7-dihydroxytryptamine labelling. Neuroscience 15: 293-307.

(36) Noble, M., and Goodman, L.J. Immunohistochemical localization of gastrin/CCK-like peptide in the brain of the honeybee. In this volume.

(37) Oertel, W.H.; Schmechel, D.E.; Mugnaini, E.; Tappaz, M.L.; and Kopin, I.J. 1981. Immunocytochemical localization of glutamate decarbxylase in rat cerebellum with a new antiserum. Neuroscience 6: 2715-2735.

(38) Pareto, A. 1972. Die zentrale Verteilung der Fühlerafferenzen bei Arbeiterinnen der Honigbiene, Apis mellifera L. Z. Zellforsch. 131: 109-140.

(39) Rehder, V.; Bicker, G.; and Hammer, M. 1986. Serotonin-immunoreactive neurons in the antennal lobes and suboesophageal ganglion of the honeybee. Cell Tissue Res., in press.

(40) Ribi, W.A. 1975. The neurons of the first optic ganglion of the bee (Apis mellifera). Adv. Anat. Embryol. Cell. Biol. 50(4): 1-43.

(41) Ribi, W.A. 1986. In this volume.

(42) Ribi, W.A., and Scheel, M. 1981. The second and third optic ganglia in the worker bee. Golgi studies of the neuronal elements in the medulla and lobula. Cell Tissue Res. 221: 17-43.

(43) Schäfer, S., and Bicker, G. 1986. Distribution of GABA-like immunoreactivity in the brain of the honeybee. J. Comp. Neurol. 246: 287-300.

(44) Schäfer, S., and Bicker, G. 1987. Common projection areas of 5-HT- and GABA-like immunoreactive fibers in the visual system of the honeybee. Brain Res., in press.

(45) Scheidler, A.; Kaulen, P.; Brüning, G.; and Erber, J. 1986. Autoradiographic localization of octopamine and serotonin binding sites in the brain of the honeybee (Apis mellifera L.). Verh. Dtsch. Zool. Ges. 79: in press.

(46) Schürmann, F.W. 1974. Bemerkungen zur Funktion der Corpora Pedunculata im Gehirn der Insekten aus morphologischer Sicht. Exp. Brain Res. 19: 406-432.

(47) Schürmann, F.W., and Elekes, K. Synaptic connectivity in the mushroom bodies of the honeybee brain: Electron microscopy and immunocytochemistry of neuroactive compounds. In this volume.

(48) Schürmann, F.W., and Klemm, N. 1984. Serotonin-immunoreactive neurons in the brain of the honeybee. J. Comp. Neurol. 225: 570-580.

(49) Storm-Mathisen, J.; Leknes, A.K.; Bore, A.T.; Vaaland, J.L.; Edminson, P.; Haug, F.S.; and Ottersen, O.P. 1983. First visualization of glutamate and GABA in neurons by immunocytochemistry. Nature 301: 517-520.

(50) Strausfeld N.J., and Bacon, J.P. 1983. Multimodal convergence in the central nervous system of dipterous insects. Fortschritte der Zoologie 28: 47-76.

(51) Snodgrass, R.E. 1956. The Anatomy of the Honeybee. Ithaca, NY: Comstock Publishing Associates.

(52) Suzuki, H. 1975. Antennal movements induced by odor and central projections of the antennal neurones in the honey bee. J. Insect Physiol. 6: 168-179.

(53) Tyrer, N.M.; Turner, J.D.; and Altman, J.S. 1984. Identifiable neurons in the Locust central nervous system that react with antibodies to serotonin. J. Comp. Neurol. 227: 313-330.

(54) Vowles, D.M. 1955. The structure and connection of the corpora pedunculata in bees and ants. Quart. J. micr. Sci. 96: 239-255.

(55) Witthöft, W. 1967. Absolute Anzahl und Verteilung der Zellen im Hirn der Honigbiene. Z. Morphol. Tiere 61:160-184.

Synaptic Connectivity in the Mushroom Bodies of the Honeybee Brain: Electron Microscopy and Immunocytochemistry of Neuroactive Compounds

Friedrich-Wilhelm Schürmann[1] and Karoly Elekes[2]

[1]Abteilung für Zellbiologie, Universität Göttingen, 3400 Göttingen, FRG

[2]Universität Konstanz, Konstanz, FRG

Abstract. Detailed morphological studies of the mushroom bodies in the brain of the worker honeybee, Apis mellifera, have led to a ground plan of their architecture and synaptic connectivity. Modern immunocytochemical studies of neuroactive compounds (serotonin, dopamine, GABA) reveal new fine details of the compartmentalization of the mushroom bodies not previously detectable. Putative transmitters can be associated with complex local synaptic circuits by immuno-electron microscopy. Functional models of the bee mushroom bodies based on morphology can be complemented and revised.

INTRODUCTION

The highly complex behavior of social insects and especially that of bees has been regarded as closely related to special structural design and equipment of sense organs and brains ever since the work of von Frisch (5). The modern neurobiological approach tries to understand behavior as being causally determined by structure and function of single neurons and restricted neural networks. Experimental studies (3, 8) have pinpointed the large mushroom bodies (MB) in the brain of worker bees as an important site for learning and memory.

Modern functional neuroanatomy can depict fine details of neurons, networks and their design not yet accessible by physiological approaches. Analysis of the fine structure, geometry and connectivity of the MB supplies a structural framework which governs their functional potential and operations. Hypotheses and models on MB functions derived from its structures (10, 14, 20) have influenced physiological approaches and have only been partially tested (4, 17). The structure of the MB in the bee brain has been well documented (17). The paired mushroom bodies (corpora pedunculata) consist of thousands of Kenyon cells which send their fine T-shaped fibres through the calyces and peduncles to the top of the alpha- and beta-lobes. The parallel arrangement of these intrinsic fibres forms the characteristic MB shape (Fig. 1). Extrinsic neurons connect the MB to various brain areas. Intrinsic and extrinsic elements compose distinct subcompartments (10, 14) (Fig. 1). Though structural peculiarities of bee MB are obvious, substantial evidence for fundamental functional differences between the MB of bees and those of other insect groups are at present not available.

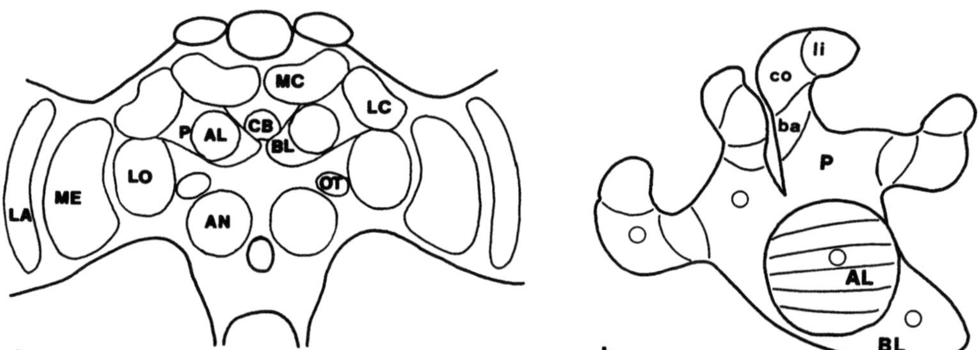

a b

Fig. 1 - a. Scheme of the bee brain with main glomerular neuropil areas, frontal view. AL = alpha -lobe, BL = beta-lobe, LC = lateral calyx, MC = medial calyx, P = peduncle of the mushroom bodies, CB = central body, OT = anterior optic tubercle, AN = antennal lobe, OL = optic lobe, LA = lamina, ME = medulla, LO = lobula. b. Scheme of one corpus pedunculatum, with subcompartments, li = lip, co = collar, ba = basal ring of the calyces, P = peduncle, AL = alpha-lobe, BL = beta-lobe. Vertical lines denote the subcompartmental layers of the AL. Circles mark samples taken for immuno-electron microscopy.

SYNAPSES AND SYNAPTIC CONNECTIVITY IN THE MUSHROOM BODIES

Studies on the synaptic fine structure of the central nervous system of bees using conventional electron microscopy have well established that the chemical synapse is asymmetric by its specific intracellular paramembranous appositions (presynaptic figures and subsynaptic web) (15). Examination of the bee MB synapses revealed a presynaptic grid of hexagonally arranged bars guiding the access of vesicles to the presynaptic membrane, surprisingly similar to the vertebrate synapse (13). Thus, the possible flow of information can be read from the polarized synaptic structure and incorporated in MB-models.

Electron microscopy of synapses combined with the analysis of position, shape and order of intrinsic and extrinsic MB neurons allowed the setting up of some general qualitative statements on input, output and crosstalk within the MB of the bee and some other selected species (14). Here, only some structural features of these studies which have been valid for functional approaches and interpretations are reported.

The MB-system receives its main inputs from a number of extrinsic sources converging into the calyces; its output sites are predominantly in the alpha- and beta-lobes by extrinsic elements, the targets of which are largely unknown. Input and output sites are located far apart and thus accessible to experimental investigation. Reciprocal chemical synapses in the stalk of worker mushroom bodies have been tentatively suggested as one substrate for crosstalk between parallel running intrinsic fibres (13). The concept of precise sequentially ordered interaction sites for parallel processing channels represents an important step enforcing a sophisticated view of modulating or changing activities between the input and output of the MB-system. Moreover, the evolutionary trend of augmentation of Kenyon cells - so predominant in bees and other social insects - could hardly be understood if it were not for refinement of information processing in intrinsic channels.

The extrinsic calycal inputs - convergent from different brain regions - convey their multisensory information in a divergent mode to dendrites of intrinsic elements which converge on output fibres in the lobes. The separation of input and output shown by micromorphology is consistent with latency differences observed in electrophysiological recordings from the calyces and lobes (4). Moreover, the mode of synaptic connectivity of a relatively small number of extrinsic input and output elements with abundant channels of intrinsic cells has led us to assume signal amplification and enhancement of signal to noise ratio by the MB-system (14) and was found in some output neurons (12).

The precise spatial alignment of extrinsic dendrites forming narrow bands arranged perpendicularly to the intrinsic parallel fibre groups is especially obvious in the MB of bees, and has been described as a structural analogue to the vertebrate cerebellum. Therefore, our hypothesis is that the MB would be especially well suited for the transposition of spatial distances into precise temporal sequences of inhibition and/or activity patterns (14). We have suggested the intrinsic fibres to be one element in a time delay line. This hypothesis was later substantially expanded by the studies of Mobbs (10) and does not conflict with electrophysiological observations. It is attractive because the suggested model is still the only one taking the special columnar structure of the MB of bees and other insects into consideration.

Complete stains of single extrinsic neurons of the MB in bees (6) and crickets (12) compared with other brain interneurons and descending nerve cells, combined with recordings after natural stimuli, corroborate the idea of parallel processing of sensory information in the central brain via a number of pathways in different neuropil areas before descending brain neurons are addressed (16, 17). We have emphasized that the MB could represent one, slow processing element in a long loop system composed of a chain of interneurons. If this long loop system is to be separated from fast, simply organized pathways to descending neurons by its time-delay features, it might be chosen for evaluating fine adjusted information flow.

CHEMONEUROANATOMY OF THE MUSHROOM BODIES

Biochemical, cytochemical and histochemical studies give valuable complementary information on the compartmentalization of MB and their chemical composition in comparison to other brain regions. Putative neuroactive compounds such as dopamine, noradrenaline, serotonin, octopamine, GABA and actylcholine have either been demonstrated for the bee MB (9) or have to be assumed (17). The non-random distribution of putative neurotransmitters is best shown by the high resolution immunocytochemical techniques. We found serotonin attributed to extrinsic fibres in two stalk compartments and the lobe compartments (Fig. 2a, b) but essentially lacking in the calyces (18). Dopamine-like immunoreactivity (Fig. 2c, d, e) is found in the calycal lips and collars but seems to be lacking in basal ring neuropil. Dopamine distribution in the stalks and lobes partially overlaps with 5-HT fibres. GABA-antibody stains (1) mark so-called feed-back neurons of the

Fig. 2 - Apis mellifera distribution of neuroactive compounds in the mushroom bodies, immunoreactive stains with the peroxidase-antiperoxidase reaction.

(a) Serotonin-like immunoreactivity, note differential staining in the pedunculus (P) and beta-lobes (BL), calyces (CA) free of immunoreactivity. Strong immunoreactivity in fibres with variable fine morphology of the central body (CB) and in nonglomerular neuropil, frontal section. Scale 100 um.

(b) Serotonin-like immunoreactivity in the alpha-lobe (AL) layers, arrowheads mark a ventral layer with strong immunoreactivity, frontal section. Scale 100 um.

(c) Dopamine-like immunoreactivity. Staining in the calycal collar (stars) and lip (li), the basal ring (triangles) appears unstained, horizontal section. Scale 100 um.

(d) Dopamine-like immunoreactivity, frontal section. Blebbed fibres in the calycal collar. Scale 20 um.

(e) Dopamine-like immunoreactivity, frontal section. Immunoreactive fine dots (arrowheads) in a stratum of the P upper peduncle, frontal section. Scale 100 um.

(f) GABA-like immunoreactivity. Immunoreactive blebs and boutons in all calyx compartments, KC = Kenyon cells, P = peduncle, frontal section.

(g) GABA-like immunoreactivity. Immunoreactivity in the calyx and alpha-lobe (stars), stained fibres (arrows) represent PCT-fibres, frontal section. Scale 100 um.

(h) GABA-like immunoreactivity. Immunoreactive boutons of the calyx collar. Scale 20 um.

Fig. 3 - Apis mellifera, mushroom bodies, immuno-electron microscopy of neuroactive compounds in the mushroom bodies.

(a) Serotonin-like immunoreactivity in a fibre with presynaptic (arrow) and postsynaptic sites, unstained fibres with presynaptic figures (arrowhead), peduncle of mushroom bodies. Scale 0.5 um.

(b)&
(c) Dopamine-like immunoreactivity in fine fibres (asterisks) with synaptic vesicles and presynaptic sites (arrows), presynaptic figures (arrowheads) in unstained fibres which occasionally synapse with immunoreactive elements, upper peduncle of mushroom body. Scale 0.5 um.

(d) GABA-like immunoreactivity. Calyx collar with stained extrinsic presynaptic elements (triangles), which can be presynaptic to unstained extrinsic boutons and/or fine intrinsic fibre dendrites. Scale 2 um.

(e) GABA-like immunoreactivity. Same area as in d., Immunoreactive fibre with presynaptic site (arrow) adjacent to an extrinsic bouton (star) with presynaptic vesicles. Scale 1 um.

(f) GABA-like immunoreactivity. Immunoreactive fibre with presynaptic site (arrow), dorsal alpha-lobe. Scale 0.25 um.

(g) GABA-like immunoreactivity. Immunoreactive PCT-fibre, postsynaptic to several small unstained fibres with presynaptic sites (arrowheads), median alpha-lobe. Scale 0.25 um.

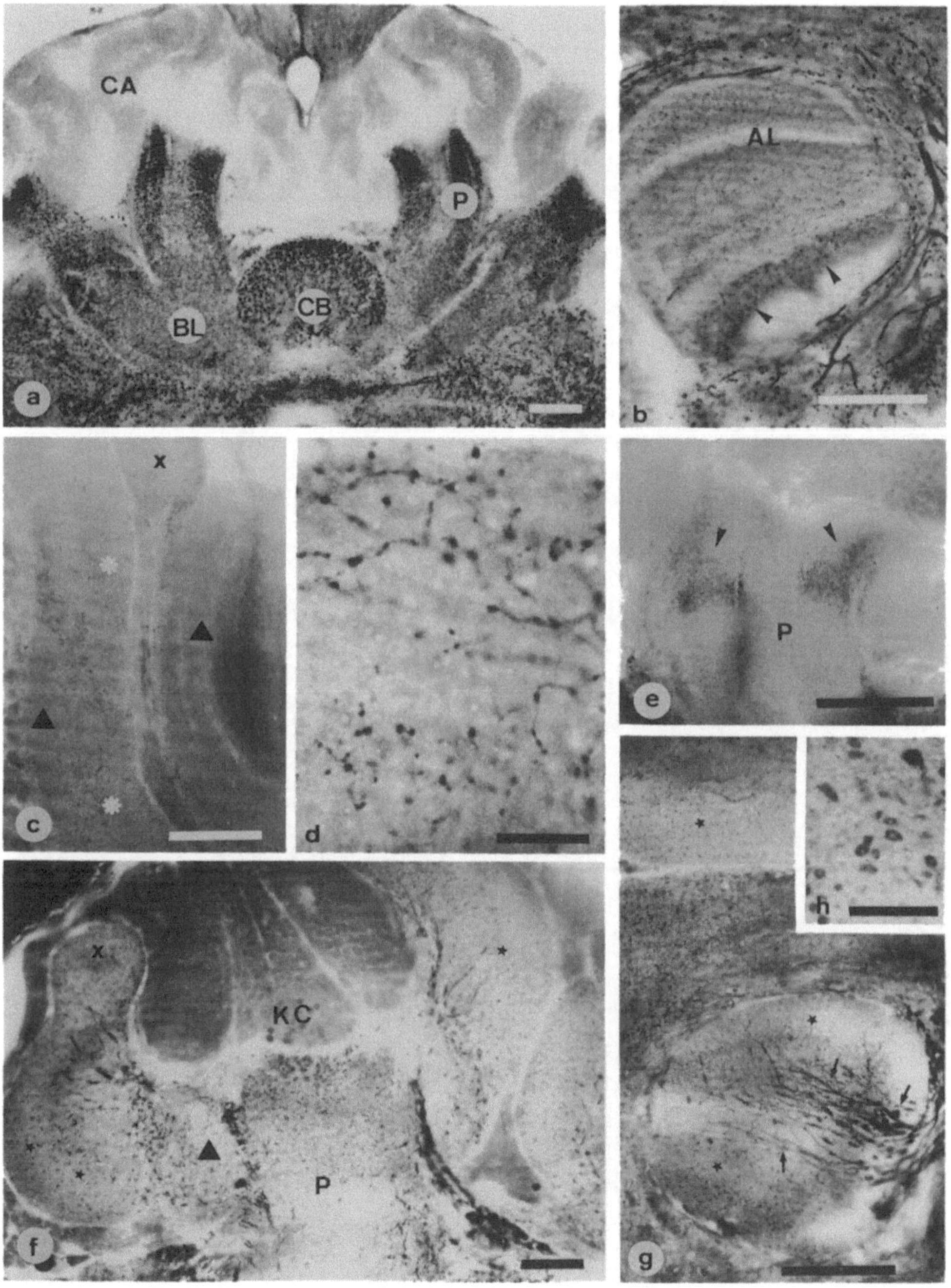

Fig. 2

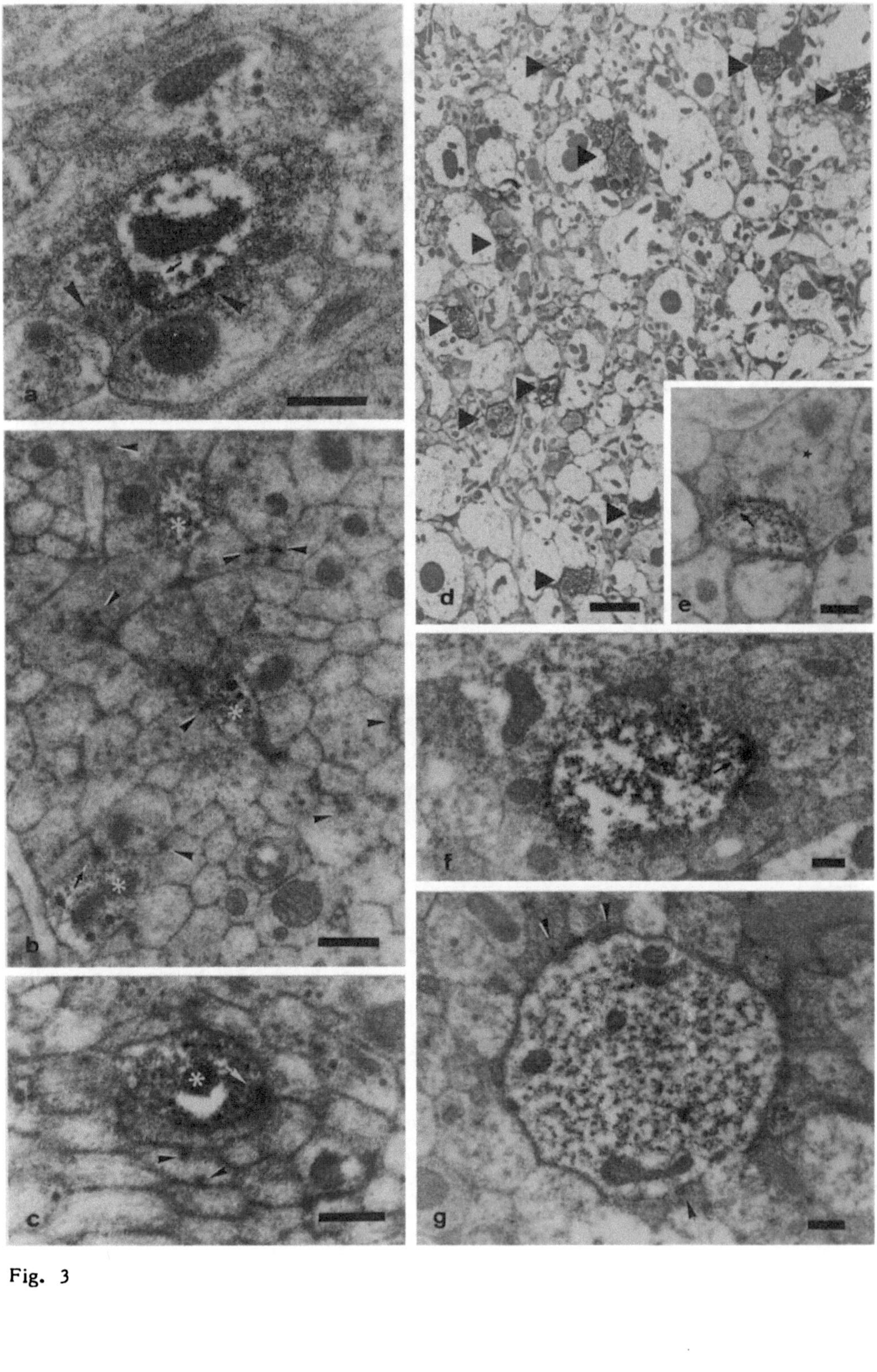

Fig. 3

protocerebral-calycal tract (PCT) connecting the calyces and the lobes (Fig. 2f, g, h). Bicker et al. (1) report a tracing of these neurons to four dorsal alpha-lobe layers and depict immunoreactivity in the calycal zones. We detected stained boutons in all the three calyx compartments and fibres in the alpha- and beta-lobes as well, stemming from the protocerebral-calycal tract, and corresponding to Mobbs (10) Golgi stains. GABA-like immunoreactivity in the ventral alpha-lobe could not be safely attributed to feedback neurons. If the ventral bands of the alpha-lobe (corresponding to the calycal lip neuropil of intrinsic fibres) are not invaded by PCT-neurons, then the marked GABA-boutons in the lip region could mean feed-back from different intrinsic fibre bundles (collar and basal ring intrinsic cells) or from PCT-connections outside the MB. Based on our immunocytochemical studies, the following points - important for functional assumptions in general - should be emphasized: 1) The micromorphology of 5-HT, dopamine, or GABA-containing fibres is neither uniform in the gross compartments of the bee MB nor in their smaller subcompartments. 2) Fibres with these neuroactive compounds partially overlap in the subcompartments. 3) All neuroactive substances indicated by immunocytochemistry are considered as extrinsic MB elements. The nature of transmitters in intrinsic cells so far remains unknown.

IMMUNO-ELECTRONMICROSCOPY OF THE MUSHROOM BODIES

Light microscopy of the distribution of putative transmitters is indispensable for the electron microscopy of synapses in chemically different fibres. We have chosen some samples for immuno-electronmicroscopy which we regard as selected windows into the complex MB-system. Nevertheless, we can offer some new details on synaptic wiring for discussion. All fibres containing 5-HT, dopamine or GABA show synaptic organelles suitable for synaptic modeling. Interestingly, we found marked presynaptic boutons indicating GABA or dopamine in the calyces. Putative GABA-ergic boutons seem to contact other extrinsic presynaptic boutons of different size and intrinsic dendrites as well (Fig. 3d, e). Therefore, in the bee MB, we do not only have simple microglomeruli with a divergent mode of synaptic connections, but also complex ones, as recently indicated (16). Complex glomeruli are often found in vertebrates (2, 19). We are confronted with complex interaction of extrinsic elements with at least two transmitters in one glomerulus, and with additional direct or indirect effects on intrinsic elements. The functional significance of these complex glomeruli, abundant in the calyces, is unknown. In the alpha- and beta-lobes (Fig. 3g) we found presynaptic sites in unstained fibres coupled to the putatively GABA-ergic PCT-fibres, which we attribute to intrinsic elements. Moreover, we detected presynaptic blebs of GABA-ergic elements in the lobes as well (Fig. 3f). This finding should not be considered contradictory to a feed-back mode of PCT-neurons but rather as further information on detailed functions of these specialized cells. We tentatively suggest functional separation (excitation or inhibition) of lobe subcompartments valid for the selection of intrinsic and extrinsic channels. Putative dopamine-containing fibres organized as a characteristic band in the MB stalk appear pre-and post-synaptic (Fig. 3b, c). 5-HT-fibres in the stalk and the lobes show pre- and postsynaptic sites in close vicinity (Fig. 3a) to each other and, therefore, appear to be suitable for local interaction of intrinsic and extrinsic cells, as stated for extrinsic elements in the MB-stalks of crickets (14). Pharmacological experiments with 5-HT should bring about an overall effect in the stalks and lobes and may probably be important to the output side of the MB and related brain parts. Our preliminary studies on the synaptic equipment of cells, defined by their transmitter candidates, do not yet cover all corners of the MB-system, but simplified views of synaptic circuitry can now be revised and the knowledge of potential interaction of fibre types completed.

CONCLUSIONS AND OUTLOOK

A number of recent investigations by both morphologists and physiologists trying to riddle the mushroom body problem have supplied some interesting results, especially on the MB of bees, thus contributing to a mosaic-like knowledge. Many of the structural and physiological features are not unique to the MB but can be attributed to single neurons or neuronal networks of brain areas and other ganglia. The special characteristics of the MB are possibly due to the combination of accumulated features. If the MB are understood as a specialized local brain center which can be best hypothesized from their structure, then their specific functional roles have to be unraveled by systematic comparative description of the functions of the differentially designed surrounding brain neuropils. Clear cut comparisons based on delicate electrophysiology have not yet been performed. From a morphological standpoint, we have stated that the MB represent one station in a long loop for elaborate processing of sensory information among a multitude of central sensory pathways involving most parts of the central brain before descending brain cells can be modulated (7, 16). Subsequent comparative research on these mutually competing pathways in relation to brain output neurons will be rewarding.

The multitude of MB cell types in the bee (5 intrinisic cell types, more than 10 extrinsic tracts and many solitary extrinsic cell types) divide the MB into subcompartments (10) which are not fully described at the light microscopical level. In accordance with structural complexity, the existence of at least six neuroactive substances in the mushroom bodies of bees implicates a variety of combinations in synaptic connectivity which await further description; first, mainly by electron microscopy and immunocytochemistry. Simplified, reduced views of synaptic nets - not excluding additional modes of connectivity (14, 17) - will now be substantially extended through new data gained by advanced morphological techniques. Using immuno-electron microscopy, we have detected a number of synaptic combinations, including synaptic contact between extrinsic fibres which fit into the concept of microcircuits suggested for our studies on synapses in the MB (11). We emphasize that structural analysis of the MB interdependent with experimental approaches has stimulated the development of a number of useful models and hypotheses on the meaning of the MB. As investigations have taught us, in complex wiring there is still no way to focus on one model only. Considering that behavioral studies of the bee are well advanced, we expect progress especially in the bee MB research.

Acknowledgments. We thank Drs. J. Hildebrand and T. Kingan from Tuscon, Arizona and M. Geffard / Bordeaux for their gifts of antibodies. Supported by the DFG (Schu 374/8).

REFERENCES

(1) Bicker, G.; Schäfer, S.; and Kingan, T.G. 1985. Mushroom body feedback interneurons in the honey bee show GABA-like immunoreactivity. Brain Res. 360:397.

(2) Elekes, K., and Szabo, T. 1985. The mormyrid brain stem. III. Ultrastructure and synaptic organization of the medullary pacemaker nucleus. Neurosci. 15: 431-443.

(3) Erber, J. 1983. The search for neural correlates of learning in the honeybee. In Neuroethology and Behavioral Physiology, eds. F. Huber and H. Markl. Berlin, Heidelberg, New York: Springer-Verlag.

(4) Erber, J.; Homberg, U.; and Gronenberg, W. 1986. The functional roles of the mushroom bodies in insects. In Arthropod Brain: Its Evolution, Development, Structure, and Function, ed. A.P. Gupta. New York: John Wiley & Sons, in press.

(5) Frisch, K.v. 1965. Tanzsprache und Orientierung der Bienen. Berlin, Heidelberg, New York: Springer-Verlag.

(6) Homberg, U. 1984. Processing of antennal information in extrinsic mushroom body neurons of the bee brain. J. Comp. Physiol. A 154: 825-836.

(7) Hörner, M., and Gras, H. 1985. Physiological properties of some descending neurons in the cricket brain. Naturwiss. 72: 603.

(8) Menzel, R.; Erber, J.; and Masuhr, T. 1974. Learning and memory in the honeybee. In Experimental analysis of insect behaviour, ed. L. Barton Browne, pp. 195-217. Berlin: Springer-Verlag.

(9) Mercer, A.R.; Mobbs, P.G.; Davenport, A.P.; and Evans, P.D. 1983. Biogenic amines in the brain of the honeybee, Apis mellifera. Cell Tissue Res. 234: 655-677.

(10) Mobbs, P.G. 1982. The brain of the honeybee Apis mellifera. I. The connections and spatial organization of the mushroom bodies. Phil. Trans. R. Soc. 298: 309-354.

(11) Pearson, K.G. 1979. Local neurons and local interactions in the nervous systems of invertebrates. In The Neurosciences, Fourth Study Program, eds. F.O. Schmitt and F.G. Worden, pp. 145-157. Cambridge, Massachusetts, and London, England: The MIT Press.

(12) Schildberger, K. 1984. Multimodal interneurons in the cricket brain: properties of identified extrinsic mushroom body cells. J. Comp. Physiol. A 154: 71-79.

(13) Schürmann, F.W. 1971. Synaptic contacts of association fibers in the brain of the bee. Brain Res. 26: 169-176.

(14) Schürmann, F.W. 1974. Bemerkungen zur Funktion der Corpora pedunculata im Gehirn der Insekten aus morphologischer Sicht. Exp. Brain Res. 19: 406-432.

(15) Schürmann, F.W. 1980. Methods for special staining of synaptic sites. In Neuroanatomical Methods - Experimental Entomology. Vol. 1A, eds. N. J. Strausfeld and T.A. Miller, pp. 241-262. New York, Heidelberg, Berlin: Springer-Verlag.

(16) Schürmann, F.W. 1985. Aspekte neuronaler Verknüpfung im zentralen Hirn der Insekten. In Schriftenreihe der Westfälischen Wilhelms-Universität Münster, pp. 51-93, Neue Folge, Heft 4.

(17) Schürmann, F.W. 1986. The architecture of the mushroom bodies and related neuropils in the insect brain. In Arthropod Brain: Its Evolution, Development, Structure, and Functions, ed. A.P. Gupta. New York: John Wiley & Sons, in press.

(18) Schürmann, F.W., and Klemm, N. 1984. Serotonin-immunoreactive neurons in the brain of the honeybee. J. Comp. Neurol. 225: 570-580.

(19) Szentagothai, J. 1970. Glomerular synapses, complex synaptic arrangements, and their operational significance. In The Neurosciences, Second Study Program, ed. F.O. Schmitt, pp. 427-442. New York: The Rockefeller University Press.

(20) Vowles, D.M. 1955. The structure and connexions of the corpora pedunculata in bees and ants. Quart. J. Micros. Sc. 96(2): 239-255.

Immunohistochemical Localization of a Gastrin/CCK-like Peptide in the Brain of the Honeybee

Michael J. Noble and Lesley J. Goodman

School of Biological Sciences, Queen Mary College, Mile End Road, London E1 4NS, U K

Abstract. The characteristics and distribution of gastrin/CCK-like immunoreactivity in the brain of the honeybee are described. Gastrin/CCK-like immunofluorescence is localized in bands within the peduncular and lobular parts of the mushroom bodies and is also present in the central body. Additional immunoreactivity is demonstrated in the ocellar tracts, optic lobes, lateral protocerebrum and antennal lobes following in vivo pretreatment with colchicine. Immunoreactive cell bodies are present in the pars intercerebralis and anteromedial protocerebrum. These are also demonstrated using the peroxidase antiperoxidase (PAP) technique, but staining of neuropil is poor compared to that obtained by indirect immunofluorescence. Staining at the EM level revealed immunoreactivity in synaptic terminals. The sensitivity of the different immunohistochemical procedures used to localize gastrin/CCK-like immunoreactivity is discussed. In the mushroom bodies and central body, the pattern of immunoreactivity closely resembles the distribution of biogenic amines such as dopamine and serotonin, with which the peptide may be co-localized. This peptide could play a role in mediating or modulating neural transmission in the bee brain.

INTRODUCTION

Neuropeptides are widely distributed in the peripheral and central nervous systems of both vertebrates and invertebrates. Often, there are little or no alterations in the amino acid sequences of peptides in widely separated phylogenetic groups, and despite the enormous catalogue of peptides and their tissues of origin which now exists, there is always a fresh sense of intrigue when a familiar molecule is localized in a novel neuropil. This is particularly true for insects, in which a number of studies have localized vertebrate-like, as well as invertebrate-specific peptides in nervous and endocrine tissues. Peptides resembling mammalian gastrointestinal hormones such as insulin, pancreatic polypeptide, cholecystokinin (CCK), gastrin and somatostatin have been identified in dipteran, orthopteran and lepidopteran nervous systems (5, 6, 7, 11, 18). Groups of peptide-containing neuroendocrine cells are scattered throughout different regions in the brain, nerve cord and retrocerebral complex in the species examined. This has made analysis of peptide function difficult in all but a small number of examples (1, 5, 6). There is, however, evidence to suggest that similar molecules have comparable roles in different species (4, 5, 7).

The hymenopteran brain, and in particular, that of the honeybee, has received detailed attention from anatomists (15), physiologists (10) and neurochemists (14). These disciplines have been successfully combined in analysing the biological roles of biogenic monoamines in identified neuronal networks such as those of the mushroom bodies (12, 13). Detailed immunohistochemical studies have also mapped the distribution of serotonin-like (20) and gamma-amino butyric acid (GABA)-like immunoreactivity in bee brains (16, 20). Information about neuropeptides in the bee is scarce. We have screened a wide range of peptide antisera on honeybee brains and found large amounts of gastrin/CCK-like immunoreactivity in a number of central neuropils (16). Here, we discuss some important characteristics of the immunoreactivity and describe its anatomical distribution.

ANTIBODY SPECIFICITY AND IMMUNOHISTOCHEMICAL TECHNIQUES

The IgG fractions of polyclonal antisera which are widely used in immunohistochemical studies are known to have the potential for cross-reacting with tissue antigens resembling the original antigenic determinant (19). It is clear, therefore, that adsorption controls are only a first step in confidently identifying a particular molecular site demonstrated by immunohistochemistry. More cross-reactivity occurs as the size of the original antigen used to raise the antiserum increases, either by conjugation of the molecule of interest with a larger protein, or because the protein of interest is itself large. This is due not only to the greater number of antigenic determinants present, but also to the mobility of certain peptide sequences within protein molecules.

Short sequence peptide molecules which are just large enough to induce an immune response without requiring conjugation are likely to give rise to the most specific antibodies. However, this step or even the use of monoclonal antibodies, does not overcome all of the problems of cross-reactivity. Tissues may contain similar molecules which share peptide sequences but which have different biochemical roles. The expression of different peptide molecules may also vary from time to time within a single cell type (17), and the peptides can be derived from the same, or different precursor polypeptides. The peptides gastrin and CCK provide a good example of where the active part of the peptide sequence is shared by both molecules. These molecules have an identical COOH-terminal pentapeptide sequence recognized by the polyclonal antibody raised against CCK octapeptide (CCK-8) (6, 7). Other forms of CCK such as those with 12, 33 or 39 residues (4) and other gastrin-like molecules will also bind this antibody. The immunoreactivity obtained is, therefore, described as gastrin/CCK-like.

Four different procedures were used in the investigation of gastrin/CCK-like immunoreactivity in the bee brain. These were indirect immunofluorescence (21) with and

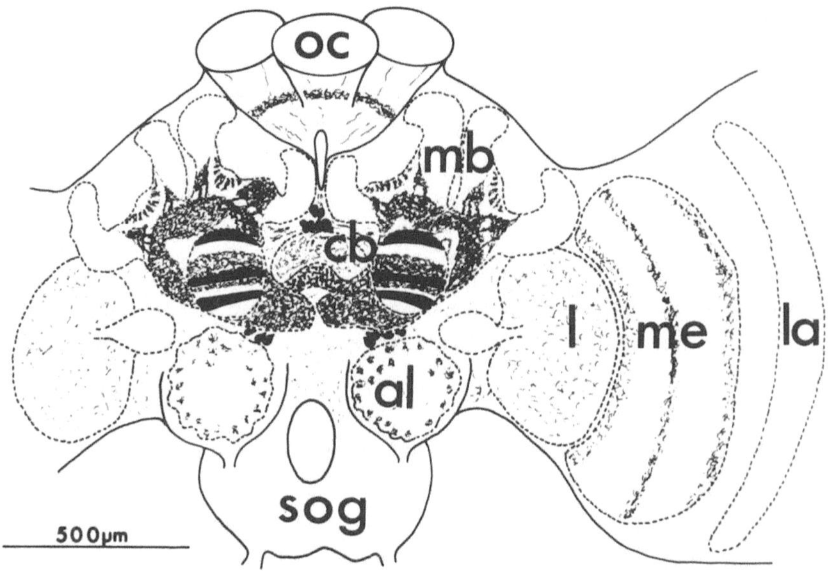

Fig. 1 - Distribution of gastrin/CCK-like immunoreactivity in the honeybee brain seen in frontal view. The density of shading reflects the intensity of immunofluorescence observed following pretreatment with colchicine. al = antennal lobe; cb = central body; l = lobula; la = lamina; me = medulla; mb = mushroom body; oc = ocelli; sog = sub-oesophageal ganglion.

without in vivo colchicine pretreatment, PAP histochemistry (5) and colloidal gold immunohistochemistry for EM analysis.

GASTRIN/CCK-LIKE IMMUNOREACTIVITY IN THE BRAIN OF THE WORKER BEE

Pattern of immunofluorescence

Large amounts of immunofluorescence are present within the mushroom bodies and central body. Specific fluorescence is not observed in controls, but tracheal autofluorescence is observed in all specimens. Immunofluorescence is first detectable midway through pupal development and is not present in adult drones. The mushroom body neuropil is divided into two dorsally-placed cup-shaped calyces connected by short, fused pedunculi to an anteriorly-projecting (alpha) and ventro-medially projecting (beta) lobe (15). The calyces are sites of relay fibre input to intrinsic interneurons (K-cells) each of which project single fibres into the lobes where synapses are made with extrinsic output or feedback neurons. The synaptic neuropil in the lobes is arranged into layers. The alpha lobes contain immunofluorescence arranged in horizontal bands (Fig. 1). The character of the immunofluorescence is homogenous in the bands but differs in intensity between bands. Eight bands are identified, three containing intense immunofluorescence, two moderate immunofluorescence and three no immunofluorescence. An identical banding pattern is seen in the beta lobes viewed in sagittal section. Pedunculi viewed in horizontal section contained rings of immunofluorescence which extend dorsally to the cone-shaped core of the calyces. No immunofluorescence is present in the lip, collar or basal ring zones of calycal neuropil, or in the columns of K-cell processes projecting into the pedunculi. No immunoreactive cell bodies are present.

The neuropil of the central body is divided into a dorso-posterior part and a ventro-anterior part. Large amounts of immunofluorescence are present in varicose fibres in the ventro-anterior part. Less intense immunofluorescence is also present in the dorso-posterior part.

The effect of colchicine pretreatment on the pattern of immunofluorescence

Pretreatment with colchicine increases the intensity of the immunofluorescence already described in the mushroom bodies and central body and unmasks gastrin/CCK-like immunofluorescence in other brain regions (Figs. 1 and 2). No specific fluorescence is observed in controls. Immunofluorescence is present in a group of seven cell bodies located on the anteromedial aspect of the brain. The primary neurites of these cells project towards the ventromedial aspect of the beta lobes. There is no immunofluorescence in the calycal neuropil. Eleven cell bodies lying dorsoposterior to the central body in the region of the pars intercerebralis also contain immunofluorescence. Processes from these neurons project into the undifferentiated neuropil of the proto- and deutocerebrum and are not seen to penetrate the neuropil of the mushroom bodies or central body. Fine plexuses of immunofluorescent fibres are distributed diffusely throughout the undifferentiated protocerebral neuropil. Weak homogenous immunofluorescence is present in the macroglomeruli of the antennal lobes. Immunofluorescence in the sub-oesophageal ganglion(SOG) and tritocerebrum is confined to a very small number of fine fibres.

Immunofluorescent fibres are present in the ocellar tracts. A small number of fibres running in the ocellar tract give rise to extensive arborisation in the sub-retinal ocellar plexus. No immunofluorescence is present in L-neurons or the ocellar retina. In the optic lobe, fine immunofluorescent fibres are present throughout the lobula and in three strata of the medulla, but not in the lamina, retina or anterior optic tubercule. No immunofluorescent cell bodies are observed in the optic lobes.

Immunoreactivity using the PAP technique

Large amounts of immunoreactivity are present in the two groups of cell bodies already described. Immunoreactivity in the mushroom body neuropil is also present in a pattern identical to that described above. No other areas contain immunoreactivity.

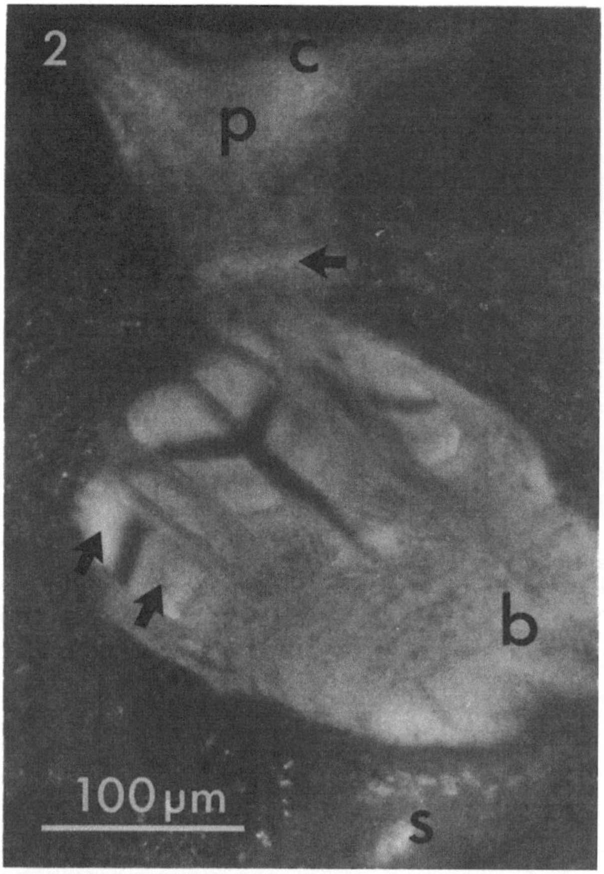

Fig. 2 - Vertical section of the brain at the level of the origin of the alpha and beta lobes of the right mushroom body. Horizontal bands of gastrin/CCK-like immunofluorescence of variable intensity are present at the distal end of the pedunculus and proximal part of the alpha lobe (arrows). One dark band containing no immunofluorescence is present near the dorsal margin of the alpha lobe root, and several are present running along the axis of K-cell projections. Immunofluorescence is present in the pedunculus (p) and extends into the core of the calyx (c). A fine plexus of varicose immunofluorescent fibres are present in the protocerebral neuropil ventro-lateral to the mushroom body. A small group of immunoreactive fibres of large diameter are located between the ventro-medial margin of the beta lobe (b) and a cell body (s). Cryostat section of a specimen fixed by immersion in paraformaldehyde and stained with the indirect immunofluorescence technique.

Ultrastructural localization of gastrin/CCK-like immunoreactivity

Electron dense reaction product confirmed as gold particles by EDAX is present in terminals in the alpha and beta lobes of the mushroom bodies and in the central body. Immunoreactivity is characteristically seen on accumulations of small vesicles (Fig. 3) and is never observed in terminals containing predominantly large, dense-cored vesicles. Immunoreactivity is also absent from inter-terminal segments of varicose fibres.

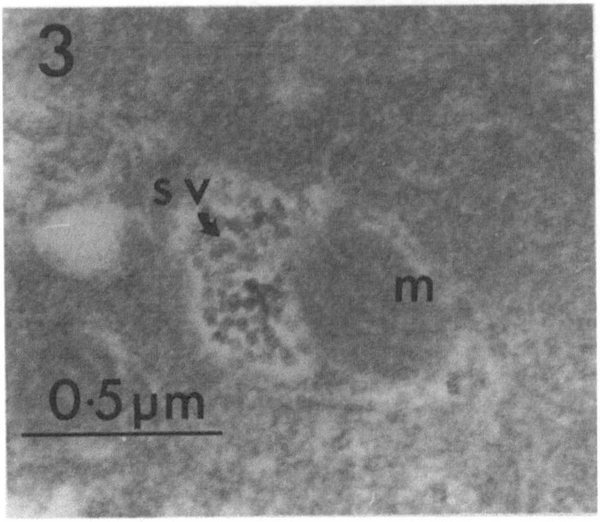

Fig. 3 - Gastrin/CCK-like immunoreactivity in a terminal in the ellipsoid part of the central body. Immunoreactivity is localized to small vesicles (sv). Mitochondrion, m. Ultrathin section of a resin-embedded specimen fixed by immersion with a glutaraldehyde: paraformaldehyde mixture and stained with a colloidal gold technique.

DISCUSSION

Techniques

Differences in patterns of immunoreactivity obtained by immunofluorescence, both with and without colchicine pretreatment, and PAP, are due to alterations of the distribution and character of antigenic sites following tissue fixations and preparation. Previous studies of the distribution of peptidergic neurons in insect tissues have relied mainly on the PAP method. Cell bodies and large neurites are stained consistently well using this technique but it is less useful than immunofluorescence for mapping immunoreactivity in neuropil. This does not seem to be the case with GABA-like immunoreactivity, the technique for which one requires glutaraldehyde that reduces specific immunofluorescence (16), or serotonin-like immunoreactivity. It is possible, therefore, that the efficacy of PAP staining for peptides is more dependent on preserved antigen concentration than previously recognized. The PAP technique is theoretically more sensitive than indirect immunofluorescence because of an additional antibody step, but this advantage can be offset by the more elaborate tissue fixation and processing involved. The property of fluorescence may also contribute to the high sensitivity of the immunofluorescence technique where small amounts of antigen are present in plexuses of very small fibres such as those of the mushroom bodies. It is unlikely that the honeybee is the only species with extensive plexuses of peptide containing fibres within central synaptic neuropil, and the future use of colchicine in immunohistochemical studies may help in identifying the location of other peptides in insect brains.

Gastrin/CCK-like peptide in the mushroom bodies and central body

Dopamine, octopamine, serotonin and GABA are neurotransmitters known to occur in high concentration in the mushroom bodies (14, 20, 21). Octopamine has been indirectly implicated as the transmitter used by K-cells, and dopamine, serotonin and GABA occur in mainly extrinsic neurons. The inter-connecting pathways within the mushroom bodies are known to be complex (14, 15) and extrinsic neurons to function as input, output and feedback routes. Transmitters in extrinsic neurons are likely, therefore, to be identified anywhere within mushroom body neuropil. These findings concur also with the distribution of gastrin/CCK-like immunoreactivity. The banding patterns in the pedunculi and lobes are characteristic of the arrangement of some plexuses of extrinsic mushroom body cells (15). The location of the anteromedial group of cell bodies with primary neurites projecting towards the beta exit point supports this hypothesis. The immunofluorescence properties of the calyces are unaffected by colchicine pretreatment. It is unlikely, therefore, that the patterns of immunoreactivity represent selective terminal localization of peptide in K-cells.

In the mushroom bodies and central body, the peptide is localized within terminals containing accumulations of small vesicles, around which immunoreactive product is concentrated. This evidence suggests that the peptide may play a role in neurotransmission, but the exact nature of this role is unclear. Peptidergic transmission (3), and proctolin cotransmission with L-glutamate (1) have both been postulated in invertebrates.

Gastrin/CCK-like peptide may also co-exist with monoamines or amino acids in the bee brain. Double labelling studies are required to determine such a relationship. CCK is present in aminergic neurons in the mammalian CNS (9) where it has been shown to modify the actions of both dopamine and glutamine. Neuronal pathways containing CCK are known to be involved in olfaction, feeding behavior and locomotion. In the bee, there is no information on the role of brain peptides. Monoaminergic pathways in the mushroom bodies of bees are known to be important in the control of olfactory-orientated behaviors (12, 13). The types of electrophysiological and behavioral paradigms used in these studies may be appropriate in analysing the role of this peptide in the mushroom bodies.

Gastrin/CCK-like peptide in other brain areas

The origins of peptide-containing fibres in other regions of the brain are less clear. It is possible that not all immunoreactive cell bodies have been identified. A large proportion of fibres are likely to be the fine arborisations of complex neuroendocrine cells originating in the pars intecerebralis or elsewhere in the brain (6, 7). Only the peptide-containing fibres in the ocelli have easily identifiable patterns of arborisation. These are likely to be the efferent processes of small ocellar neurons, the cell bodies of which may belong to the lateral members of the group of cell bodies lying dorsoposterior to the central complex (8). GABA-like immunoreactivity has also been demonstrated in this plexus (20). Efferent innervation of the lateral eyes of Limulus by aminergic and peptidergic neurons is well documented (2). It is unclear in the bee whether the peptidergic projections represent a connection between the ocellar tract and neuroendocrine system originating in the pars intercerebralis or are circuits involved in local control of ocellar function.

We feel that the gastrin/CCK-like peptide described here plays an important role in a number of neuronal pathways in the bee brain. To our knowledge, this is the first neuropeptide to be localized in the synaptic neuropil of the mushroom bodies and central body (16). Further characterization of the biochemical and physiological properties of the peptide are needed. There are likely to be other peptides present and the expression of these peptides may vary during the life of the animal. The importance of using a number of histochemical and analytical techniques when describing immunoreactive staining patterns is apparent.

Acknowledgements. We are very grateful to Dr. B. Walcott, S.U.N.Y. at Stony Brook for the use of facilities and antisera.

REFERENCES

(1) Adams, M.E., and O'Shea, M. 1983. Peptide cotransmitter at a neuromuscular junction. Science 221: 286-289.

(2) Batelle, B.A. 1984. Efferent innervation to Limulus eyes. T.I.N.S. 7: 277-281.

(3) Boer, H.H.; Schot, L.P.C.; Reichelt, D.; Brand, H.; and Maat, A. ter. 1984. Ultrastructural immunocytochemical evidence for peptidergic neurotransmission in the pond snail Lymnaea stagnalis. Cell Tiss. Res. 238: 197-201.

(4) Dockray, G.J. 1984. Cholecystokinin. In Brain Peptides, eds. D.T. Krieger, M.J. Brownstein and J.B. Martin, pp. 851-869. New York: John Wiley and Sons.

(5) Duve, H., and Thorpe, A. 1980. Localisation of pancreatic polypeptide (PP)-like immunoreactive material in neurons in the brain of the blowfly, Calliphora erythrocephala (Diptera). Cell Tiss. Res. 210: 101-109.

(6) Duve, H., and Thorpe, A. 1981. Gastrin/cholecystokinin (CCK)-like immunoreactive neurones in the brain of the blowfly, Calliphora erythrocephala (Diptera). Gen. Comp. Endocrinol 43: 381-391.

(7) Duve, H., and Thorpe, A. 1984. Immunocytochemical mapping of gastrin/CCK-like peptides in the neuroendocrine system of the blowfly, Calliphora vomitoria (Diptera). Cell Tiss. Res. 237: 309-320.

(8) Goodman, L.J. 1981. Organization and physiology of the insect dorsal ocellar system. In Handbook of Sensory Physiology, Volume VII/C6. Comparative Physiology and Evolution of Vision in Invertebrates, ed. H. Autrum, pp. 201-286. Berlin, Heidelberg, New York: Springer-Verlag.

(9) Hokfelt, T.; Skirbol, L.; Rehfeld, J.F.; Goldstein, M.; Morley, K.; and Dann, Q. 1980. A subpopulation of mesencephalic dopamine neurons projecting to limbic areas contains a cholecystokinin-like peptide. Evidence from immunohistochemistry combined with retrograde tracing. Neuroscience. 5: 1093-2124.

(10) Homberg, U., and Erber, J. 1979. Response characteristics and identification of extrinsic mushroom body neurons of the bee. Z. Naturforsch. 34c: 612-615.

(11) Lavenseau, L.; Gadenne, C.; and Trabelsi, M. 1984. Immunofluorescent localisation of a substance immunologically related to insulin in the protocerebral neurosecretory cells of the European corn borer. Cell Tiss. Res. 238: 207-208.

(12) Mercer, A.R., and Erber, J. 1983. The effects of amines on evoked potentials recorded in the mushroom bodies of the bee brain. J.Comp. Physiol. A. 151: 469-476.

(13) Mercer, A.R., and Menzel, R. 1982. The effects of biogenic amines on conditioned and unconditioned responses to olfactory stimuli in the honeybee. Apis mellifera. J. Comp. Physiol. A. 145: 363-368.

(14) Mercer, A.R.; Mobbs, P.G.; Davenport, A.P.; and Evans, P.D. 1983. Biogenic amines in the brain of the honeybee, Apis mellifera. Cell Tiss. Res. 234: 655-677.

(15) Mobbs, P.G. 1982. The brain of the honeybee, Apis mellifera. I. The connections and spatial organization of the mushroom bodies. Phil. Trans. Roy. Soc. B298: 309-354.

(16) Noble, M.J. 1985. Immunofluorescence studies on the brain of the honeybee, Apis mellifera. J. Anat. 140(3): 518-519.

(17) Petrics-Gesser, B., and Larsson, L.I. 1985. Changes from enkephalin-like to gastrin/cholecystokinin-like immunoreactivity in snail neurons. J. Neurosci. 5(6): 1412-1417.

(18) Romoef, M., and Remy, C. 1984. Early immunohistochemical detection of somatostatin-like and methionine-enkephalin-like neuropeptides in the brain of the migratory locust embryo. Cell Tissue Res. 236: 289-292.

(19) Schot, L.P.C.; Boer, H.H.; and Montagne-Wajer, C. 1984. Characterization of multiple immunoreactive neurons in the central nervous system of the pond snail Lymnaea stagnalis with different fixatives and antisera adsorbed with the homologous and the heterologous antigens. Histochem. 81: 373-378.

(20) Schafer, S., and Bicker, G. 1986. Distribution of GABA-like immunoreactivity in the brain of the honeybee. J. Comp. Neurol. 246: 287-300.

(21) Schürmann, F.W., and Klemm, N. 1984. Serotonin-immunoreactive fibres in the brain of the honeybee. J. Comp. Neurol. 225: 500-580.

Biogenic Amines and the Bee Brain

Alison Mercer
University of Otago, Department of Zoology, Box 56, Dunedin, New Zealand

Abstract. Dopamine, noradrenaline, 5-hydroxytryptamine (serotonin) and octopamine have been detected in the brain of the honeybee, Apis mellifera. Although the distribution of biogenic amines in the brain neuropil is well documented, the physiological functions of brain amines remain unclear. It is hoped that the coordinated multidisciplinary studies currently underway in the honeybee will help to reveal the functional roles played by biogenic amines in the insect brain.

INTRODUCTION

It has been 20 years since the first histochemical demonstration of catecholamine-containing neurones in the insect brain (11). Although there is a wealth of information available to us now on the quantities and cellular distribution of amines in the insect nervous system (7, 13), the functional roles of biogenic amines in the insect brain remain unclear. Evidence to suggest that amines function as neurotransmitters, neuromodulators, and neurohormones in insects is derived primarily from studies of the peripheral nervous system (2, 7, 8, 23). The central nervous system (CNS), less accessible to detailed neurophysiological analysis, has received much less attention. Functions of biogenic amines in the insect brain has been inferred largely from information on the cellular distribution of amines in specific regions of the brain neuropil. Such inferences are of limited value. Extrapolation of functional roles from anatomical data alone can be misleading (7). Furthermore, the distribution of neurones containing catecholamines and indolealkylamines in the insect brain varies from species to species (13). It is difficult, therefore, to extrapolate information about the possible physiological functions of biogenic amines in the insect brain from one species of insect to another. For this reason, studies aimed at elucidating the roles played by biogenic amines in the insect brain, and the mechanisms through which they operate, should focus on particular species of insects, but which insects do we focus upon, and how can the problems inherent in working with the CNS, in particular the insect brain, be overcome?

Evans (7) suggests that a multidisciplinary approach is required to provide insight into the roles of biogenic amines in the insect brain. Such an approach should prove fruitful for whatever species of insect is focused upon. The honeybee, however, is particularly well suited to such an investigation. The neuroanatomy of the bee brain is well understood (21, 22), and the distribution of biogenic amines in the brain of this insect well documented (12, 13, 18, 26). The role of biogenic amines in the control of behavior in the honeybee is of particular interest. The rich behavioral repertoire of the honeybee has excited a great deal of attention over the years, and the stereotyped nature of much of the bee's behavior makes this animal particularly accessible to analysis. Our extensive knowledge of the honeybee, its brain and behavior, provides an excellent basis for investigation of the physiological functions of biogenic amines in the brain of this insect.

Distribution of Biogenic Amines in the Bee Brain

The dye, neutral red, has been used to stain amine-containing cells in the insect nervous system (3, 9, 10, 20). The mechanism of staining is unclear, but several types of biogenic amine-containing neurones are known to take up the dye. In whole mounts of the bee brain treated with neutral red (Fig. 1), intense staining can be seen in cell bodies in and around the cup-shaped calyces of the mushroom bodies, and in the alpha-lobes of the mushroom body neuropil. Staining is also apparent at the boundary between the protocerebrum and deutocerebrum of the brain, and in the optic lobes. Some proctolin-containing cells in the insect nervous system, which have not yet been demonstrated to contain a biogenic amine, are reported to stain specifically with neutral red also (24). Staining is not selective for amine-containing neurones. Results obtained using neutral red staining techniques, therefore, must be supplemented with information from biochemical analyses of the brain tissue.

In the honeybee, octopamine (OA), dopamine (DA), noradrenaline (NA), and 5-hydroxytryptamine (5-HT, serotonin), have been detected in the brain using high performance liquid chromatography and radioenzymatic assay techniques (20, see Table 1). The levels of biogenic amines in the brain of the honeybee are very similar to those reported for the brain of the cockroach, Periplaneta americana, and the locust, Schistocerca gregaria (3, 10, 27). The cerebral ganglion (brain minus optic lobes), contains more DA than OA, approximately the same amounts of DA and 5-HT, and very low levels of NA. Adrenaline has not been detected in the brain of the honeybee, nor indeed conclusively, in any region of the insect nervous system (7). The cellular distribution of catecholamines (DA and NA) and indolalkylamine (5-HT) in the brain of the honeybee has been determined using fluorescence histochemistry techniques (12, 13, 18). After treatment with formaldehyde gas (12, 13), or glyoxylic acid (20), monoamine-containing neurones can be detected throughout the cerebral ganglion, concentrated in the highly structured central body and mushroom body neuropils (see Fig. 2). In the antennal lobes of the honeybee, slow fading green fluorescence typical of catecholamines is found in fibres restricted to the inner margins of the peripherally located 'olfactory glomeruli' (12, 13, 20; see Fig. 3), where sensory receptor inputs converge on

TABLE 1 - Biogenic amine content in the brain of the honeybee.

Brain Structure	Biogenic Amine			
	DA	NA	5-HT	OA
Cerebral ganglion	25.0	1.1	21.4	7.6
Optic lobes (per pair)	15.1	1.0	19.4	5.0
Retina	5.1	n.d.	3.1	0.2
Lamina	0.4	n.d.	1.4	0.5
Medulla	n.d.	n.d.	1.5	1.1
Lobula	0.3	0.3	2.6	0.5
Calyx	0.5	0.2	1.0	0.3
Alpha-lobe	0.9	0.2	3.3	1.3
Antennal lobe	0.8	n.d.	3.0	0.5

*Values are expressed as concentration in pmoles per structure. DA = dopamine, NA = noradrenaline, 5-HT = 5-hydroxytryptamine, OA = octopamine, n.d. = none detectable. Data reproduced from Mercer et al., 1983. Information concerning standard errors, number of observations, and detection methods used can be obtained from the original manuscript.

intrinsic interneurones and on extrinsic fibres that project to the calyces of the mushroom bodies in the protocerebrum of the brain (25, 29). In the visual ganglia, yellow fluorescence that fades rapidly under excitation light is found after treatment with glyoxylic acid (20; see Fig. 4). Such fluorescence is characteristic of the fluorophore derived from the indolalkylamine, 5-HT. 5-HT-immunoreactive fibres have been detected recently in the optic lobes of the honeybee using immunocytochemical staining techniques (26, see Fig. 4b, see Bicker et al. this volume).

Brain Activity, Behavior and Biogenic Amines

OA has a marked effect on the input of visual information to the mushroom bodies of the bee brain. Iontophoretic application of octopamine to the optic lobes, for example, causes rapid and long-term enhancement of light-evoked potentials recorded in the alpha-lobes of the mushroom body neuropil (18). OA has been detected in all regions of the optic lobes in the bee (20). As in the cockroach and the locust (10), amounts of OA present in the visual ganglia are highest in the medulla (see Table 1). Evans suggests that OA in the medulla of the locust may be involved in central modulation of activity in the locust visual system (7, 8). Although the evidence of a central modulatory role for OA in the locust is limited at present, there is good evidence that OA functions as a neuromodulator in the peripheral nervous system of this insect (7, 8). OA injected into the protocerebrum of the bee brain enhances the bee's

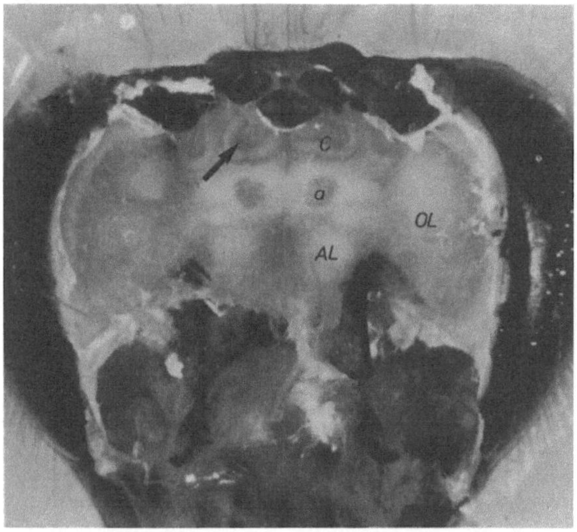

Fig. 1 - The brain of the honeybee stained with neutral red. Staining is intense in cell bodies in and around the calyces (c) of the mushroom bodies (arrow) and in the alpha-lobes (a) of the mushroom body neuropil. Staining is also apparent in the optic lobes (OL), and between the deutocerebrum, which includes the antennal lobes (AL), and protocerebrum of the brain.

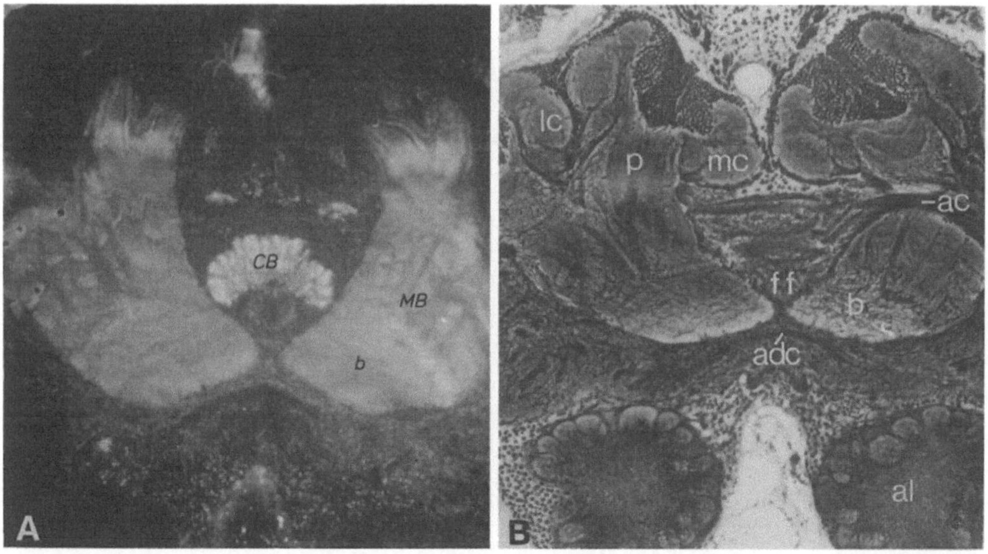

Fig. 2 - A. Vertical section showing intense fluorescence in the highly structurd neuropils of the mushroom bodies (MB) and central body (CB) in the protocerebrum of the bee brain after treatment with glyoxylic acid. B. Normal histological section stained with protargol included for orientation purposes. ac = anterior commissure, adc = anterior deutocerebral commissure, al = antennal lobe, CB = central body, ff = frontal flange of central body, lc = lateral calyx of mushroom body, MB = mushroom body, mc = median calyx of mushroom body, p = pedunculus.

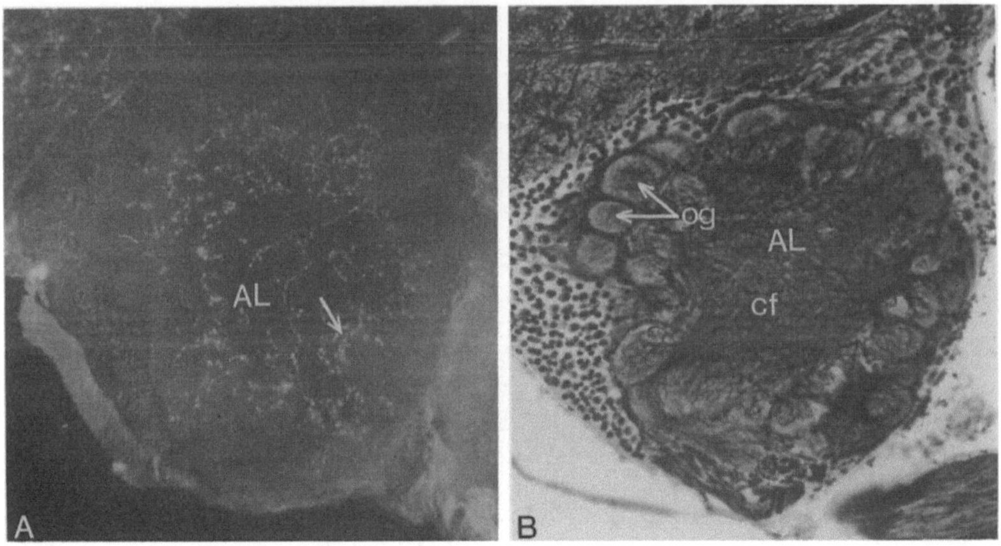

Fig. 3 - A. Distribution of catecholamine containing neurones in the antennal lobe (AL) of the bee brain. After treatment with glyoxylic acid, intense green fluorescence (arrow) is apparent in fibres that project along the inner margins of the peripherally located 'olfactory glomeruli' (og). B. A normal histological section stained with protagol included for orientation purposes. cf = central feltwork of the antennal lobe.

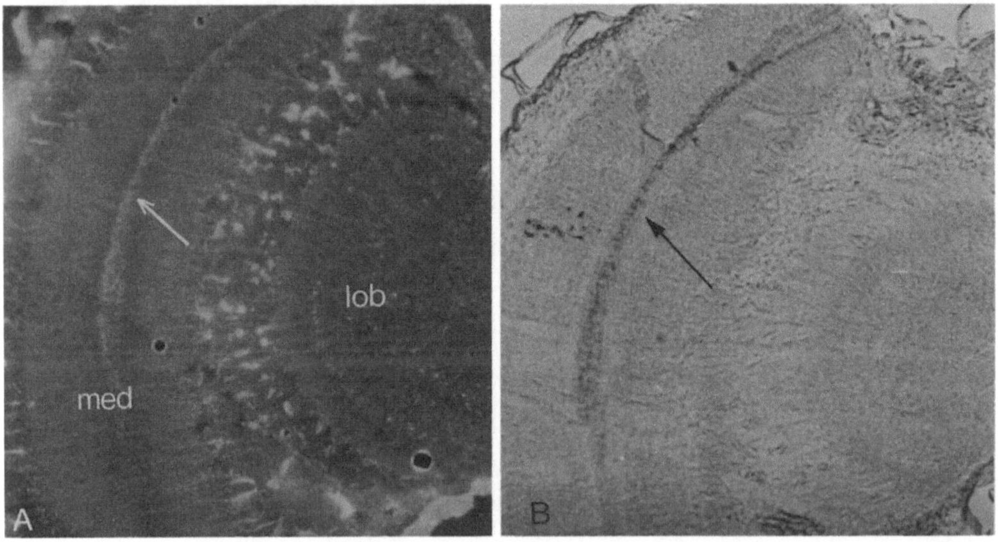

Fig. 4 - A. Fluorescence in the medulla of the optic lobe of the honeybee after treatment with glyoxylic acid. B. 5-HT-immunoreactive fibers detected in the medulla of the optic lobe using the PAP method of Sternberger (1979) (Jack and Mercer, unpublished observation). lob = lobula, med = medulla.

responsiveness to olfactory stimuli at the behavioral level (19). The effect closely resembles sensitization induced by stimulation of the bee with sugar water (4). At the cellular level, however, the effects of OA on responses to olfactory inputs recorded in the mushroom bodies of the bee brain are variable. OA reduces the size of potentials evoked by stimulation of the antennae with air or scent in some animals, but enhances responses to olfactory stimuli in others (18). As yet we know very little about the receptors mediating the effects of biogenic amines in the insect brain, so interpretation of results such as these is difficult at present. In future studies, high priority must be given to the investigation of receptor mechanisms operating in the insect brain. Unlike OA, iontophoretic application of DA to the brain of the honeybee does not alter the size of potentials evoked by light stimuli recorded extracellularly in the mushroom body neuropil (18). The effects of DA on responses to olfactory inputs recorded in the mushroom bodies of the bee brain, however, are much more consistent than those of OA. Iontophoretic application of DA into the mushroom body neuropil reduces the size of potentials evoked by stimulation of the antennae with air or scent (18). Full recovery of responses is apparent within 30 minutes of DA application. Recovery of responses to olfactory stimuli, following an initial reduction after treatment with DA, is apparent at the behavioral level also. DA injected into the protocerebrum of the bee brain reduces the percentage of bees responding to a conditioned olfactory stimulus (19). Sixty minutes after treatment, responses have returned to a level similar to that observed in untreated controls. Recovery of responses to conditioned olfactory stimuli does not occur, however, if DA is applied to the antennal lobes of the bee brain immediately prior to conditioning (15). The effects of applying dopamine to the antennal lobes of the bee brain are side specific. Using the proboscis conditioning paradigm (14), bees can be conditioned to orange scent in a single conditioning trial with only one antenna exposed to the conditioned stimulus. Applying DA to the antennal lobe ipsilateral to the 'conditioned antenna' 14 minutes after conditioning causes a marked reduction in the percentage of bees responding to the conditioned stimulus in subsequent tests, whereas DA applied to the antennal lobe contralateral to the 'conditioned antenna' has no effect on the level of responses to the conditioned stimulus (15). It is particularly interesting that the reduction in percent response to a conditioned olfactory stimulus is significantly smaller in bees conditioned to the scent stimulus in multiple conditioning trials prior to treatment of the antennal lobes with DA (15). First order olfactory interneurones connect the antennal lobes with the calyces of the mushroom bodies, higher brain centers believed to play an important role in the formation of olfactory learning in the honeybee (5, 16). Evidence suggests that dopaminergic interneurones influence the output of information from primary olfactory centers of the bee brain, affecting indirectly processes of olfactory learning in this insect (17). The effects of DA on output of information from the antennal lobes of the bee brain are now being investigated at the cellular level. It appears that the effects of biogenic amines on response characteristics of deutocerebral output neurones are as complex as the responses themselves (Flanagan, pers. comm.). This is hardly surprising in view of the complex integrative nature of the antennal lobes in the insect brain (1; see Masson this volume), and the fact that dopaminergic neurones form only one small subpopulation of interneurones identified in the antennal lobes of the honeybee that are likely to influence sensory processing in the deutocerebrum of the bee brain.

Investigation of the role of biogenic amines in the brain of the honeybee is in its preliminary stages. Results so far are suggestive, but inconclusive. Potential for identification of specific amine-containing neurones in the brain of the honeybee accessible to detailed analysis is offered by the highly sensitive immunocytochemical staining techniques now available (28). However, raising antibodies specific to a particular amine has proved difficult. Antibodies to 5-HT are available commercially and have been used to investigate the distribution of 5-HT-containing neurones in the brain of the honeybee (26, see Bicker et al. this volume), but success to date with antibodies raised against other biogenic amines, such as the primary catecholamine DA, and the phenolamine OA, has been limited (30). Detailed physiological, pharmacological, and biochemical analysis of aminergic neurones identified in the brain promises rapid advancement of our knowledge and understanding of brain amines in insects. Until this is possible, however, we must rely on a less direct approach, using coordinated multidisciplinary studies such as those underway in the honeybee, to reveal functional roles of biogenic amines in the insect brain.

REFERENCES

(1) Boeckh, J.; Ernst, K.D.; Sass, H.; and Waldow, U. 1984. Anatomical and physiological characteristics of individual neurones in the central antennal pathway of insects. J. Insect Physiol. 30: 15-26.

(2) Brown, C.S., and Nestler, C. 1985. Catecholamines and indolalkylamines. In Comprehensive Insect Physiology, Biochemistry and Pharmacology, eds. G.A. Kerkut and L.I. Gilbert, Vol. 11, pp. 435-497. Oxford: Pergamon Press.

(3) Dymond, G.R., and Evans, P.D. (1979). Biogenic amines in the nervous system of the cockroach, Periplaneta americana: association of octopamine with mushroom bodies and dorsal unpaired median (DUM) neurones. Insect Biochem. 9: 535-545.

(4) Erber, J., and Schildberger, K. 1980. Conditioning of an antennal reflex to visual stimuli in bees (Apis mellifera L.) J. Comp. Physiol. 135: 217-225.

(5) Erber, J.; Masuhr, T.; and Menzel, R. 1980. Localization of short-term memory in the brain of the bee, Apis mellifera. Physiol. Entomol. 5: 343-358.

(6) Evans, P.D. 1978. Octopamine distribution in the insect nervous system. J. Neurochem. 30: 1009-1013.

(7) Evans, P.D. 1980. Biogenic amines in the insect nervous system. Adv. Insect Physiol. 15: 317-473.

(8) Evans, P.D. 1985. Octopamine. In Comprehensive Insect Physiology, Biochemistry and Pharmacology, eds. G.A. Kerkut and L.I. Gilbert, Vol. 11, pp. 499-530. Oxford: Pergamon Press.

(9) Evans, P.D., and O'Shea, M. 1977. An octopaminergic neurone modulates neuromuscular transmission in the locust. Nature 270: 257-259.

(10) Evans, P.D., and O'Shea, M. 1978. The identification of an octopaminergic neurone and the modulation of a myogenic rhythm in the locust. J. Exp. Biol. 73: 235-260.

(11) Frontali, N., and Norberg, K.A. 1966. Catecholamine-containing neurons in the cockroach brain. Acta Physiol. Scand. 66: 243-244.

(12) Klemm, N. 1974. Vergleichend-histochemische Untersuchungen über die Verteilung monoamin-haltiger Strukturen im Oberschlundganglion von Angehörigen verschiedener Insektenordnungen. Ent. germ. 1: 21-49.

(13) Klemm, N. 1976. Histochemistry of putative transmitter substances in the insect brain. Prog. Neurobiol. 7: 99-169.

(14) Kuwabara, M. 1957. Bildung des bedingten Reflexes von Pavlovs Typus bei der Honigbiene, Apis mellifica. J. Fac. Sci. Hokkaido Univ. (Ser 6) 13: 458-464.

(15) Macmillan, C.S., and Mercer, A.R. An investigation of the role of dopamine in the antennal lobes of the honeybee, Apis mellifera. Submitted for publication.

(16) Menzel, R.; Erber, J.; and Masuhr, T. 1974. Learning and memory in the honeybee. In Experimental Analysis of Insect Behavior, ed. L. Barton Browne, pp. 195-217. Berlin, Heidelberg, New York: Springer-Verlag.

(17) Mercer, A.R. 1986. Biogenic amines in the insect brain. In Arthropod Brain: Its Evolution, Structure and Functions, ed. A.P. Gupta. New York: Wiley & Sons, in press.

(18) Mercer, A.R., and Erber, J. 1983. The effects of amines on evoked potentials recorded in the mushroom bodies of the bee brain. J. Comp. Physiol. 151: 469-476.

(19) Mercer, A.R., and Menzel, R. 1982. The effects of biogenic amines on conditioned and unconditioned responses to olfactory stimuli in the honeybee Apis mellifera. J. Comp. Physiol. 145: 363-368.

(20) Mercer, A.R.; Mobbs, P.G.; Davenport, A.P; and Evans, P.D. 1983. Biogenic amines in the brain of the honeybee, Apis mellifera. Cell Tissue Res. 234: 655-677.

(21) Mobbs, P.G. 1982. The brain of the bee Apis mellifera. I. The connections and spatial organisation of the mushroom bodies. Phil. Trans. R. Soc. Lond. B 298: 309-354.

(22) Mobbs, P.G. 1985. Brain structure. In Comprehensive Insect Physiology, Biochemistry, and Pharmacology, (Vol. 5, Nervous System, Structure and Motor Function) eds. G.A. Kerkut and L.I. Gilbert, Vol. 5 pp. 299-370. Oxford: Pergamon Press.

(23) Orchard, I. 1982. Octopamine in insects: neurotransmitter, neurohormone and neuromodulator. Canad. J. Zool. 60: 659-669.

(24) O'Shea, M., and Adams, M.E. 1981. Pentapeptide (Proctolin) associated with an identified neuron. Science 213: 567-569.

(25) Pareto, A. 1972. Die zentrale Verteilung der Fuhlerafferenz bei Arbeiterinnen der Honigbiene, Apis mellifera. L. Z. Zellforsch. mikrosk. Anat. 131: 109-140.

(26) Schürmann, F.W., and Klemm, N. 1984. Serotonin-immunoreactive neurons in the brain of the honeybee. J. Comp. Neurol. 225: 570-580.

(27) Sloley, B.D., and Owen, M.D. 1982. The effects of reserpine on amine concentrations in the nervous system of the cockroach (Periplaneta americana). Insect Biochem. 12: 469-476.

(28) Sternberger, L.A. 1974. Immunocytochemistry. New Jersey: Prentice Hall Inc.

(29) Suzuki, H. 1975. Antennal movements induced by odour and central projection of the antennal neurons in the honeybee. J. Insect Physiol. 21: 831-847.

(30) Vieillemaringe, J.; Duris, P.; Geffard, M.; Le Moal, M.; Delaage, M.; Bensch, C.; and Girardie, J. 1984. Immunohistochemical localization of dopamine in the brain of the insect Locusta migratoria migratorioides in the comparison with the catecholamine distribution determined by the histofluorescence technique. Cell Tissue Res. 237: 391-394.

Neural Signal Processing in the Median Protocerebrum of the Bee

Jochen Erber and Uwe Homberg
Institut für Biologie der Technischen Universität Berlin, Franklinstr. 28/29,
D-1000 Berlin 10, FRG

INTRODUCTION

As in most animals, the major sense organs of the bee, the compound eyes, the ocelli and the antennae are located on the head of the animal. Therefore, large parts of the head ganglion, in particular the optic and antennal lobes, are primarily concerned with the processing of sensory information. We will not deal with the neurophysiology of these sensory neuropils of the brain here and the reader is referred to the chapters by Ribi, Hertel and Goodman in this volume. However, the various sensory information is funnelled into the median protocerebrum and from there via descending interneurons to motor centers of the thoracic ganglia. The various sensory inputs are integrated primarily in the lateral parts of the median protocerebrum and linked to specific descending pathways. In addition, the brain contains two structures, the paired mushroom bodies (MB) and the central complex (cc) (Fig. 1), which have no equivalents in the ganglia. They seem to be hierarchically parallel structures in that they are largely superimposed on the sensory to motor-center pathways in the lateral protocerebrum. Recordings and stainings of single cells in the various brain areas, as well as field potential measurements, more detailed anatomical analyses, and recently immunocytochemical and autoradiographic investigations have specified our knowledge of the physiological roles and relationships of the mushroom bodies, the central complex and the 'diffuse' protocerebral lobes in the brain of the honeybee.

THE MUSHROOM BODIES

Many different hypothetical functions have been attributed to the mushroom bodies in insects (5). The spectrum of hypotheses ranges from purely sensory signal processing to the control of complex behavioral patterns. In bees and flies there is considerable convergence of experimental data concerning the important role of the MB in olfactory memory formation (6, 8, 12; see also the chapter by Menzel in this volume).

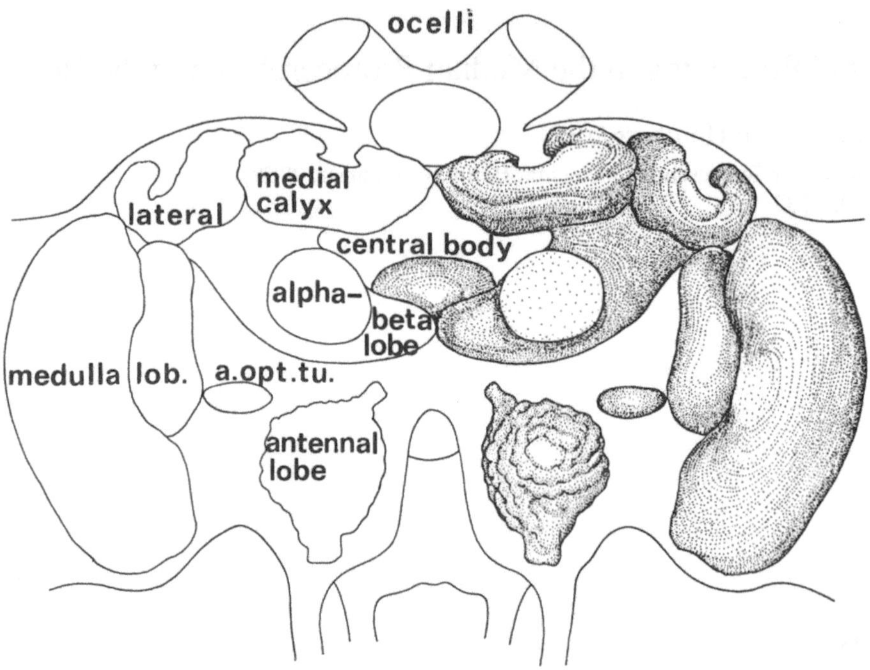

Fig. 1 - Frontal diagram of the bee brain showing the main neuropils of the proto- and deutocerebrum. a. op. tu = anterior optic tubercle, lob. = lobula. Scale: 100 um.

The neurons of the MB system can be divided into two groups, the intrinsic neurons which form the MB and give them their peculiar shape and the extrinsic neurons which represent inputs, outputs and connections of intrinsic neurons. The neurons connecting the lobes of the MB with the calyces are often regarded as feedback neurons, but as these cells often also have projection areas in the protocerebrum and, as there is so far no solid proof for a true feedback function, the term 'connecting neurons' appears to be more appropriate.

INPUT NEURONS OF THE MUSHROOM BODIES

Physiologically and neuroanatomically the inputs to the calyces of the MB differ in the insect orders. The most massive inputs arise from the antenno-glomerular tract (AGT), which is also termed antenno-cerebral tract (ACT) or tractus olfactorio-glogularis (TOG). Cells of this tract innervate one glomerulus in the antennal lobe and project to the calyces and the lateral protocerebral lobe of the brain. The structure of these input neurons suggest that they feed sensory information from the antenna to the MB and in parallel to the projection sites in the lateral protocerebrum. The physiological recordings of single neurons of the AGT in the bee and in the cricket reveal that these simple neuroanatomical interpretations are only partly correct (10, 18). Most neurons of the AGT display multimodal characteristics, responding to olfactory, mechanical, and chemical stimuli applied to the ipsilateral antenna. But these cells can also signal sensory stimulation from sensory organs which are not located on the antenna. Therefore, we have to conclude that the calyces receive multimodal inputs via the AGT.

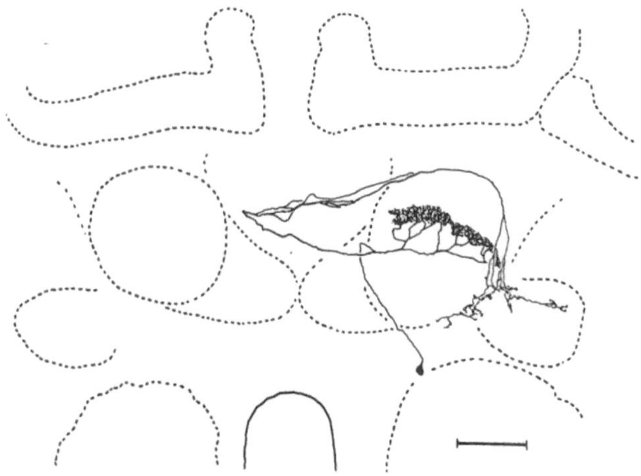

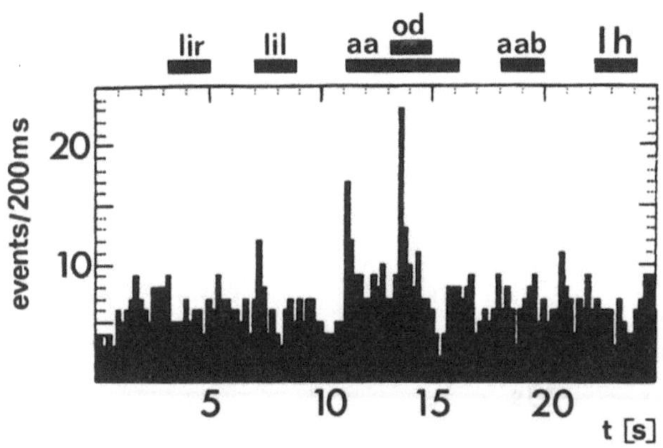

Fig. 2 - Frontal reconstruction of presumable MB output cell and peristimulus time histogram. lil = light left; lir = light right; aa = air puff applied to the antennae; od = odor mixture; aab = air puff applied to thorax and abdomen; lh = removal of leg holder. Scale: 100 um.

In the honeybee, several tracts connect the optic lobes with the calyces. Neurons of these tracts respond to visual stimulation. Some of the cells recorded so far were movement sensitive and direction selective (7). Very little is known about the physiology of other neurons projecting from the protocerebrum to the calyces of the MB. These presumable input cells show differing and often multimodal response characteristics.

OUTPUT AND CONNECTING NEURONS OF THE MUSHROOM BODIES

In bees, output neurons with arborizations in the lobes of the MB often have more complex, multimodal characteristics than calycal input neurons. These cells often also respond to visual stimuli, suggesting convergence of sensory information from the AGT neurons and from the visual neurons connecting the optic lobes with the calyces (Fig. 2, Fig. 3A).

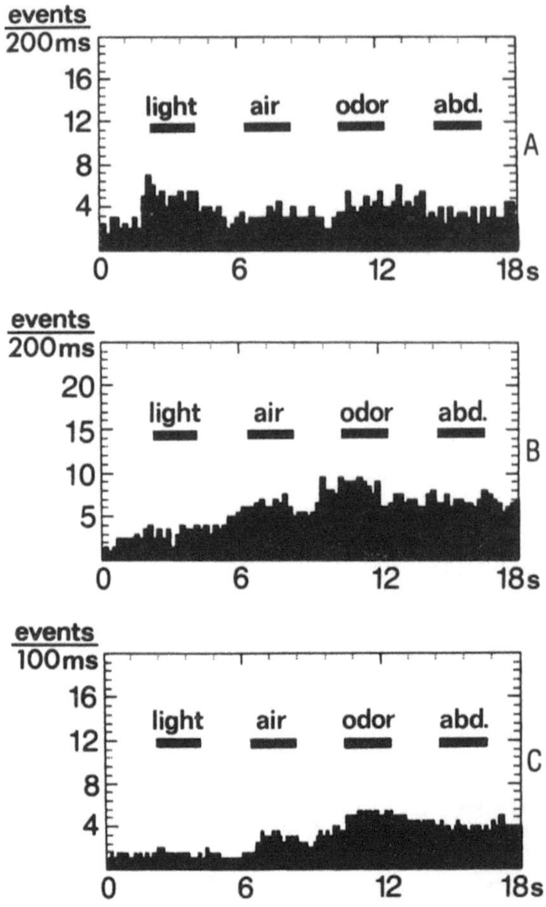

Fig. 3 - Peristimulus time histograms of 3 connecting neurons. Light = light flash; air = air puff applied to antennae; odor = olfactory stimulation; abd = mechanical stimulation of thorax and abdomen. Neurons B and C display pronounced aftereffects, the spontaneous discharge rates of the cells are increased for many seconds after olfactory stimuli (7).

While sensory convergence in the outputs of the MB is not very astonishing, the very pronounced after-effects of many of these cells are a feature which seems to be characteristic for MB output cells. The after-effects can outlast the stimulus by many seconds, sometimes even minutes (Fig. 3B,C). After-effects can be regarded as a specific form of sensory memory which enables the nervous system to 'sample and hold' sensory inputs.

Another type of temporal signal processing in the MB can be found in output and connecting neurons. The temporal succession and spacing of stimuli can determine the response properties of these cells (17). This feature has not been systematically studied, but it could explain the often observed lasting response changes in MB output cells.

Signal processing within the MB can only be analysed when the multiple feedback and presumably feedforward loops of the system are opened. Recently Bicker et al. (1) have shown that connecting neurons with a possible feedback function of the protocerebral calycal tract are characterized by GABA-like immunoreactivity (see also chapter by Bicker et al. in this volume). GABA antagonists can be used to analyse the function of this loop of connecting neurons. Recent analyses in my laboratory suggest that the feedback loop is, in fact, inhibitory. Similar to single cell studies, long-lasting aftereffects can also be observed in recordings using evoked potentials. The time course of these potentials closely resembles the activity pattern of MB output neurons (Fig. 3). The duration of the aftereffects and their size is augmented when the presumable feedback loop is blocked by GABA antagonists. This makes the hypothesis that feedback neurons produce the aftereffects obsolete (14). The application of GABA antagonists suggests that the calyces are not the only site for inhibitory action of the connecting neurons. Therefore, the term 'feedback loop' probably represents an oversimplification of the system.

THE CENTRAL COMPLEX

The subdivisions of the central complex (protocerebral bridge, upper and lower division of the central body, noduli; Fig. 4) form a highly ordered three-dimensional network of interconnected neuropils in the center of the bee brain. The protocerebral bridge, the fan-shaped body and the superior arch of the upper central body division, as well as the lower division can be regarded as neuronal strata which are perpendicularly subdivided into 8 segments or columns. The connections of extrinsic central complex neurons seem to be restricted to the 'diffuse' protocerebral lobes, major projection areas being the lateral accessory lobes. Wide-field amacrine and tangential neurons innervating one or more strata can be distinguished from segmental interneurons whose arborizations are restricted to single segments. Segmental neuronal elements share characteristic anatomical features. They have their output region in the lateral accessory lobes contralateral to their dendritic inputs in the protocerebral bridge. An additional branching field in the central body is either ipsi- or contralateral.

Several cell types of the central complex have been studied electrophysiologically (9, 11, 13). Amacrine cells of the protocerebral bridge respond predominantly to stationary and moving visual stimuli, which is in good agreement with the neuroanatomical evidence of a fiber connection to optic neuropils. Recordings from segmental and tangential neurons, however, revealed no systematic differences between these groups in the response patterns to sensory stimuli. Compared to mushroom body neurons, these cells show a lesser degree of multimodiality. A relatively high percentage does not respond to any stimulus. In addition, central complex cells often exhibit only small modulation in the frequency of action potentials when a variety of sensory stimuli (visual, various mechanical, olfactory, gustatory) is presented. This indicates that the central complex gets only weak input from sense organs, probably by a few multisynaptic connections, since there is no anatomical evidence for major

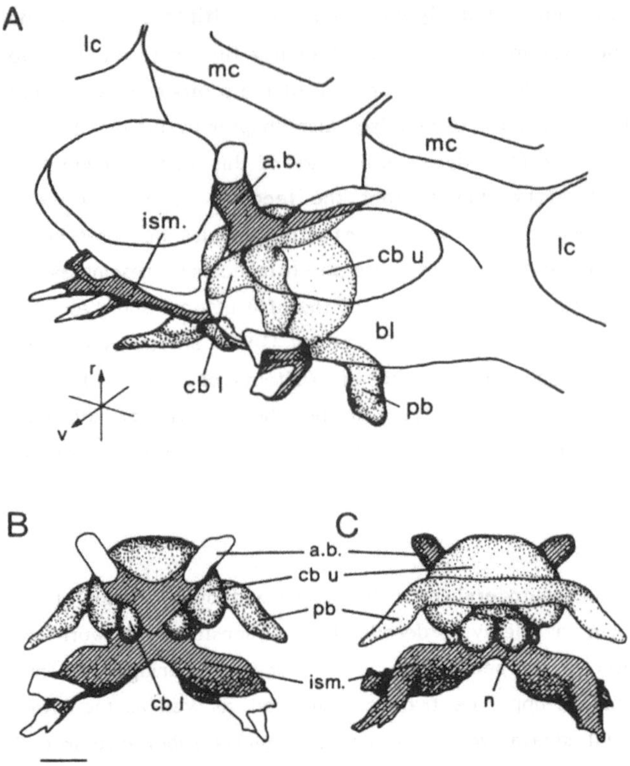

Fig. 4 - Fiber tracts (shaded) and compartments of the central complex. A. Spatial relationship to the mushroom bodies. B. Anterior, C. posterior view. r = rostral; v = ventral; a.b.= anterior bundles; bl = beta-lobe; cb 1 = central body lower division; cb u = central body upper division; ism.= isthmus tract; lc = lateral calyx; mc = medial calyx; n = nodulus; pb = protocerebral bridge. Scale: 100um.

fiber tracts connecting it to sensory neuropils. Likewise, the absence of direct connections to descending neurons and the precise bilateral fiber geometry in the central complex leads to the speculation that it has some modulatory function in regulating and balancing the flow of information in both brain halves.

Some recordings, however, revealed responses to very specific stimuli only (e.g., to a moving light source and not to stationary light or to one odor and not another (Fig.5)), indicating that these cells may be tuned to a specific sensory situation, probably with some behavioral relevance for the bee.

Recent immunocytochemical investigations using an antibody against GABA-protein conjugates found GABA-like immunoreactivity especially in the lower division, but not in the protocerebral bridge and only in a few fibers of the upper division (15). The immunoreactive neurons are probably tangential cells innervating the lower division and the lateral accessory lobes. This indicates a role of the central body in mutual inhibitory interactions of the two brain halves, but so far there are no physiological data to support this hypothesis.

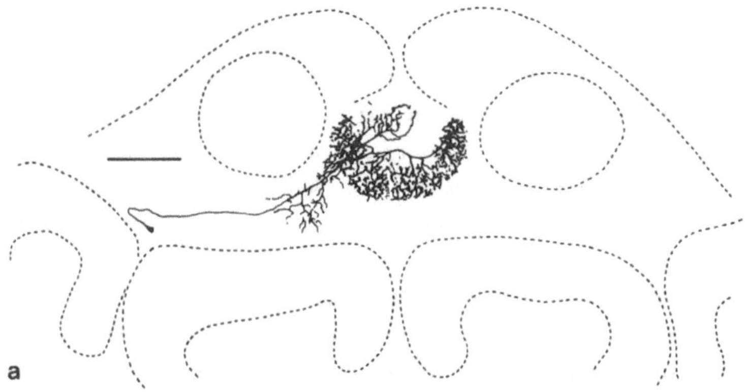

Fig. 5 - a. Tangential neuron innervating the superior arch of the upper central body division and the frontal protocerebrum medial to the alpha-lobe.

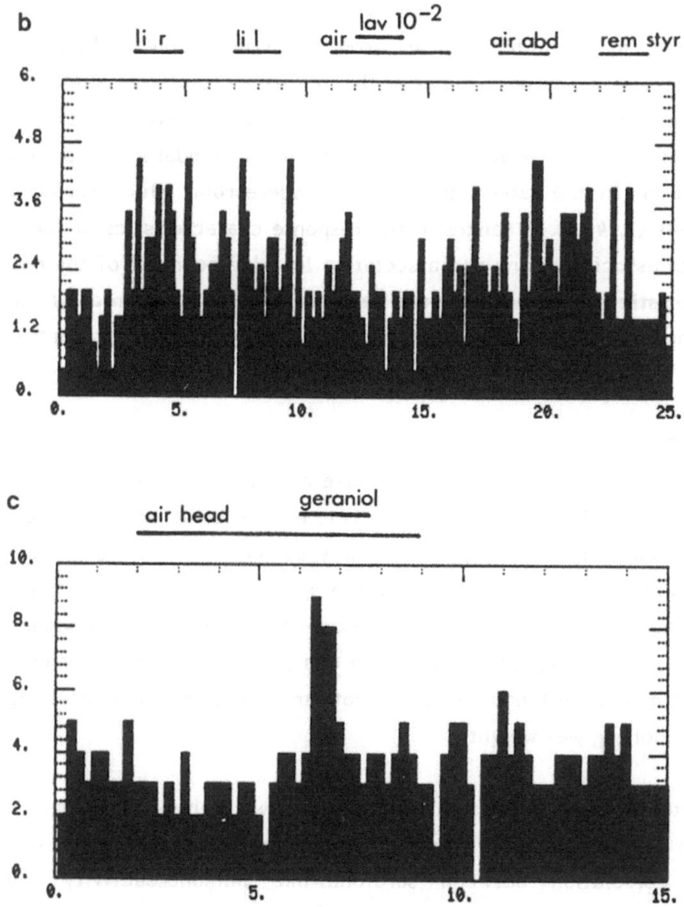

Fig. 5 - b, c: Peristimulus time histograms. Ordinate = number of action potentials per 200 ms; abscissa = time in s.; li r = light right; li l = light left; air = air puff applied to the head; lav 10^{-2} = 1% lavender oil in paraffin oil; air abd. = mechanical stimuli to the abdomen; rem. styr. = mechanical stimuli to thorax. (11) Scale: 100 um.

'DIFFUSE' PROTOCEREBRUM

The design and interpretation of electrophysiological experiments in the 'diffuse' protocerebral lobes suffer from our poor understanding of the neuroanatomical organization of these parts of the brain. The lateral protocerebrum is the major area of multimodal convergence of visual (compound eye and ocelli), olfactory and mechanosensory inputs which are ultimately transferred onto descending pathways (19, 21). Sensory inputs to the diffuse protocerebrum as well as feedback information about ongoing motor activity comes, in addition, from ascending neurons originating in the suboesophageal ganglion or the thoracic ganglia. And finally, large portions of the brain, especially dorso-posterior and lateral areas, possibly have a function comparable to the vertebrate hypothalamus, in that neurons which regulate neurosecretion have arborizations in these areas and send axons via the median bundle and nervus corporis cardiacis to the neurosecretory corpora cardiaca. As to be expected, neurons in the median bundle, therefore, hardly respond to sensory stimuli (9).

Most interneurons in the diffuse lobes seem to have a unique Gestalt and, likewise, unique physiological characteristics (7, 9); therefore, a classification of these neurons may be largely impossible. After many single cell recordings, however, some regional physiological characteristics begin to emerge. In the anterior lobes around the mushroom bodies, the response characteristics of local interneurons resemble the properties of mushroom body neurons, and poststimulus aftereffects can be observed frequently (7). Aftereffects and changes in the response characteristics have also been observed in multimodal lobula output neurons and in local interneurons in the lateral posterior protocerebrum, which probably receive inputs from lobula cells (3, 4, 7). Changes in the response characteristics of these neurons can be correlated with associative and non-associative learning behavior of the bee during the recording. These plastic phenomena have not been observed in other areas of the protocerebrum (e.g., in multimodal neurons of the anterior optic tubercle (7, 9)), or in central complex neurons (10)

TRANSMITTER BINDING SITES

Recent immunocytological investigations in the bee brain have revealed the distribution and even the Gestalt of neurons with specific transmitters (Bicker, et al.; Noble and Goodman, this volume). Although, these studies represent important progress in our understanding of the bee brain, they remain incomplete as long as the sites where specific transmitters act are unknown. Therefore, we used autoradiographic methods to localize serotonin and octopamine binding sites in the brain (16). The binding of (^{3}H)serotonin and (^{3}H)octopamine was highly specific (90-95%). The highest density of binding sites for both transmitters can be localized in the MB (approximately 160 fmol/mg wet weight).

The distribution of binding sites reveals specific patterns for the two transmitters (Fig. 6). For serotonin, the distribution can be compared with the immunocytological studies (Bicker, et al, this volume). The correlation between serotonin-like immunoreactivity and

(^{3}H)serotonin binding sites is excellent in the MB, whereas there is an obvious mismatch between high immunoreactivity and low transmitter binding in the cc. In the medulla and lobula, the binding sites for serotonin are evenly distributed, while immunoreactivity reveals specific bands of presumable serotonergic neurons.

The distribution of octopamine binding sites is different from the serotonin distribution in the medualla, the cc and, partly, in the MB. These new investigations help us to define areas where neurotransmitters or modulators possibly act, but they also pose new questions concerning the mismatch between immunoreactive neurons and binding sites.

CONCLUSIONS

The electrophysiological recordings of neural activity in the median protocerebrum of the bee has enlarged our knowledge about the functional significance of this central part of the brain. Apparently, the MB in the different insect orders process different sensory modalities. Antennal information probably is the dominant input to the MB in cockroaches (2), cercal and acoustic information seems to play an important role in the cricket MB (18), while the MB of the bee process visual, antennal and other sensory information. The MB in different insect orders probably have common neuronal principles of information processing, rather than common modalities which are processed.

Although sensory modalities converge in the MB, the primary function of this neuropil does not seem to be to combine different modalities. An important part of modality convergence already occurs in the antennal lobes and is apparent in MB input neurons. Temporal signal processing seems to be the eminent function of the MB. The generation of long-lasting aftereffects, the specific responses to specific successions of stimuli and the temporal concatenation of incoming information are characteristic features of this neuropil. These forms of temporal signal processing might be necessary prerequisites for memory formation.

Neuronal signal processing in the central complex (cc), on the other hand, is quite different from the results found in the MB. The cc receives mostly indirect inputs from many sensory organs and seems to be involved in the control of motor activity. A number of experiments, especially new neurochemical data, suggest that the lower division of the central body plays a major part in the inhibitory interactions between the two halves of the brain. The cc might, therefore, serve a role in balancing information outflow of the right and left sides of the brain.

As we learn more about the information processing and wiring diagram in the median protocerebrum, more and more functional compartmentation is discovered. On the other hand, few of these compartments can be regarded as functional units of their own. An example for this may be the MB with a great majority of intrinsic cells and few connections to other areas. However, most areas are innervated mainly by projection neurons that

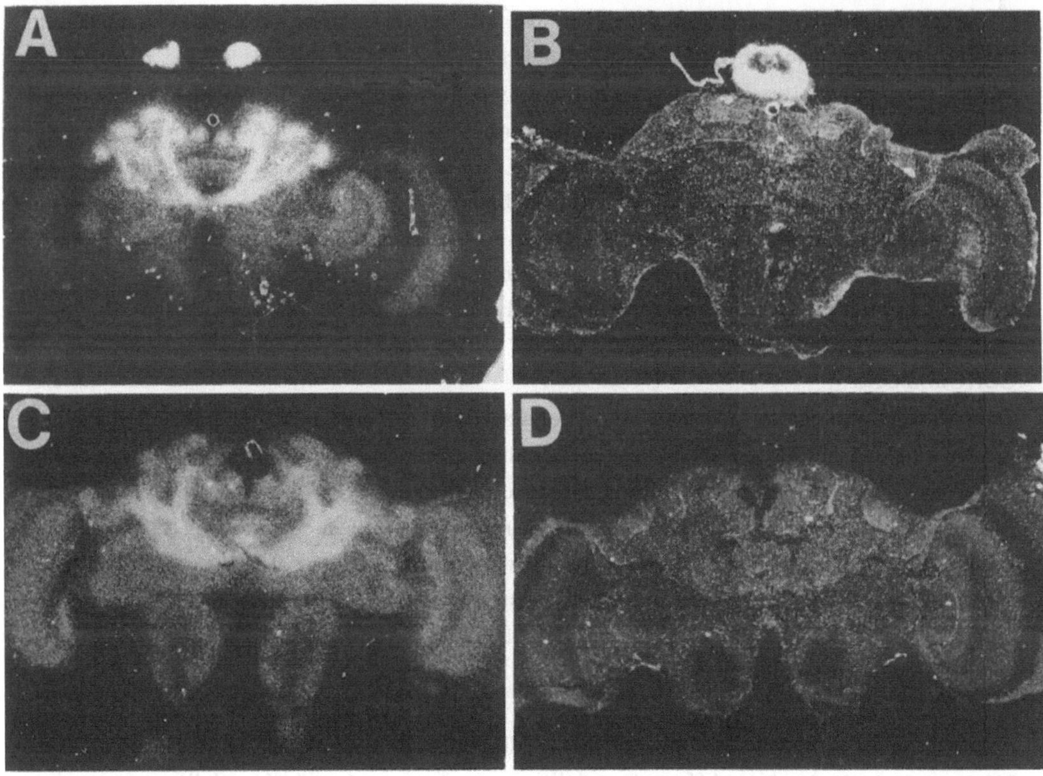

Fig. 6 - Autoradiographs for (^{3}H)serotonin and (^{3}H)octopamine binding. A = total binding for (^{3}H)serotonin (5,8 nM); B = control for unspecific binding of (^{3}H)serotonin; C = total binding for (^{3}H)octopamine (8,8 nM); D = control for unspecific binding of (^{3}H)octopamine (16).

connect them to many different other regions, examples for this are the anterior optic tubercle or the central complex. All neurons that innervate a certain neuropil like the central body probably share certain physiological characteristics, but considering the diversity of neurons, it may be difficult to find these common properties.

From biochemical aspects, and especially immunocytochemical and transmitter binding studies, a different kind of functional subdivision of the brain may arise. We can now map neurons that share the same neurotransmitter (15, 20) and we can quantitatively describe the distribution of transmitter binding sites within the insect brain (16). This complementary approach allows the formulation of new hypotheses concerning the action of specific transmitters or neuromodulators. It also helps to bridge the wide gap between behavior and neurophysiology because it is now possible, with neuropharmacological techniques, to manipulate defined pathways and neuropil areas and to test the behavioral effects of these manipulations at the same time.

SUMMARY

The mushroom bodies and the central complex, hierarchically parallel structures in the bee brain, are functionally superimposed on the more direct sensory-to-motor connections in the lateral parts of the median protocerebrum. The mushroom bodies process multimodal information. Their main physiological function seems to be neuronal signal processing in the time domain. The cc receives mostly indirect and weak inputs from many sense organs. We suggest that the cc is involved in the functional coordination of both brain halves, partly by inhibitory interactions. The lateral part of the median protocerebrum is the primary location for the convergence of sensory pathways onto descending cells. Recent immunocytological and autoradiographic studies reveal transmitter-specific neurons and binding sites in the bee brain. These findings and the existing physiological data enable new experimental approaches concerning the functional role of specific areas of the bee brain.

Acknowledgements. We thank T. Hartmann and A. Scheidler for permission to use unpublished and published data. Supported by the Deutsche Forschungsgemeinschaft grants Er 79/3-1 and Ho 950/2-1.

REFERENCES

(1) Bicker, G.; Schäfer, S.; and Kingan, T.G. 1985. Mushroom body feedback interneurons in the honeybee show GABA-like immunoreactivity. Brain Res. 360: 394-397.

(2) Boeckh, J.; Ernst, K.D.; Sass, H.; and Waldow, U. 1984. Anatomical and physiological characteristics of individual neurons in the central antennal pathway of insects. J. Insect Physiol. 30: 15-26.

(3) Erber, J. 1981. Neural correlates of learning in the honeybee. TINS 4: 270-273.

(4) Erber, J. 1983. The search for neural correlates of learning in the honeybee. In Neuroethology and Behavioral Physiology, ed. F. Huber and H. Markl, pp. 216-227. Berlin, Heidelberg, New York: Springer-Verlag.

(5) Erber, J.; Homberg, U.; and Gronenberg, W., in press. The functional roles of the mushroom bodies in insects. In Arthropod Brain: Its Evolution, Development, Structure, and Functions, ed. A.P. Gupta. New York: J. Wiley.

(6) Erber, J.; Masuhr, Th.; and Menzel, R. 1980. Localisation of short-term memory in the brain of the bee, Apis mellifera. Physiol. Entomol. 5: 343-358.

(7) Gronenberg, W. 1984. Das Protocerebrum der Honigbiene im Bereich des Pilzkörpers - eine neurophysiologisch-anatomische Charakterisierung. Dissertation, Freie Universität Berlin.

(8) Heisenberg, M.; Borst, A.; Wagner, S.; and Byers, D. 1985. Drosophila mushroom body mutants are deficient in olfactory learning. J. Neurogen. 2: 1-30.

(9) Homberg, U. 1985. Das mediane Protocerebrum der Honigbiene (Apis mellifica) im Bereich des Zentralkörpers: Physiologische und morphologische Charakterisierung. Dissertation, Freie Universität Berlin.

(10) Homberg, U. 1984. Processing of antennal information in extrinsic mushroom body neurons in the bee brain. J. Comp. Physiol. 154: 825-836.

(11) Homberg, U. 1985. Interneurons of the central complex in the bee brain (Apis mellifica, L.). J. Insect Physiol. 31: 251-264.

(12) Menzel, R.; Erber, J.; and Masuhr, Th. 1974. Learning and memory in the honeybee. In Experimental Analysis of Insect Behavior, ed. L. Barton-Browne, pp. 195-217. Berlin, Heidelberg, New York: Springer-Verlag

(13) Milde, J. 1982. Elektrophysiologische und anatomische Untersuchungen an Interneuronen erster und höherer Ordnung des Ocellensystems der Biene (Apis mellifica carnica). Dissertation, Freie Universität Berlin.

(14) Mobbs, P.G. 1982. The brain of the honeybee Apis mellifera. I. The connections and spatial organization of the mushroom bodies. Phil. Trans. Roy. Soc. Lond. Ser. B 298: 309-354.

(15) Schäfer, S., and Bicker, G. 1986. Distribution of GABA-like immunoreactivity in the brain of the honeybee. J. Comp. Neurol. 246: 287-300.

(16) Scheidler, A.; Kaulen, P.; Brüning, G.; and Erber, J. 1986. Autoradiographic localization of octopamine and serotonin binding sites in the brain of the honeybee (Apis mellifera L.) Verh. Dtsch. Zool. Ges. 79: in press.

(17) Schildberger, K. 1981. Some physiological features of mushroom body linked fibers in the house cricket brain. Naturwissenschaften 67: 623.

(18) Schildberger, K. 1984. Multimodal interneurons in the cricket brain: properties of identified extrinsic mushroom body cells. J. Comp. Physiol. 154: 71-79.

(19) Schürmann, F.W. 1982. On the synaptic connections, tracts and compartments in the brain of the honeybee. In The Biology of Social Insects, ed. M.D. Breed, C.D. Michener, and H.E. Evans, pp. 390-394. Boulder, Colorado: Westview Press.

(20) Schürmann, F.W., and Klemm, N. 1984. Serotonin-immunoreactive neurons in the brain of the honeybee. J. Comp. Neurol. 225: 570-580.

(21) Strausfeld, N.J., and Bacon, J.P. 1983. Multimodal convergence in the central nervous system of dipterous insects. Fortschritte der Zoologie 28: 47-76.

Development

Hormonal Regulation of Age Polyethism in the Honeybee, Apis mellifera

Gene E. Robinson

Department of Entomology, Cornell University, Ithaca, N.Y. 14853, USA

Abstract. This paper develops a model of hormonally regulated division of labor in honeybee (Apis mellifera) colonies. According to the model, changes in juvenile hormone (JH) titers modulate the bees' responses to stimuli associated with the tasks they perform. JH seems to act as a behavioral primer, regulating a colony's allocation of labor by altering the probabilities with which individual bees perform different tasks. JH also coordinates the tightly coupled processes of age-dependent exocrine and behavioral development. Results implicating JH in the control of age polyethism are reviewed, including the findings that JH analog methoprene causes precocious foraging, affects the timing and frequency of task performance in the nest and induces premature production of alarm pheromones. Methoprene also causes a premature decrease in the threshold sensitivity to alarm pheromones, which agrees with the prediction that JH modulates the perception of task-related stimuli. This model is consistent with the data currently available, but needs considerable testing; relevant studies are suggested.

INTRODUCTION

Division of labor among workers is fundamental to the organization of the honeybee society because it is more efficient for a colony to accomplish tasks concurrently with ensembles of specialized individuals than to perform tasks sequentially with undifferentiated workers (33). Division of labor in the honeybee society is characterized by two features. First, worker bee behavior changes dramatically with age, a phenomenon known as age polyethism (15, 48). Workers progress through four age castes during their 4- to 7-week life that are spatially segregated in the nest and are each marked by a focus on one of the following tasks: cell cleaning, brood and queen care, food storage, and foraging (46). Workers may perform more than one job at any age prior to foraging (25, 27), so transitions in the nest from caste to caste involve age-dependent changes in the relative frequency with which tasks are performed (46). In contrast, their final behavioral shift is abrupt and marks the onset of a phase devoted only to foraging.

The second important property of the honeybee colony's system of labor allocation is that individual bees are able to respond to changing colony needs by altering the trajectory of their age-dependent behavioral development, which results in great variability in the ages at which tasks are performed (28, 33). Despite the prominence of division of labor in honeybee social organization, the means by which it is regulated are poorly understood. This bears on one of the central questions in insect sociobiology (58): since individuals do not have complete awareness of all that transpires in their colony, how do adaptive patterns of colonial behavior emerge from the activities of individual members? One approach to discovering how the activities of workers in age castes are integrated into an efficiently operating colony is to first identify physiological mechanisms that underlie age polyethism. In this paper I review results supporting the hypothesis that juvenile hormone (JH) acts as such a mechanism in the honeybee. I also discuss a model of division of labor in which JH plays a central role in the workers' ability to respond to changing colony needs.

JH TITERS IN WORKER BEES

Juvenile hormones are sesquiterpenes with many fundamental roles in the postembryonic physiological and behavioral development of insects (26). JH III is the only JH homolog found in the worker honeybee (19); its titer increases with age (14, 19, 40), from about 5 pmol/100 ul hemolymph on the first day following eclosion to approximately 20 pmol/100 ul hemolymph 25 days later. The rising titer is correlated with an age-dependent increase in the volume of the corpora allata (16), the glands that produce JH.

Because JH is a small, lipophilic non-immunogenic molecule that occurs in most insects in extremely small quantities (18), its quantification is problematic. The difficulties associated with measuring JH titers have influenced the direction of research on JH's involvement in honeybee division of labor. Titers have been measured from large samples of hemolymph using the Galleria bioassay (14, 44), Hagenguth and Rembold's physico-chemical technique (19) and the Strambi (51) radioimmunoassay (40), but these methods are not sensitive enough to allow titer determinations on individual bees. This limits the ability to correlate hormone titers with behavioral status, one of the classical techniques for investigating hormonal regulation of behavior, because of the great inter-individual variability in worker behavior, even among bees of the same age (32).

Another traditional endocrinological approach that is of limited utility for studies of honeybee age polyethism is to work with individuals in which the corpora allata have been removed and exogenous JH has been introduced. This has been done to investigate JH's physiological effects (21), but it is difficult to successfully introduce surgically altered bees into full-sized colonies for behavioral observation. These constraints have led to the extensive use of a third endocrinological technique: studying the effects of exogenous hormone treatments on marked but otherwise unmanipulated workers. Although this approach generally yields evidence which is reliable in inferring hormonal involvement in behavior (57), the current absence of corroborating data for most of the treatment experiments discussed in this paper argues for a cautious acceptance of the conclusions presented.

PHYSIOLOGICAL EFFECTS OF JH

Applications of JH or JH analogs induce several changes in worker bee physiology that are associated with age-dependent behavioral development. Injections of JH I (43,44), the Law-Williams JH mimic (24) or orally administered JH analogs (3) caused a premature degeneration of the brood-food producing hypopharyngeal glands, a process that usually accompanies the shift from nest to field activities. JH's role in regulating the hypopharyngeal glands was confirmed by Imboden and Lüscher (21), who found that removal of the corpora allata blocked the hypopharyngeal glands' decline, while adding exogenous JH III reversed this effect, i.e., caused gland degeneration. Bees who work in the nest are also characterized by higher titers of vitellogenin and other hemolymph proteins and a greater percentage of dense membrane leucocytes relative to older foraging bees. JH and JH analog treatments caused the levels of these proteins and leucocytes to drop prematurely, while allatectomy prevented their age-dependent decrease (45). JH and JH analog treatments also significantly shorten lifespan. Robinson (36) found 6- and 10- day decreases in mean longevity in two field trials as a result of treatment, which could have been the result of hormonally induced precocious foraging (see next section), since bees usually have 10- to 20-day foraging careers regardless of the age at which they begin (35). However, JH apparently does exert a direct effect on lifespan; Jaycox et al. (24) reported that treated bees kept in laboratory cages rather than in free-flying colonies also displayed a significant decrease in longevity. These results suggest that rising endogenous JH titers cause worker bees to age.

The activity of exocrine glands that produce larval food, wax, and alarm pheromones is closely linked with a worker's behavioral maturation and is also age-dependent (58). The degenerative effects of JH on hypopharyngeal gland morphology suggested that exocrine gland activity may be under hormonal control. Robinson (36) investigated this by quantifying alarm pheromone production in response to methoprene, a JH analog that is used extensively because of its proven JH activity in all insect species on which it has been tested (e.g., 50, 54), including the honeybee (20). The basic method, which was used in all of my experiments described in this paper, was to topically treat one-day-old adult bees with methoprene diluted in acetone, introduce them to typical colonies and study their physiological and behavioral development. In this study bees were collected at the ages of 7, 14 and 21 days to prepare extracts for gas chromatographic analysis. As seen in Fig. 1a, 2-heptanone was not found in untreated bees or in those treated with 25 ug methoprene until day 21. Boch and Shearer (6) also found that the production of this pheromone typically begins at about three weeks of age; the mandibular glands switch from synthesizing larval food to producing 2-heptanone during the transition from nest to field activities that usually occurs at this time. In contrast, bees treated with 250 ug methoprene already contained 2-heptanone by day 14. Premature onset of 2-heptanone production is probably associated with a premature decline in the synthesis of larval food by the mandibular glands, just as the precocious degeneration of the hypopharyngeal glands induced by JH treatments discussed above likely results in a change in secretory activity, from production of larval food to production of invertase, an enzyme used to convert nectar to honey.

The honeybee's principal alarm pheremone, isopentyl acetate, is produced by a gland in the vicinity of the sting (17). On day 7, workers treated with 250 ug methoprene had significantly greater amounts of isopentyl acetate than did 25 ug-treated or control workers (Fig. 1b). There were no significant differences between groups by day 14; a similar effect of age probably would have been observed for 2-heptanone had samples been taken beyond day 21. This is because methoprene did not cause abnormal amounts of either pheromone to be present (5, 6); rather, it induced production precociously. The production of isopentyl acetate begins at 3 to 4 days of age (5) and is not associated with the nest-to-field shift. Premature synthesis of both alarm pheromones by methoprene-treated workers suggests that JH is involved in controlling exocrine events throughout the life of the bee.

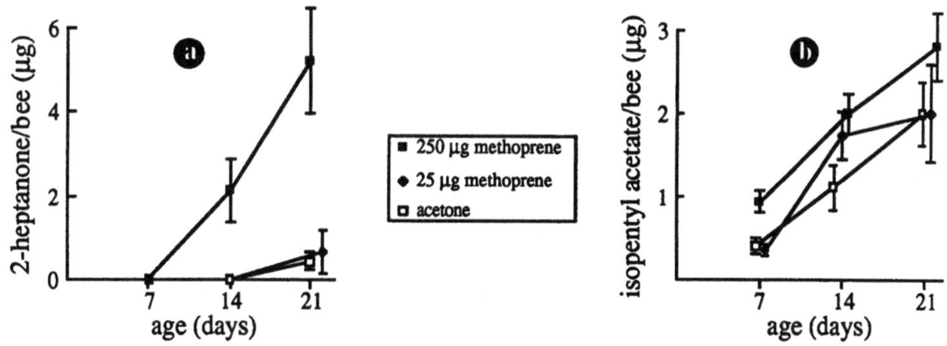

Fig. 1 - Effects of methoprene on pheromone production in honeybees: mean ± SE per bee of a) 2-heptanone and b) isopentyl acetate. ANOVA indicated that bees treated with 250 ug contained significantly more 2-heptanone on days 14 and 21 and more isopentyl acetate on day 7 than control bees or those treated with 25 ug (36).

BEHAVIORAL EFFECTS OF JH

JH's effects on age-dependent physiological processes suggested an involvement in the shift from nest activities to foraging (43). The first experiments on this subject were performed by Jaycox et al. (23) and Jaycox (22), who reported that bees injected with either the Law-Williams JH mimic or JH I apparently began foraging at younger ages and took more foraging flights relative to untreated bees. These studies did not however distinguish between specific effects on the age at which foraging began and the intensity of foraging activity. Effects on the timing of foraging would support the hypothesis that JH plays a role in temporal division of labor. Effects on foraging intensity alone would suggest that JH is involved in regulating foraging performance, and may, for example, control the differentiation of workers into scouts or recruits, two subgroups of foragers with distinct activity patterns (47). This question was resolved by Robinson (36), who found that methoprene treatments affected the age at which foraging began but not foraging intensity (Table 1). Bees treated with 250 ug methoprene began foraging about 8 days earlier than untreated individuals or those treated with lower doses, an impressive difference, considering that bees only live for about 4 to 7 weeks (35). Subsequent experiments (37) have demonstrated that premature foraging can be induced in a dose-dependent manner with applications of 50 to 250 ug. The evidence thus supports the idea that JH affects the transition from nest activities to foraging.

TABLE 1 - Effects of methoprene on the onset and intensity of honeybee foraging behavior. Four colonies were used; data were pooled for analyses because inter-colony differences were not significant. Two other parameters of foraging intensity, foraging flight time (min h^{-1} bee^{-1}) and the number of days spent foraging, were also not affected by treatments. A second trial conducted with three different colonies yielded the same results (36).

Treatment	250 μg	25 μg	2.5 μg	Acetone	Untreated
		Age at first foraging flight[1]			
Mean	13.6 A	19.1B	18.8B	22.1B	20.4B
SE	1.5	1.3	1.1	1.2	1.2
N	21	31	45	27	39
		$F = 4.65$		$p < 0.005$	
	Foraging Intensity (Number of foraging trips · h^{-1} · bee^{-1})				
Mean	1.7	1.9	1.7	1.9	1.7
SE	0.1	0.1	0.1	0.1	0.1
N	19	43	57	45	52
		$F = 1.92$		$p > 0.1$	

[1]Means followed by different letters are significantly different at alpha = 0.05; Tukey's honestly significant difference test.

JH and JH analog treatments also influence the age-dependent spatial distribution of bees in the hive prior to foraging (24, 36), causing them to prematurely shift from the broodnest region, where younger bees typically engage in cell cleaning and brood and queen care (46), to the peripheral regions of the hive, where food storage tasks occur (46). Coupled with methoprene's effects on the production of isopentyl acetate, a developmental process that begins independently of the nest-to-field shift, these results suggested that JH may be involved in the regulation of age polyethism throughout the life of the bee, not only during the shift to foraging.

Robinson (37) tested the hypothesis that age polyethism is hormonally mediated by conducting blind observations of one-day-old individually marked bees that were treated with different doses of methoprene to simulate premature increases in JH titer of varying magnitudes. Groups of hormonally distinct workers were thus created to determine whether they displayed dose-dependent patterns of age-dependent behavior, despite their identical ages. Dose-dependent treatment effects would suggest an association between naturally rising endogenous JH titers and the relative frequency with which age-dependent behaviors are performed.

Methoprene affected task performance in two ways. There were dose-dependent telescopic effects on the age polyethism schedule, i.e., significant decreases in the number of days engaged in brood and queen care, food storage and nest maintenance and a premature onset of foraging (as in 36). Hormone treatments also strongly affected the age-dependent frequency with which acts of brood and queen care, food storage and nest maintenance were performed, again in a dose-dependent manner. The effects of methoprene combined to alter temporal caste structure in all three trials of this experiment, as indicated by significant dose-dependent differences in the relative frequency with which the principal tasks of cell cleaning, brood and queen care, food storage and foraging were performed. In trial 3 (Fig. 2), for example, acetone-treated bees passed through three age castes, that is at each age they performed one of the principal tasks more often than the other two (46). Based on the results of other trials (37), they also would have eventually been observed in the fourth caste as foragers had the experiment continued. Bees treated with 50 ug displayed typical age caste differentiation (i.e., four age castes), but brood and queen care activity was less prominent relative to the control group. This effect was intensified at higher doses (150 and 200 ug) so that at virtually no age did the performance of brood and queen care prevail over the other three tasks. In other words, they essentially skipped the brood and queen care caste; they passed through a phase of typical cell cleaning behavior (which was not affected by methoprene), to a premature food storage phase, and then began foraging precociously. Results varied strikingly between trials: treatments caused bees to skip the food storage caste in addition to the brood and queen care caste in trial 1 (not shown), presumably because there was less need for food storage activity at that time, as suggested by a relatively low observed frequency for this task in the control group. Methoprene thus did not induce invariant labor patterns, but rather modified behavior within a context of environmentally mediated changes in colony need. Furthermore, treatments did not elicit responses outside of the normal range of honeybee behavior: untreated bees may also display similarly altered age polyethism schedules under stressful environmental and colony conditions (e.g., 31). These observations suggest that: 1) changes in JH levels underlie the bees' ability to effectively respond to changing colony needs, and 2) methoprene's effects were physiologically relevant;

these subjects will be discussed later in this paper. Methoprene exerted its strongest behavioral influences on brood and queen tending and foraging behavior, which are among the tasks most closely associated with age-dependent exocrine gland development (58). Other tasks, such as cell cleaning, are unaffected, perhaps because their performance is apparently independent of glandular activity. This again points to JH's involvement in coordinating exocrine and behavioral development, processes which are so tightly linked in the worker bee.

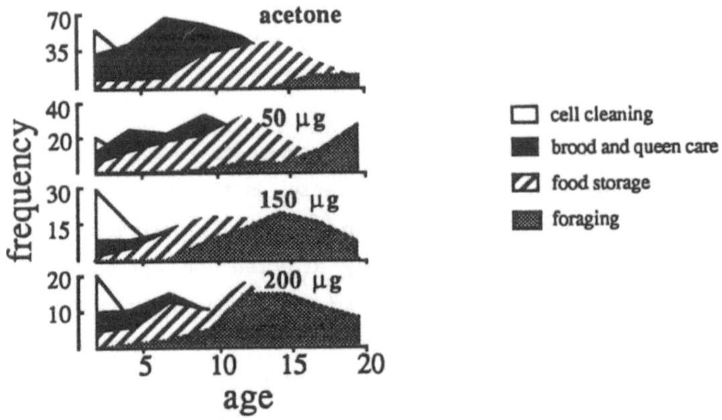

Fig. 2 - Effects of methoprene on honeybee temporal caste structure. Chi-square tests revealed significant ($p < 0.05$ — 0.0005) dose-dependent differences in the relative apportionment of labor among the four principal tasks at all ages in this and two other trials of the same experiment. Note that behavioral curves overlap. Absolute frequencies declined with increasing doses of methoprene because treated bees began taking orientation and foraging flights at relatively younger ages; this decreased their probability of being observed in the hive and shortened their lifespan (37).

MODE OF ACTION OF JH ON AGE POLYETHISM

Because bees older than a few days are capable of accomplishing many different tasks (25, 27) it is logical to consider age polyethism as a probabilistic process (58), dilineated by age-dependent differences in the probabilities that tasks will be performed. This suggests that worker bees undergo age-dependent changes in their response thresholds to the stimuli that elicit the performance of tasks. Robinson (37) invoked one of the principal means by which hormones regulate behavior (2) and hypothesized that JH modulates the bees' response thresholds. For example, a young bee with a low JH titer may be more responsive to the stimuli associated with developing larvae that elicit brood care than to those involved with foraging, and vice versa for an older bee with a higher JH titer. This hypothesis was tested (38) by examining the effects of methoprene on alarm pheromone perception, because olfactory stimuli are of central importance in mediating task performance. Alarm pheromones were chosen as model stimuli because: 1) their chemical identity is known; 2) they are associated with an important task, nest defense (11) and 3) age-dependent increase in responsiveness to these odors (10) parallel the ontogeny of defensive behavior (7, 52). The prediction was that methoprene would prematurely reduce the threshold sensitivity of bees to alarm pheromones.

Using a behavioral assay based on the one developed by Collins and Rothenbuhler (12) and a blind experimental protocol, the result was that methoprene significantly lowered response thresholds (Fig. 3a). Treated bees did not become hypersensitive to alarm pheromones; rather the development of maximum sensitivity to these odors was hastened so that it was already exhibited by 5- to 8-day-old bees, while untreated bees did not display fully mature behavioral responses until 16 days of age. In contrast, peripheral perception, as measured by the electroantennogram technique (41), was not affected by treatments (Fig 3b), suggesting that JH affects processes that occur in the bee's central nervous system (CNS). This is consistent with the fact that most hormonal effects on perception occur in the CNS (55).

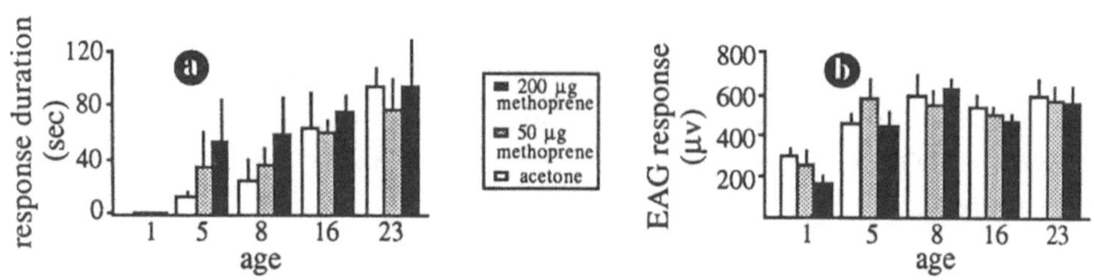

Fig. 3 - Effects of methoprene on honeybee alarm pheromone perception: mean (+SE) responses to isopentyl acetate (IPA). a) behavioral assay: 10 ug IPA; N=9(except N=6 for day 23); b) electroantenogram (EAG) assay: 2 ug IPA; N=10(day 1), 22(day 5), 20(day 8), 22(day 16) and 15(day 23). ANOVA indicated significant age-dependent effects only of 200 ug methoprene on alarm pheromone sensitivity in the behavioral assay on days 5 and 8 but no effect on the EAG response at any age. Not shown are the results for two additional parameters of the behavioral response, latency and intensity, as well as behavioral and EAG responses to two concentrations of 2-heptanone and a second concentration of IPA, in this and a second trial; all of these data agree with those presented (37).

It is widely assumed that caste-specific differences in sensitivity to task-associated stimuli underlie division of labor in insect societies (62), despite limited supporting evidence (59, 62). Since alarm pheromone perception is a component of colonial nest defense (11), a task that is allocated to an age-specific subgroup of a colony's workers (27), these results provide additional support for this view of division of labor. More importantly, they provide evidence in favor of the hypothesis that differences in caste-specific response thresholds can be hormonally modulated.

MODELS EXPLAINING THE ROLE OF JH IN REGULATING DIVISION OF LABOR

Two models of hormonally mediated age polyethism have been proposed. Bühler et al. (8) hypothesize that a single (untested) mechanism, JH-induced temperature preferences in the hive, affects both the physiological development of "summer" vs. "winter" bees (13) and division of labor. This model seems more appropriate for JH's involvement in the former rather than in division of labor during the active season, because as discussed elsewhere (39), it does not adequately describe JH's behavioral effects on age polyethism. According to Robinson's model (37), the probability that a worker will perform a particular task is determined by: 1) a genetically programmed change in CNS response thresholds to task-associated stimuli that is mediated by rising JH titers, and 2) prevailing environmental and colony conditions, which determine the magnitude of a colony's need for the task to be performed (Fig. 4). Experimental colony perturbations (33) elicit behavioral responses similar to those caused by methoprene, suggesting that extrinsic conditions also influence division of labor by modulating the JH titer of individual bees, thus changing their response thresholds. Age polyethism is sensitive to changes in several environmental and colony conditions (see Fig. 4), which may regulate JH via neurosecretory hormonal systems. Diapause induction (53) and phase determination in locusts (9) are examples of the man JH-controlled processes that are regulated by specific environmental cues in this manner. At present the evidence for extrinsic regulation of honeybee JH titers is limited to Bühler et al.'s (8) report that temperature and CO_2 concentration can affect the JH titers of caged bees in the laboratory. Robinson et al. (40) found variation in the age-specific JH titers of bees in free-flying colonies, most likely because of seasonal differences, but potential effects on age polyethism were not examined.

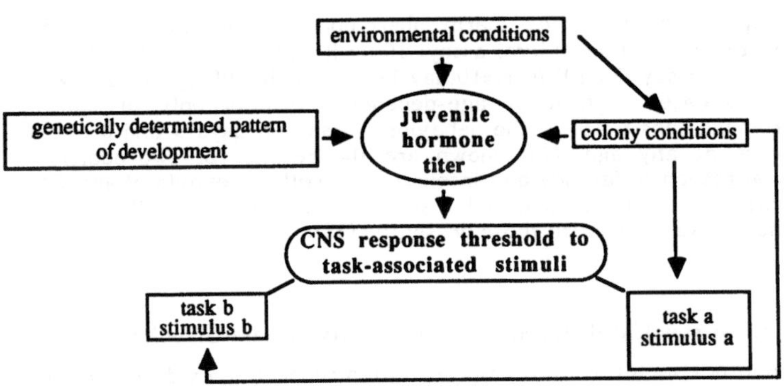

Fig. 4 - Model explaining the role of JH in regulating honeybee division of labor. The probability that a worker bee will perform a given task is determined by: 1) JH-dependent response thresholds that determine the probability of responding to stimuli that elicit the performance of a task, and 2) environmental and colony conditions that determine the probability of encountering a task, by shaping colony needs and determining the relative magnitude of the tasks (depicted here as the relative size of "Task A" and "Task B" boxes). Environmental and colony factors known to affect age polyethism are food availability (49), colony population (63), colony age structure (e.g., 29), amount of storage comb (42) and amount of brood (64); the level of queen pheromones circulating in the colony (22) influences worker foraging intensity but possible effects on age polyethism have not been studied. According to the model, JH titers increase with worker age due to a genetically determined pattern of development; in addition, JH titers (and therefore response thresholds) may be modulated by environmental and colony conditions, enabling individual workers to respond to changing colony needs (36).

According to this model, JH regulates individual bee behavior by influencing the probability that a worker will perform a particular task. In addition, extrinsic modulation of JH titers may underlie a colony's ability to efficiently allocate its labor resources in response to changing environmental and colony conditions.

FURTHER STUDIES

JH's role in the differentiation of morphologically distinct castes is well-known (30), but the honeybee is the first species in which a hormonally mediated system of temporal caste determination has been found. The present case for JH's involvement in age polyethism rests largely on the results of treatment experiments with methoprene. The results of experiments with radiolabelled methoprene (4) and a structurally similar JH analog with essentially no hormonal activity (1, 37), and the previously noted observation that methoprene did not cause aberrant bee behavior or pheromone production all suggest (see also 37) that the high doses of methoprene used relative to endogenous JH titers indeed induced physiologically relevant responses. Nevertheless, correlations between JH titer and behavioral status, if possible, would provide important supportive evidence for JH's role in regulating age polyethism.

Two lines of research are suggested by the model discussed above. First, the identification of environmental and colonial factors that affect division of labor may be accomplished by searching for extrinsic cues that modulate JH titers. It would also be desirable to determine whether other mechanisms that have been hypothesized to help mesh the activities of individual bees with the needs of their colony, which involve "patrolling" behavior (27) and/or trophallaxis (35), act (if at all) on JH titers or are independent of JH. Studies aimed at elucidating mechanisms of integration in insect societies are needed; despite the fact that colonies of many social insect species exhibit great resiliency to changes in colony and environmental conditions (e.g., 60, 61) the specific stimuli perceived by individuals that result in adaptive colony responses have not been identified. A second direction for future research is to investigate precisely how JH exerts its presumed effects on the bee's CNS. A great deal is known about the interactions between hormones and the nervous system for simple endocrine-controlled insect behaviors (56), but relatively little information is available about the neural basis of more complex social behaviors such as age polyethism.

Currently there is great interest in unraveling the behavioral and physiological mechanisms underlying caste differentiation and division of labor. Much progress has been made in understanding behavioral aspects of colony regulation (see chapter by Seeley in this volume; 34). Equally impressive have been the results of studies on the physiology of reproductive division of labor (30). In contrast, it is apparent that the study of physiological bases of worker age caste differentiation has only just begun. Although it is likely these studies will expand to other species, the honeybee, because of its remarkably intricate and flexible system of age polyethism, made especially accessible to thorough study by established techniques of culture and experimental manipulation, will continue to be a model organism for mechanistic studies of division of labor.

Acknowledgements. G.B. Staal, Zoecon Corp., Palo Alto, CA, has kindly provided me with JH analogs throughout my studies. I thank G.C. Eickwort, H.H. Hagedorn, R. Nowogrodzki, P.W. Sherman and P.K. Visscher for stimulating discussion and comments that improved this manuscript. My experimental work was supported by a Lady Davis Fellowship, Cornell University-USAID Title XII Strengthening Grant, Cornell University Summer Research Fellowship, Sigma Xi Grants-in-Aid (one Cornell chapter, one national), and the generosity of R.A. Morse, for which I am deeply grateful.

REFERENCES

(1) Baker, F.C.; Hagedorn, H.H.; Schooley, D.A.; and Wheelock, G. 1983. Mosquito juvenile hormone: identification and bioassay activity. J. Insect Physiol. 29: 465-470.

(2) Beach, F.A. 1983. Hormones and psychological processes. Can. J. Psych. 37: 193-210.

(3) Beetsma, J., and Ten Houten, A. 1974. Effects of juvenile hormone analogues in the food of honeybee colonies. Z. Ang. Ent. 77: 292-300.

(4) Bigley, W.S., and Vinson, S.B. 1979. Degradation of ^{14}C methoprene in the Imported Fire Ant, Solenopsis invicta. Pestic. Biochem. Physiol. 10: 1-13.

(5) Boch, R., and Shearer, D.A. 1966. Iso-pentyl acetate in stings of honeybees of different ages. J. Apic. Res. 5:65-70.

(6) Boch, R., and Shearer, D.A. 1967. 2-heptanone and 10-hydroxy trans dec-2-enoic acid in the mandibular glands of worker honey bees of different ages. Z. Vergl. Physiol. 54:1-11.

(7) Breed, M.D. 1983. Correlations between aggressiveness and corpora allata volume, social isolation, age and dietary protein in worker honeybees. Insectes Soc. 30:482-495.

(8) Bühler, A.; Lanzrein, B.; and Wille, H. 1983. Influence of temperature and carbon dioxide concentration on juvenile hormone titre and dependent parameters of adult worker honey bees (Apis mellifera L.). J. Insect Physiol. 29:885-893.

(9) Chapman, R.F. 1976. A Biology of Locusts. London: Edward Arnold Ltd.

(10) Collins, A.M. 1980. Effect of age on the response to alarm pheromones by caged honey bees. Ann. Ent. Soc. Amer. 73:307-309.

(11) Collins, A.M.; Rinderer, T.E.; Tucker, K.W.; Sylvester, H.A.; and Lackett, J.J. 1980. A model of honeybee defensive behaviour. J. Apic. Res. 19: 224-231.

(12) Collins, A.M., and Rothenbuhler, W.C. 1978. Laboratory test of the response to an alarm chemical, isopentyl acetate, by Apis mellifera. Ann. Ent. Soc. Amer. 71:906-909.

(13) Fluri, P.; Wille, L.; Gerig, L.; and Lüscher, M. 1977. Juvenile hormone and the determination of winter bee physiology (Apis mellifera). Proc. 8th Cong. IUSSI, Wageningen, Holland, pp 28-29.

(14) Fluri, P.; Lüscher, M.; Wille, H.; and Gerig, L. 1982. Changes in weight of the pharyngeal gland and haemolymph titres of juvenile hormone, protein and vitellogenin in worker honey bees. J. Insect Physiol. 28: 61-68.

(15) Free, J.B. 1965. The allocation of duties among worker honeybees. Symp. Zool. Soc. Lond. 14: 39-59.

(16) Gast, R. 1967. Untersuchungen über den Einfluss der Königinnensubstanz auf die Entwicklung der endokrinen Drüsen bei der Arbeiterin der Honigbiene (Apis mellifica). Insectes Soc. 14: 1-12.

(17) Ghent, R.L., and Gary, N.E. 1962. A chemical alarm releaser in honey bee stings (Apis mellifera L.). Psyche 69: 1-6.

(18) Granger, N.A., and Goodman, W.G. 1983. Juvenile hormone radioimmunoassays - theory and practice. Insect Biochem. 13: 333-340.

(19) Hagenguth, H., and Rembold, H. 1978. Identification of juvenile hormone 3 as the only JH homolog in all developmental stages of the honey bee. Z. Naturforsch. 33 C: 847-850.

(20) Hussein, M.H., and Abdel-Aal, Y.A.I. 1978. Effect of ZR-515 on honey bee, Apis mellifera L. Z. Ang. Ent. 87: 109-111.

(21) Imboden, H., and Lüscher, M. 1975. Allatektomie bei adulten Bienen-Arbeiterinnen (Apis mellifica). Rev. Swisse Zool. 82: 694-698.

(22) Jaycox, E.R. 1970. Honey bee queen pheromones and worker foraging behavior. Ann. Ent. Soc. Am. 63: 222-228.

(23) Jaycox, E.R. 1976. Behavioral changes in worker honey bees (Apis mellifera L.) after injection with synthetic juvenile hormone (Hymenoptera:Apidae). J. Kans. Ent. Soc. 49: 165-170.

(24) Jaycox, E.R.; Skowronek, W.; and Gwynn, G. 1974. Behavioral changes in a worker honey bee (Apis mellifera) induced by injections of a juvenile hormone mimic. Ann. Ent. Soc. Am. 67: 529-534.

(25) Kolmes, S.A. 1985. A quantitative study of the division of labour among worker honey bees. Z. Tierpsychol. 68: 287-302.

(26) Laufer, H., and Borst, D.W. 1983. Juvenile hormone and its mechanism of action. In Endocrinology of Insects, eds. G.H. Downer and H. Laufer, pp. 203-216. New York: Liss, Inc.

(27) Lindauer, M. 1952. Ein Beitrag zur Frage der Arbeitsteilung im Bienenstaat. Z. Vergl. Physiol. 34: 299-345.

(28) Michener, C.D. 1974. The Social Behavior of the Bees: A Comparative Study. Cambridge: Belknap Press of Harvard University.

(29) Milojevíc, B.D. 1940. A new interpretation of the social life of the honeybee. Bee World 21: 39-41.

(30) Nijhout, H.F., and Wheeler, D.E. 1982. Juvenile hormone and the physiological basis of insect polymorphisms. Quart. Rev. Biol. 57: 109-133.

(31) Nolan, W.J. 1924. The division of labour in the honeybee. N.C. Bkpr. (Oct.): 10-15.

(32) Nowogrodzki, R. 1983. Individual differences and division of labor in the honey bees. Ph.D. Dissertation, Cornell University, Ithaca, New York.

(33) Oster, G.F., and Wilson, E.O. 1978. Caste and Ecology in the Social Insects. Princeton: Princeton University Press.

(34) Reeve, H.K., and Gamboa, G.J. 1983. Colony activity integration in primitively eusocial wasps: the role of the queen (Polistes fuscatus, Hymenoptera: Vespidae). Behav. Ecol. Sociobiol. 13: 63-74.

(35) Ribbands, C.R. 1952. Division of labour in the honeybee community. Proc. R. Soc. Lond. 140: 32-43.

(36) Robinson, G.E. 1985. Effects of juvenile hormone analogue on honey bee foraging behaviour and alarm pheromone production. J. Insect Physiol. 31: 277-282.

(37) Robinson, G.E. Submitted a. Regulation of honey bee age polyethism by a juvenile hormone analog.

(38) Robinson, G.E. Submitted b. Alarm pheromone perception in the honey bee:evidence for division of labor based on hormonally modulated response thresholds.

(39) Robinson, G.E. Submitted c. Does temperature and carbon dioxide concentration in the nest of the honey bee regulate division of labor?

(40) Robinson, G.E.; Strambi, A.; Strambi, C.; Paulino-Simoes, Z.L.; Tozeto, S.O.; and Barbosa, J.M.N. Submitted. Juvenile hormone titers in European and African honey bees.

(41) Roelofs, W.L. 1984. Electroantennogram assays: rapid and convenient screening procedures for pheromones. In Techniques in Pheromone Research, eds. H.G. Hummel and T.A. Miller, pp. 131-160. New York:Springer-Verlag.

(42) Rösch, G.A. 1930. Untersuchungen über die Arbeitsteilung im Bienenstaat II. Die Tätigkeiten der Arbeitsbienen unter experimentell veränderten Bedingungen. Z. Vergl. Physiol. 12: 1-71.

(43) Rutz, W.; Gerig, L.; Wille, H.; and Lüscher, M. 1974. A bioassay for juvenile hormone (JH) effects of insect growth regulators (IGR) on adult worker honeybees. Mitt. Schweiz. Ent. Ges. 47: 307-313.

(44) Rutz, W.; Gerig, L.; Wille, H.; and Lüscher, M. 1976. The function of juvenile hormone in adult worker honeybees, Apis mellifera. J. Insect Physiol. 22: 1485-1491.

(45) Rutz, W.; Imboden, H.; Jaycox, E.R.; Wille, H.; Gerig, L.; and Lüscher, M. 1977. Juvenile hormone and polyethism in adult worker honeybees (Apis mellifera). Proc. 8th Cong. IUSSI, Wageningen, Holland, pp. 26-27.

(46) Seeley, T.D. 1982. Adaptive significance of the age polyethism schedule in honeybee colonies. Behav. Ecol. Sociobiol. 11: 287-293.

(47) Seeley, T.D. 1983. Division of labor between scouts and recruits in honeybee foraging. Behav. Ecol. Sociobiol. 12: 253-259.

(48) Seeley, T.D. 1985. Honeybee Ecology. Princeton: Princeton University Press.

(49) Sekiguchi, K., and Sakagami, S.F. 1966. Structure of foraging population and related problems in the honey bee, with consideration on the division of labour in bee colonies. Hokkaido Natn. Agric. Exp. Stn. Rep. 69: 1-65.

(50) Staal, G.B. 1975. Insect growth regulators with juvenile hormone activity. Ann. Rev. Ent. 20: 417-460.

(51) Strambi, C.; Strambi, A.; De Reggi, M.L.; Hirn, M.H.; and Delaage, M.A. 1981. Radioimmunoassay of insect juvenile hormones and their diol derivatives. Europ. J. Biochem. 118: 401-406.

(52) Szabo, T.I., and Townsend, G.F. 1974. Behavioural studies on queen introduction in the honeybee. 1. Effect of the age of workers (from a colony with a laying queen) on their behaviour towards an introduced virgin queen. J. Apic. Res. 13: 19-25.

(53) Tauber, M.J.; Tauber, C.A.; and Masaki, S. 1986. Seasonal Adaptations of Insects. Oxford University Press, New York.

(54) Tobe, S.S., and Stay, B. 1979. Modulation of juvenile hormone synthesis by an analogue in the cockroach. Nature 281: 481-482.

(55) Truman, J.W. 1978. Hormonal control of invertebrate behaviour. Horm. and Behav. 10: 214-234.

(56) Truman, J.W., and Dominick, O.S. 1983. Endocrine mechanisms organizing invertebrate behavior. BioScience 33: 546-551.

(57) Truman, J.W., and Riddiford, L.M. 1974. Hormonal mechanisms underlying insect behaviour. In Advances in Insect Physiology Vol. 10., eds. J.E. Treherne, M.J. Berridge, and V.B. Wigglesworth, pp. 297-352. New York: Academic Press.

(58) Wilson, E.O. 1971. The Insect Societies. Cambridge: Belknap Press of Harvard University.

(59) Wilson, E.O. 1978. Division of labor in fire ants based on physical castes (Hymenoptera: Formicidae: Solenopsis). J. Kans. Ent. Soc. 51: 615-636.

(60) Wilson, E.O. 1983. Caste and division of labor in leaf-cutter ants (Hymenoptera:Formicidae:Atta). III. Ergonomic resiliency in foraging by A. cephalotes. Behav. Ecol Sociobiol. 14: 47-54.

(61) Wilson, E.O. 1984. The relation between caste ratios and division of labor in the ant genus Pheidole (Hymenoptera: Formicidae). Behav. Ecol. Sociobiol. 16: 89-98.

(62) Wilson, E.O. 1985. Between-caste aversion as a basis for division of labor in the ant Pheidole pubiventris (Hymenoptera: Formicidae). Behav. Ecol. Sociobiol. 17: 35-37.

(63) Winston, M.L., and Neilson-Punnett, E. 1982. Factors determining temporal division of labour in honeybees. Can. J. Zool. 60: 2947-2952.

(64) Winston, M.L., and Fergusson, L.A. 1985. The effect of worker loss on temporal caste structure in colonies of the honeybee (Apis mellifera L.) Can. J. Zool. 63: 777-780.

Organization and Plasticity of the Olfactory System of the Honeybee, Apis mellifera

Claudine Masson and Gérard Arnold

Laboratoire de Neurobiologie Comparée des Invertebres, INRA-CNRS (UA 1190), 91440 Bures-sur-Yvette, France

Abstract. From a neurobiological point of view, the olfactory system of the honeybee is of considerable interest. Many adult behavioral responses, such as olfactory conditioning through food reward, suggest plasticity of the nervous system involved in olfactory processing. It seems likely that adult olfactory plasticity may be dependent on the olfactory history of individuals. Here we have selected recently obtained data which suggest that the olfactory system in the bee is especially suitable for an analysis of neuronal plasticity during post-embryonic development. Both normal development, and the role of epigenetic factors in the stabilization of the synapses are considered with respect to their impact on adult behavior. The organization of the antennal system is described in detail to provide a reference point for the developmental studies.

THE ANTENNAL SENSORY SYSTEM

In the bee, as in all insect species studied to date, olfactory information is collected by primary receptor neurons housed in specialized sensilla. The most complete study of the number and distribution of the sensilla on the antennae of the honeybee is that of Esslen and Kaissling (19). There is a notable dimorphism between the antenna of the worker and drone with respect to both the relative number of sensilla of each type, and the total number of sensory cells present. The antenna of the worker has 6,400 sensilla, 2,600 of which are sensilla placodea (41%), whereas the drone antenna has 19,700 sensilla, 18,600 of which are s. placodea (94%). Only 1,600 s. placodea are found on the antenna of the queen. The majority of sensory cells (97% in the worker and 99% in the drone) appear to be olfactory cells. Pores in the cuticle of the sensilla provide gateways for odorant molecules to reach the dendritic membranes of the underlying receptor cells, where sensory transduction takes place. The olfactory receptor cells are typical bipolar neurons. A single dendrite extends distally from the soma and terminates, often with several ramifications, in the sensillum liquor within the cuticular region of the sensillum (24). Proximally, the receptor cell axon projects to the deutocerebrum of the brain. It is generally believed that the olfactory receptor cells function as independant sensory units (18, 26, 28). These neurons are responsible for the selectivity and specificity of detection, and for olfactory discrimination.

It appears that inter- or intra-specific chemicals that induce changes in the behavior and/or physiology of individuals are more or less complex mixtures of several components. This is true of pheromones, for example, the queen pheromone (7, 13), the Nasanoff pheromone (41) and the alarm pheromone (10), and true also of allelochemicals, such as the plant aromas used as attractants for forager bees (39, 40). It appears that for each effective chemical blend, there is a corresponding peripheral sensory "image" resulting from the activity of particular sensory neurons. Identification of specific signals, therefore, involves the integration of the various signal components. Such "integrator mechanisms" consist of a convergence of neuroreceptors onto target neurons in the central nervous system. There is extensive convergence of the peripheral afferents onto the deutocerebral output neurons (9, 27, 28, 31). The mean ratio of this convergence, estimated in various insects, is circa 1,000 afferents for 1 efferent. For the pheromonal sex pathway in the cockroach Periplaneta americana a convergence of 5,000:1 has been estimated (18).

There are 2 categories of deutocerebral neurons. The deutocerebral output neurons which send their processes from the deutocerebrum to higher centres in the brain, mainly in the protocerebrum (mushroom bodies and lateral lobe), and the local interneurons which are confined to the antennal lobe. Local interneurons appear to be closely involved in the processing of the large amount of incoming olfactory information (9, 12, 18, 27, 28, 31, 32). The immunocytochemical distribution of gamma-aminobutyric acid (GABA) and its biosynthetic enzyme 1-glutamic acid decarboxylase (GAD) in the honeybee deutocerebrum (6,44) suggests that inhibitory mechanisms may be involved in the processing of data in this region of the bee brain. The antennal lobe contains other neurotransmitters (Mercer et al.), (46). Dopamine seems to be restricted to the centripetal periphery of the glomeruli (25), serotonin (5-HT) is found in varicose nerve fibres that project around the central core of the glomeruli (46), and acetylcholine is believed to be the principal neurotransmitter released by afferent neurons in the antennal lobe of some insects, for example, Manduca sexta (21).

Peripheral olfactory coding appears to be quite different for pheromones and allelochemicals (8, 28, 30, 31). In most species, chemical information concerning the sex pheromones, and interspecifically acting pheromones, is conveyed to the brain via separate, non-overlapping primary axons. The increase of activity in any single axon encodes for the quality of one particular odorous compound. This coding is termed a "labelled lines" pattern. In contrast, analyses of olfactory cell responses to food odors show, for example, that these cells respond to several constituents and thus are less specialized than pheromone receptor cells. Here, information about the quality of the odor is mainly transmitted to the brain via overlapping lines, the information encoded in an "across fiber" pattern.

If we consider these different chemicals with their specific mode of coding and the behaviors they trigger, it is interesting to note that the stereotype behavioral responses, generally elicited by specific pheromones via a "specialist system" of receptor cells, may be considered as genetically preprogrammed, involving an innate releasing mechanism. This is not true of some of the more adaptive behavioral responses, for example, to volatile food sources, themselves chemically unstable (40). These adaptive behavioral responses may involve experience as demonstrated by conditioning experiments in honeybees. These responses are elicited through a more "generalist system" of receptor cells. In the worker, these cells belong to different "reaction groups" with overlapping response spectra (26, 50).

The convergent organization of the antennal lobes allows selection of adequate stimulus components through integrative, amplifying and enhancement mechanisms, and adjustments towards variations in the biological signal composition (quality and/or intensity). An appreciation of neuronal organization at the deutocerebral level may be crucial to understanding the rules underlying the neural basis of olfactory plasticity.

SPATIAL AND QUANTITATIVE ORGANIZATION OF THE ADULT ANTENNAL LOBE

There have been a number of anatomical descriptions of the antennal lobe system in the honeybee (3, 4, 34, 38, 48, see Fig. 1 and 2). With local antennal applications of cobalt ions, Arnold et al. (2) made a morphological and quantitative analysis of the antennal pathway. A comparative study has been made in the workerbee and the drone (3, 4) and in the queen (5, Fig.1). In the workerbee, the drone, and the queen the antennal sensory axons at their entrance into the brain are subdivided into three branches. Of these 3 branches, one goes straight towards the protocerebrum in the region of the giant ocellar fibers, one projects to the ipsilateral side of the suboesophageal ganglion by passing contralaterally, and the last branch projects into the postero-median area of the protocerebrum. The diameters of bundles of sensory neurones in the drone are greater than those of homologous bundles in the worker because of the larger number of sensory cells in the antenna of the drone (19), whereas, in the queen, afferent bundles are smaller than in workers. This is certainly due to the fact that there are fewer antennal sensilla in the queen than in the worker (Mac Indoo, 1922).

The neuropile of the antennal lobe is an egg-shaped mass oriented along an antero-ventral, postero-dorsal axis. A comparison between the three castes shows that size differences exist with a mean volume of 9,900 - 800 x 10^3 um^3 for the worker, 12,200 - 2,200 x 10^3 um^3 for the drone, and 7,170 - 599 x 10^3 um^3 for the queen. There is a slight variability due to the conditions of postembryonic development (i.e. different colonies, different seasons).The glomerular neuropile located at the periphery of the antennal lobe (Fig.1) represents 46%, 44%, and 43% of the total volume of the deutocerebrum in the worker, the drone, and the queen respectively. The large majority of the glomeruli are egg-shaped. A thin, discontinuous layer (probably made up of glial cell processes) surrounds the glomeruli. Four main regions of the glomerular neuropile (anterior and dorsal; ventral; intermediate; and posterior), can be distinguished according to corresponding afferent bundles in the 3 castes. Despite the very similar appearance of the glomeruli in the worker and the queen, fundamental differences in the organization of each of the 4 regions of the glomerular neuropile exist between the

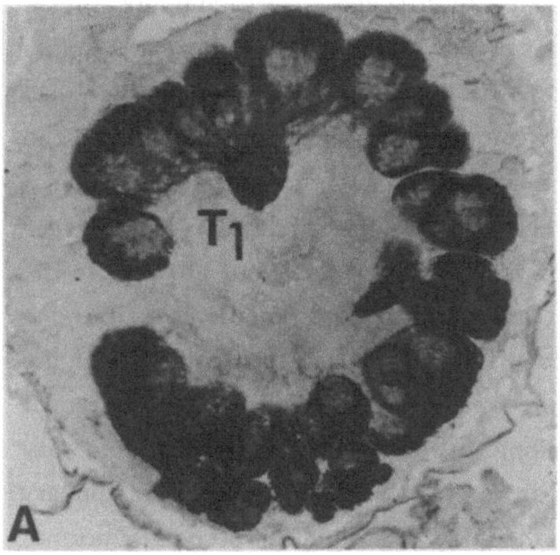

Fig. 1 - A, B, C. Frontal sections of the antennal lobe of a workerbee (A), a queen bee (B) and a drone (C). In the 3 castes, 4 main regions of the glomerular neuropile have been distinguished according to corresponding afferent bundles. The number and the pathway of these bundles are very similar. The anterior and dorsal regions are the most developed of all the glomerular regions, and receive their afferents from the T1 bundle. Compared with the worker, the diameter of the antennal lobe is bigger in the drone and smaller in the queen; this is due to the larger number of sensory cells in the drone antenna, and smaller number in the case of the queen. The organization of the antennal lobe is very similar for the queen (Fig. 1B) and the workerbee (Fig. 1A) except for a glomerulus in the dorsal region which is relatively more developed in the queen and could be a macroglomerulus (arrow). In the drone, the antennal lobe contains 4 voluminous glomerular complexes (arrow), 3 in the dorsal region (Fig. 1C) and 1 in the intermediate region.

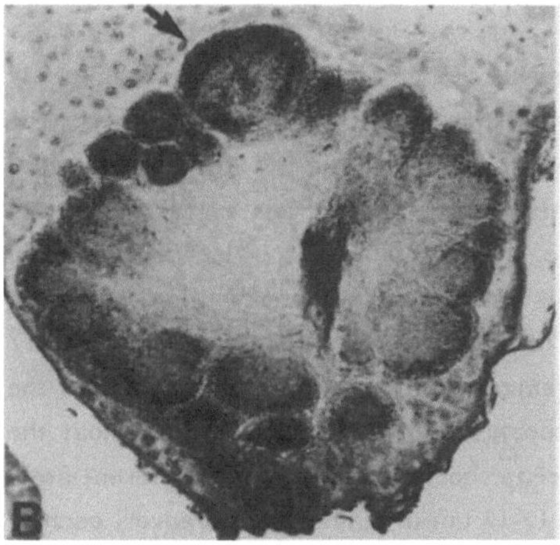

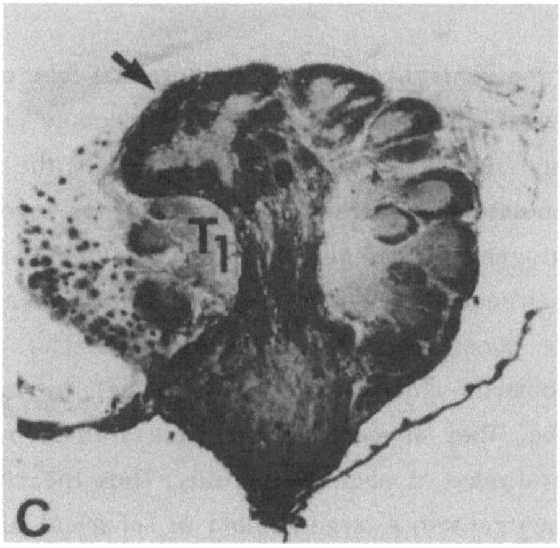

two sexes. On the basis of Golgi-stained receptor axons, Mobbs (34) divides the glomeruli into at least 5 distinct types. Generally, each glomerulus receives input from only one kind of receptor axon. However, occasional bi-glomerular endings are encountered. In the worker and the queen, all but 7 of the glomeruli have a characteristic intensely stained cortical layer which is thick in the upper part of each glomerulus, and diminishes towards the inner part. This layer represents about 55% of the glomerular volume. It is in this area that the synaptic connections between the sensory axons and the deutocerebral neurons take place. Microscopic observations show that this layer contains spherical sub-units (3-5um) the functional significance of which remains to be demonstrated but which suggest very complex microcircuitry at this level. In the drone, there are two types of glomeruli that are morphologically different. On the one hand, normal glomeruli identical to those described for the worker with a cortical layer densely stained. On the other hand, 4 voluminous glomerular complexes (3 in the dorsal region, 1 in the intermediate region) more or less irregular in shape. They have a cortical layer with a thickness of 10-45 um. Moreover, the sub-units in this layer are larger (10-30 um) than in the workerbee glomeruli. The antennal lobe of the honeybee answers to the concept of glomerular invariance which requires that the glomeruli are homologous from one insect to the next (Chambille et al, 1980). Three conditions must be satisfied to fulfil the requirements for glomerular invariance: (i) a constant number of glomeruli in each antennal lobe, (ii) a constant position of the identified glomeruli between individuals, and (iii) comparable dimensions of the identifiable glomeruli from one insect to the next. It appears that the workerbee has an average of 166 glomeruli, the queen 155, and the drone 103 normal glomeruli and 4 glomerular complexes. The volume of the glomerular complexes is 9 to 40 times greater than that of other glomeruli. The mean volume of the glomeruli is smaller in the queen than in the worker (Fig.2) except for one glomerulus located in the dorsal region of the antennal lobe that is larger in the queen. This glomerulus, and its homologue in the worker, is found in the same position as one of the 3 dorsal glomerular complexes in the drone. This raises the interesting question of the female sex dimorphism and needs further investigation.

In the ventral regions of the antennal lobe of the worker bee and the queen, there is an easily identifiable group of glomeruli (a "lobule",5) recessed slightly from the mass of others. The only significant variability found in the number of glomeruli among the experimental population of workerbees analysed has involved this distinct group. This suggests that the autogeny of the glomeruli of this lobule might be strongly under the influence of certain environmental factors not yet known. Such a group is not present in the drone. In the worker, the queen, and the drone, the posterior region of the sensory antennal lobe includes 7 glomeruli which are different in their intrinsic organization to those in other regions of the lobe. They appear less intensely stained by the cobalt which is distributed throughout the total mass of each glomerulus. Thus the characteristic cortical layer is not differentiated. They contain a large number of spherical sub-units (5-12 um in diameter). Moreover, each of these seven glomeruli is innervated by a single, thin, well defined bundle of receptor neurons suggesting that each of the 7 glomeruli has a different function. Such an arrangement might be very useful for investigating the functional significance of the synaptic structures in the antennal lobe.

The deutocerebral output neurons have glomerular dendritic fields that often appear like an almost solid ball because of the density of the dendritic branches within the glomerulus. The main deutocerebral efferents project into the protocerebrum via the antenno-glomerular tract (AGT) (23). Only a few fibers project towards the contralateral antennal lobe. The

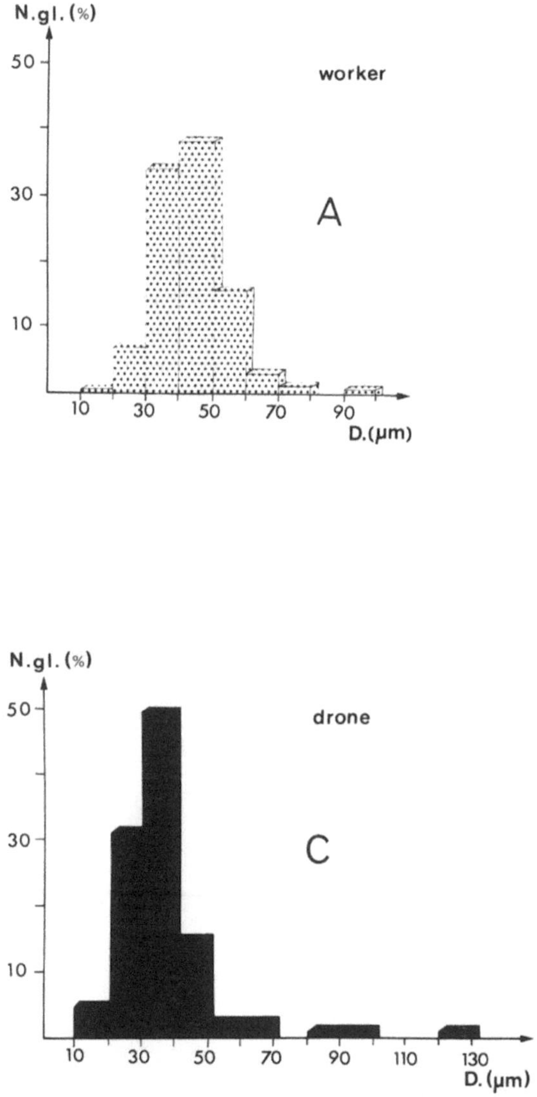

Fig. - 2 A, B, C. Comparison of the distribution and frequency of glomerular diameters in the worker (A), the queen (B), and the drone (C).

organization of efferents is very similar between the 3 castes, despite slight differences in trajectory and projectional areas. There are 4 main tracts projecting towards the ipsilateral protocerebrum, the median tract, the lateral tract, the anterior and the posterior mediolateral tracts. Their projectional areas are the lip of the calyces of the mushroom bodies and the lateral lobe of the protocerebrum (4, 35). (This region seems to be an important area of deutocerebral afferent projections. Its dorsal part is a true intersection of fibers ascending to, and descending from, the mushroom bodies.)

POST-EMBRYONIC DEVELOPMENT

The antennal olfactory pathway changes drastically during post-embryonic development, especially in Holometabola, such as the bee, where metamorphosis results in an important structural and morphogenic reorganization. In such insects, the adult antenna develops during metamorphosis from imaginal discs (16, 42, 43). The functional maturation of the sensory olfactory neurons of the workerbee has been studied using the classical electroantennogramm (EAG) recording technique. This technique has been used to investigate insects at different ages, from the day of emergence to the 22 day old adult. The experiments were performed on individuals of strictly known age classes, identified and controlled since egg-laying (29). Such experiments revealed a notable increase in response between 0 and 4 days old for all qualities and intensities of odorants tested. The maximum response was attained at day 4, and stayed more or less at this level until the bees were 8 days old. A slow decrease in the amplitude of the EAGs took place between day 8 and day 15 (Fig.3). If the maximal value of the response at day 4 is termed 100%, at emergence the value is about 30%, and at day 2 it is 75%. At day 15 the average response is 80%, and thereafter a steady state is reached which is maintained throughout the life of the individual. It is remarkable that the amplitude of the response at emergence was never zero. Recent experiments show that functional maturation begins in the three days before emergence (unpublished). This has been demonstrated in another Holometabola, the moth Manduca sexta (47).

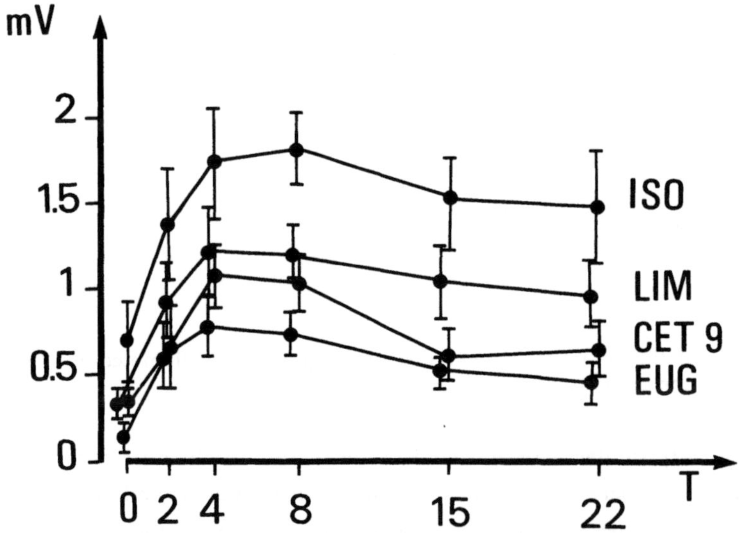

Fig. 3 - Changes in the electrophysiological response of the olfactory antennal sensory cells (EAG) with aging. Olfactory maturation takes place during the the first four days after emergence, and is independent of the odorant used. The EAG becomes smaller again after the 8th day. CET 9: Trans-9-oxo-2 decenoic acid, EUG: eugenol, ISO: isoamyl acetate, LIM: limonene.

A detailed analysis of the organizational development of the antennal lobe has been made for the workerbee, Apis mellifera (1, 29, 37). In the workerbee, the total developmental duration between egg-laying and eclosion is 21 days.

Pupal ecdysis occurs 12 days after egg-laying; pupal metamorphosis takes 9 days. During pupal development, the differentiating antennal olfactory neurons elaborate dendrites which enter developing sensilla and send their sensory axons to their target neurons in the ipsilateral antennal lobe of the deutocerebrum. The deutocerebral neurons are formed as a result of mitotic divisions of a number of large neuroblasts; solitary neuroblasts produce varying cellular groups in the adults, the others, grouped together in a compact region actively develop until the fourth day of nymphal development, and form the principal cellular group in the adult. As the antennal lobe increases in size during the pupal period, it also changes its form. The imaginal antennae begin to develop in the prenymph; the axons reach the antennal lobe during this period, forming two different tracts, the only differentiated structures in the lobe (37).

The developmental formation of the antennal afferent pathway was investigated using passive axonal transport of cobalt ions on each day of pupal development under controlled conditions (1, 29) (Fig.4). The development of the synaptic fields (evidenced by the glomeruli) between the endings of the axons of the antennal neuroreceptors and the processes of the second order neurons has been analysed. On the first day of pupal development (i.e. 9 days before emergence), cobalt ions migrate along the antennal axons towards a black-filled area in the position of the future organized antennal lobe. No soma are stained and the axons do not project anywhere else in the central nervous system. On the second day, the 3 main antennal sensory bundles appear. On the third day (7 days before emergence), the first glomerular-like structures (or "pre-glomeruli") appear. Their intrinsic structure is quite different from that of the adult, they are more spherical and appear to be homogeneous in texture, being stained completely black. When the developing pre-glomeruli first appear, (i) the deutocerebral neurons become arranged into small groups and some of the cell bodies can be filled with cobalt ions, (ii) a group of fibers in the AGT is clearly filled by the stain. These fibers can be followed into different centers in the brain (the lips of the mushroom bodies and the lateral lobe of the protocerebrum, and the contralateral side of the deutocerebrum). Immediately after this period, during a short interval between the 5th and 4th days before emergence, the entire AGT appears to be established. At the same time there is a marked increase in the number of pre-glomeruli which extend into the subsequent period. Simultaneously, the main group of deutocerebral neurons, located in the dorso-lateral antennal lobe of the adult brain rapidly acquires its definitive organization. On the 7th day, 3 days before emergence, the general synaptic organization of the antennal afferent pathway seems to be complete. The adult-like appearance is seen not only in the general spatial organization of the glomeruli, but also in the specific intrinsic structure of each glomerular entity. Thus the shape and volume of each glomerulus are very similar to that of the adult; the characteristic cortical layer to which the synapses are confined fills intensely with cobalt. The adult appearance of the glomeruli therefore arises during the 24 hours between the 4th and the 3rd day before emergence. Apart from the precise timing, there are strong similarities between the development of the system in the bee and in the moth, Manduca sexta. In Manduca, synaptic acitivity has been observed before the neuroreceptors transmit sensory information. In Holometabola, therefore, the establishment of synaptic connections and maturation of the response properties of the deutocerebral neurons appears to occur after the arrival of afferent fibers, but before the establishment of the "true" functioning of the olfactory system.

PLASTICITY

In terms of neural development and plasticity, therefore, the olfactory system of the bee is particularly interesting. On the one hand, the bulk of connections between the first order neurons and efferent deutoneurons seems to be established 5 days before emergence. On the other hand, maturation of neuroreceptors occurs during the first days (mainly the 4th day) after emergence. The rapid and extensive development of the final organization of the synaptic fields in the antennal lobes (i.e. the characteristic synaptic cortex of glomeruli) confined to a few hours 3 days before emergence, could be closely related to the huge increase in stabilization of local interneuron connections. As the development of local interneurons could be dependent largely on the functioning of the sensory antennal system (49) an important question arises: are all glomerular synapses already stabilized before emergence, or is the final stabilization of these specific connections under the influence of epigenetic criteria and olfactory stimulation of antennae during a specific period (critical period)?.

It is clear that the presence of antennal afferents is crucial for the development of the antennal lobe. In the moth Manduca sexta (22, 45, 47), removal of the antennae before the birth of sensory neurons results in lobes of reduced volume and irregularly formed deutocerebral neuropile. In the male moth, no macroglomerular structure develops in the deprived antennal lobe. Moreover, grafting experiments indicate a remarkable plasticity in the development of the sexual characteristics of the antennal system of Manduca. In the workerbee, very similar results have been established. When the antennal lobe is deprived of its normal sensory innervation during pupation, the setting up of the glomeruli and the volume of the lobe are closely related to the time of the surgery. Removal of the antennae after connections of afferent terminals onto their output target deutocerebral neurons have been made (i.e. 4 days before emergence), prevents the setting up of the cortical synaptic layer in the glomeruli . This reinforces the important role of afferent inputs in the organization of the lobe. To investigate the plasticity of the antennal system in Apis mellifera, we have developed techniques of social deprivation in workerbees that cause sensory deprivation (29). The preliminary results strongly suggest that there is a critical period of several days before and after emergence. Deprivation during the week immediately following the day of

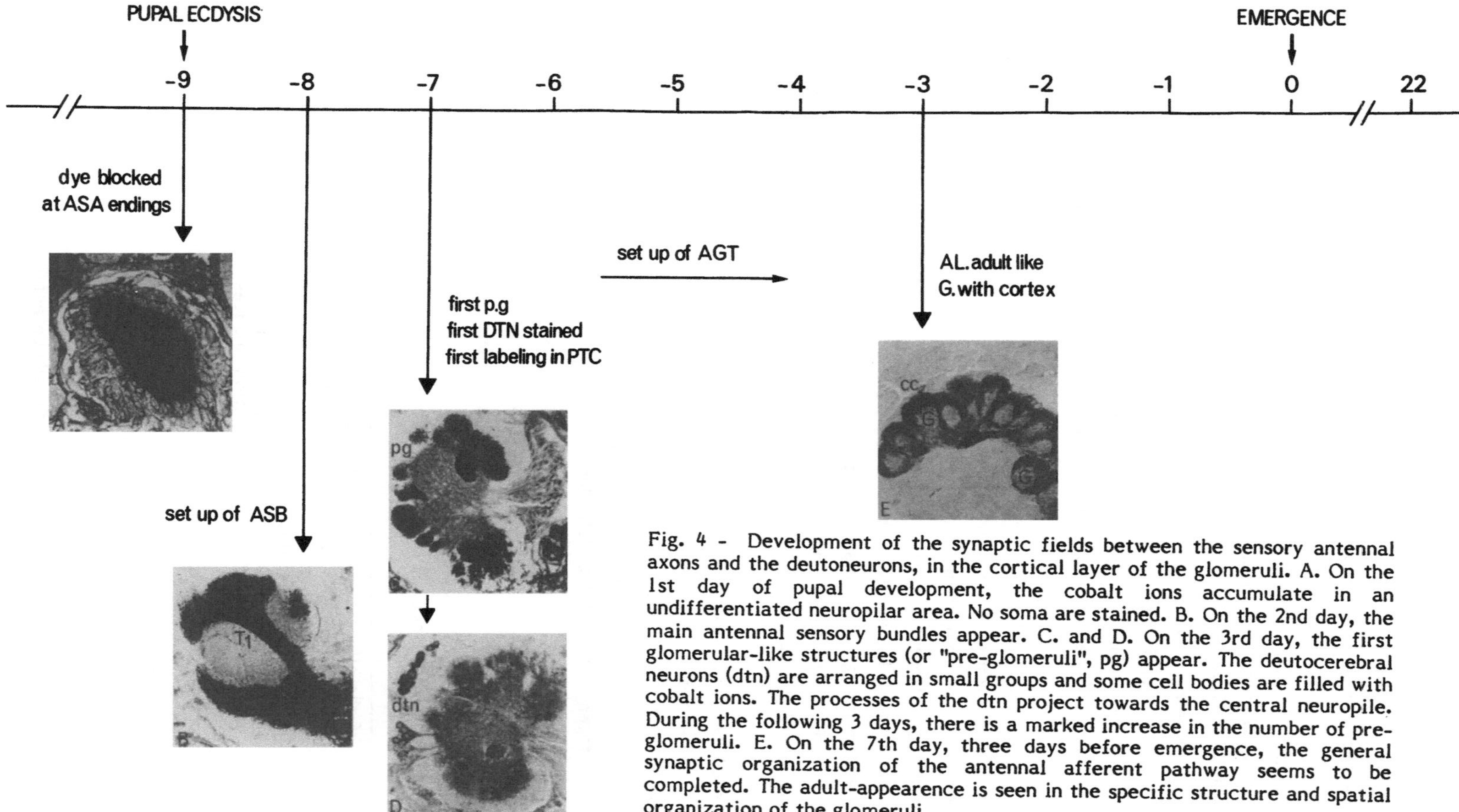

Fig. 4 - Development of the synaptic fields between the sensory antennal axons and the deutoneurons, in the cortical layer of the glomeruli. A. On the 1st day of pupal development, the cobalt ions accumulate in an undifferentiated neuropilar area. No soma are stained. B. On the 2nd day, the main antennal sensory bundles appear. C. and D. On the 3rd day, the first glomerular-like structures (or "pre-glomeruli", pg) appear. The deutocerebral neurons (dtn) are arranged in small groups and some cell bodies are filled with cobalt ions. The processes of the dtn project towards the central neuropile. During the following 3 days, there is a marked increase in the number of pre-glomeruli. E. On the 7th day, three days before emergence, the general synaptic organization of the antennal afferent pathway seems to be completed. The adult-appearence is seen in the specific structure and spatial organization of the glomeruli.

emergence induced a modification of the global antennal sensitivity measured by EAG recordings. The deprived bees remained 20-30% less responsive than bees reared in normal conditions (29) (Fig. 5B). Moreover, such social isolation induces important morphological modifications in the synaptic fields of connections between the two main neuronal networks, neuroreceptors and deutocerebral neurons : (i) the cortical layer of the glomeruli is affected by a decrease in volume of circa 20 % and, (ii) the total volume of the glomeruli is also smaller than that of bees reared in normal conditions. In contrast, the volume of the central body is not affected by deprivation (Fig.5A). These results strongly support the hypothesis of a critical period in the development of the olfactory system of the workerbee, especially in the stabilization of the connections between the two main neuronal networks in the antennal lobes.

The functional significance of these morphological data in terms of behavior is now being analysed, as are data concerning olfactory imprinting. Experiments using specific imprinting with geraniol during different periods (1,4, and 8 days) from the day of emergence of workerbees tested later in dynamic flow choices olfactometer are now in progress. Results so far indicate that imprinting during less than 8 days is enough to induce a modification of the normal attractive behavior of the adult bee towards the imprinting odorant used at its behavioral threshold (Fig.5C).

The plasticity of neuronal structures is certainly one of the most exciting domains in neurobiology (36). The bee brain and sensory systems seem to be particularly good candidates to test the hypothesis of selective stablilization of synapses (14). Not only the olfactory system appears to be under the control of epigenetic factors, but also the visual system (20). Moreover, the ontogeny of complex behaviors (i.e. nursing, foraging) involving different sensory modalities induce changes in the morphology of dendritic spines of calycal interneurons (15, 11). It is known that adult workerbees have sensory, short-term and long-term memory phases, and that they can learn very rapidly and recall a learnt odor after only one food reward (33). Attempts have been made to identify neural correlates of learning in the bee (17). A good knowledge of the rules of functional stabilization of the synapses

Fig. 5 - Plasticity of the olfactory system. Schematic diagram representing the main results concerning the existence of a critical period in the development of the olfactory system of the workerbee.
A. and B. Sensory deprivation: Experiments on social deprivation (SD) during (A) the whole nymphal period and the first 6 days after emergence of the adult life and (B) from emergence until the 6th day of adult life. A. This deprivation induces important morphological modifications of the synaptic fields of connections with the glomeruli. The volume of both the glomeruli and cortical layer is smaller in the isolated bees, than those of bees reared under normal conditions (G). The volume of the central body (used as reference) is not affected by this deprivation. B. This deprivation induces a modification of the global antennal sensitivity as measured by the EAG's recordings. C. Olfactory imprinting. Olfactory imprinting was undertaken using geraniol, and was applied at various intervals (1, 4 and 8 days) after the day of emergence. The 12 day old workerbees were then tested in an olfactometer. Imprinting undertaken during days 4 to 8 of the adult life, increases the normal attractive behavior of the adult bee towards the imprinted odorant.

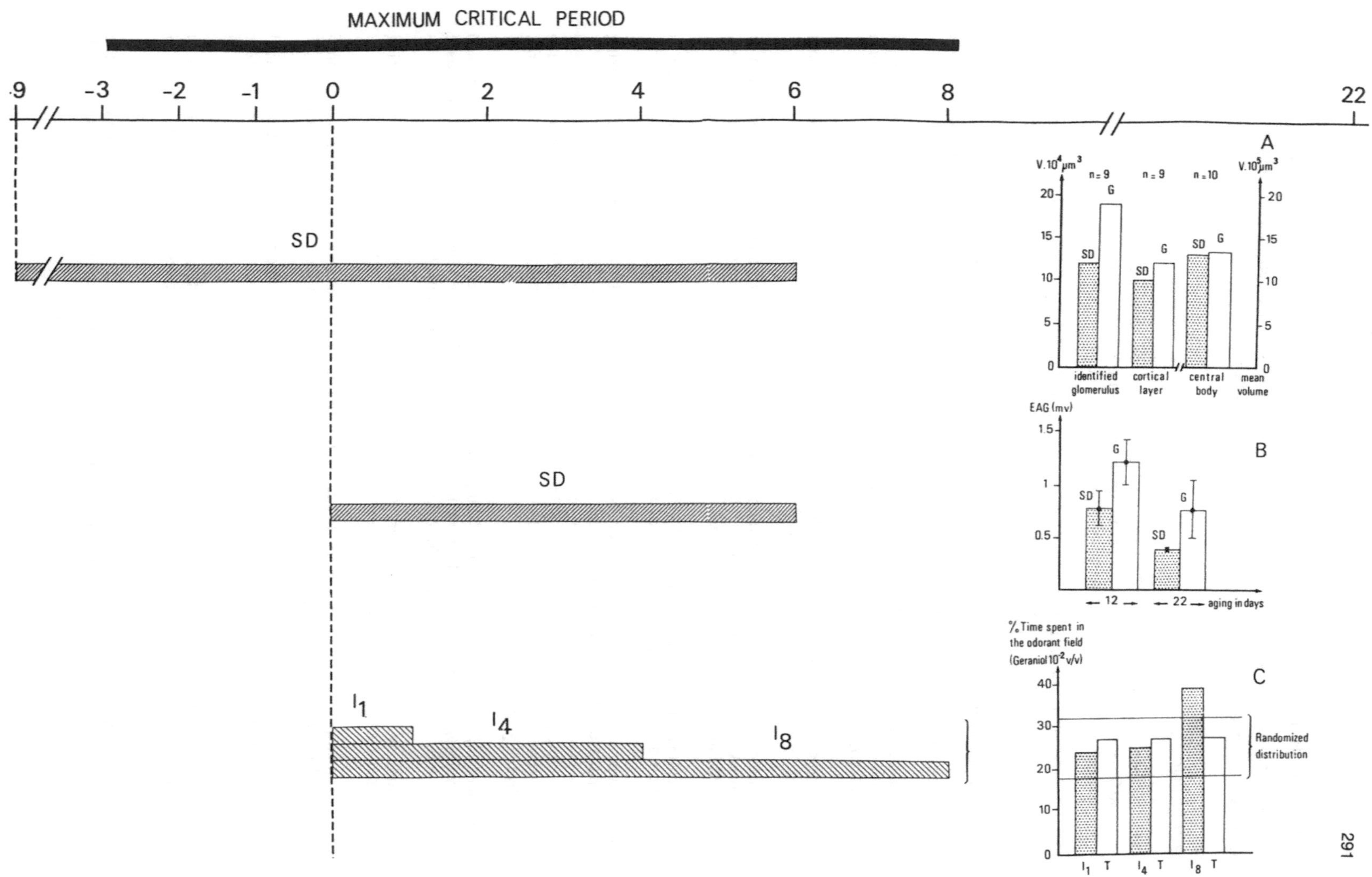
MAXIMUM CRITICAL PERIOD
·9
-3
-2
-1
0
2
4
6
8
22
SD
SD
I1
I4
I8
A
V.10⁴μm³
n = 9
n = 9
n = 10
V.10⁵μm³
SD
G
identified glomerulus
cortical layer
central body
mean volume
EAG (mv)
B
12
22
aging in days
% Time spent in the odorant field (Geraniol 10⁻² v/v)
C
Randomized distribution
I1 T
I4 T
I8 T

involved in odor learning may allow us to analyse with more precision the neural basis of odor learning and plasticity, and to understand to what degree adult behavior triggered by odorant cues is under the control of the olfactory history of the individual.

REFERENCES

(1) Arnold, G., and Masson, C. 1983. Mise en place des connexions synaptiques de la voie afférente antennaire au cours du développement nymphal de l'ouvrière d'abeille Apis mellifica ligustica. C.R. Acad Sc Paris III: 131-136.

(2) Arnold, G.; Masson, C.; and Budharugsa, S. 1983. Organisation spatiale du système nerveux antennaire de l'abeille étudiée au moyen d'une technique de marquage aux ions cobalt. Apidologie 14(2): 127-135.

(3) Arnold, G.; Masson, C; and Budharugsa, S. 1984. Demonstration of a sexual dimorphism in the olfactory pathways of the drones (Apis mellifica L., Hymenoptera, Apidae). Experientia 40: 723-725.

(4) Arnold, G.; Masson, C.; and Budharugsa, S. 1985. Comparative study of the antennal afferent pathway of the workerbee and the drone (Apis mellifera L.) Cell Tiss. Res. 242: 593-605.

(5) Arnold, G.; Masson, C.; and Budharugsa, S. 1986. Spatial organization of the antennal lobe in the queen honeybee. Int. J. Insect Morphol. Empryol., in press.

(6) Arnold, G.; Masson, C.; and Denizot, J.P. 1986. Immunocytochemical demonstration of GABA in the honeybee brain. In Proc. Symp. Invertebrate Peptides and Amines. Bordeaux: Soc. Exp. Biol., in press.

(7) Barbier, M., and Lederer, E. 1960. Structure chimique de la substance royale de la reine d'abeille. C.R. Acad. Sc. Paris 250: 4467-4469.

(8) Blum, M.S.; Fales, H.M.; Tucker, K.W.; and Collins, A.M. 1978. Chemistry of the sting apparatus of the worker honeybee. J. Apic. Res. 17(4): 218-221.

(9) Boeckh, J., and Boeckh, V. 1979. Threshold and odor specificity of pheromone sensitive neurons in the deutocerebrum of Antherea pernyi and Antherea polyphemus. J. Comp. Phys. 132(3): 235-242.

(10) Boeckh, J.; Boeckh, V.; and Kühn, A. 1977. Further data on the topography and physiology of central olfactory neurons in insects. In Inter. Symp. Olfaction and Taste VI, eds. J. Le Magnen and P. Mac Leod, pp. 315-322. London: IRL.

(11) Blum, M.S.; Fales, H.M.; Tucker, K.W.; and Collins, A.M. 1978. Chemistry of the sting apparatus of the worker honeybee. J. Apic. Res. 17(4): 218-221.

(12) Brandon, J.G., and Coss, R.G. 1982. Rapid dendritic spine stem shortening during one-trial learning: the honeybee's first orientation flight. Brain Research 252: 51-61.

(13) Burrows, M.; Boeckh, J., and Esslen, J. 1982. Physiological and morphological properties of interneurones in the DTC of male cockroaches which respond to female pheromones. J. Comp. Physiol. 145: 447-457.

(14) Callow, R.K.; Chapman, J.R.; and Paton, P.N. 1964. Pheromones of the honeybee: chemical studies of the mandibular gland secretion of the queen. J. Apic. Res. 3(2): 77-89.

(15) Chambille, I.; Rospars, J. P. ; and Masson, C. 1980. The deutocerebrum of the cockroach Blaberus craniifer Burm. Spatial organization of the sensory glomeruli. J. Neurobiol. 11: 1-23.

(16) Changeux, J.P.; Heidmann, T.; and Patte, P. 1984. Learning by selection. In The Biology of Learning, eds. P. Marler and H.S. Terrace, pp. 115-133. Berlin: Springer-Verlag.

(17) Coss, R.G.; Brandon, J.G.; and Globus, A. 1980. Changes in morphology of dendritic spines on honeybee calycal interneurons associated with cumulative nursing and foraging experiences. Brain Research 192: 49-59.

(18) Eassa, Y.E.C. 1963. Metamorphosis of the cranial capsule and its appendages in the cabbage butterfly, Pieris brassicae. Ann. Entomol. Soc. Amer. 56: 510-521.

(19) Erber, J. 1981. Neural correlates of learning in the honeybee. Trends in Neurosci. 4(11): 270-273.

(20) Ernst, K.D., and Boeckh, J. 1983. A neuroanatomical study on the organization of the central antennal pathways in insects. Cell Tissue Res. 229: 1-22.

(21) Esslen, J., and Kaissling, K.E. 1976. Zahl und Verteilung antennaler Sensillen bei der Honigbiene. Zoomorph. 83: 227-251.

(22) Hertel, H. 1983. Change of synapse frequency in certain photoreceptors of the honeybee after chromatic deprivation. J. Comp. Physiol. 151: 477-482.

(23) Hildebrand, J.G., and Maxwell, G.D. 1980. Neurochemical explorations of the central nervous system of the moth Manduca sexta and especially of the antennal and visual pathways. In Insect Neurobiology and Pesticide Action (NEUROTOX 79), pp. 101-107. London: Society of Chemical Industry.

(24) Hildebrand, J.G.; Hall, L.M. and Osmond, B.C. 1979. Distribution of binding sites for 125 I- labelled bungarotoxin in normal and deafferented antennal lobes of Manduca sexta. Proc. Natl. Acad. Sci. USA 76(1): 499-503.

(25) Jawlowski, H. 1957. Nerve tracts in bee (Apis mellifica) running from the sight and antennal organs to the brain. Ann. Univ. Mariae Curie Sklodowska XII, 22: 307-322.

(26) Kaissling, K.E., and Thorson, J. 1980. Insect olfactory sensilla: structural chemical and electrical aspects of the functional organization. In Receptors for Neurotransmitters, Hormones and Pheromones in Insects, eds. O.B. Satelle et al., pp. 261-281. Amsterdam: Elsevier/North Holland Biomedical Press.

(27) Klemm, N. 1974. Vergleichend-histochemische Untersuchungen über die Verteilung monoamin-haltiger Strukturen im Oberschlundganglion von Angehörigen verschiedener Insektenordungen. Ent. germ. 1: 21-49.

(28) Lacher, V. 1964. Elektrophysiologische Untersuchungen an einzelnen Rezeptoren für Geruch, Kohlendioxid, Luftfeuchtigkeit und Temperatur auf den Antennen der Arbeitsbienen und der Drohne (Apis mellifica L.). Z. vergl. Physiol. 48: 587-623.

(29) Mc Indoo, N. E. 1922. The auditory sense of the honeybee. Neurol. 34: 173-199.

(30) Masson, C. 1977. Central olfactory pathways and plasticity of responses to odorous stimuli in insects. In Int. Symp. Olfaction and Taste VI, eds. J. LeMagnen and P. MacLeod, pp. 315-322. London: IRL.

(31) Masson, C. 1984. Neural basis of olfaction in insects. In Comparative Physiology: Sensory Physiology, eds. K. Schmidt-Nielsen, L. Bolis, and S.H.P. Maddrell, pp. 245-255. Cambridge: University Press.

(32) Masson, C., and Arnold, G. 1984. Ontogeny, maturation and plasticity of the olfactory system in the workerbee. J. Insect Physiol. 30: 7-14.

(33) Masson, C., and Brossut, R. 1981. La communication chimique chez les insectes. La Recherche 121: 406-416.

(34) Masson, C., and Mustaparta, H. 1986. Chemical information processing in the olfactory systems of insects. Physiological Reviews, in press.

(35) Matsumoto, S.G., and Hildebrand, J.G. 1981. Olfactory mechanisms in the moth manduca sexta: response characteristics and morphology of central neurons in the antennal lobes. Proc. Roy. Soc. Lond. B. 213: 249-277.

(36) Menzel, R.; Erber, J. and Masuhr, T. 1974. Learning and memory in the honeybee. In Experimental Analysis of Insect Behaviour, ed. L. Barton Browne, pp. 195-217. Berlin, Heidelberg, New York: Springer-Verlag.

(37) Mercer, A. R.; Mobbs, P. G.; Davenport, A. P. and Evans, P. D. 1983. Biogenic amines in the brain of the honeybee. Cell Tissue Res. 234: 655-677.

(38) Mobbs, P.G. 1982. The brain of the honeybee Apis mellifica. I. The connections and spatial organization of the mushroom bodies. Phil. Trans. R. Soc. Lond. 298: 309-354.

(39) Mobbs, P.G. 1984. Neural networks in the mushroom bodies of the honeybee. J. Insect Physiol. 30(1): 43-58.

(40) Palka, J. 1984. Precision and plasticity in the insect nervous system. Trends in Neurosci. 7(12): 455-456.

(41) Panov, A.A. 1961. The structure of the insect brain at successive stages in postembryonic development. 4. The olfactory center. Ent. Rev. 40: 140-145.

(42) Pareto, A. 1972. Die zentrale Verteilung der Fühlerafferenz bei Arbeiterrinnen der Honigbiene Apis mellifera L. Z. Zellforsch. Micro. Anat. 131: 109-146.

(43) Pham-Delegue, M.H.; Fonta, C.; and Masson, C. 1983. L'apprentissage olfactif chez l'abeille et le bourdon: une étude comparée par conditionnement associatif. C.R. Acad. Sci. Paris, III, 296: 501-506.

(44) Pham-Delegue, M.H.; Masson, C.; and Etievant, P. 1986. Selective olfactory choices among food scents by honeybee, a study by coupled associative conditioning and chemical analysis. J. Chem. Ecol. 12(3): 781-793.

(45) Pickett, J.A.; Williams, I.H.; Martin, A.P. and Smith, M.C. 1980. Nasonov pheromone of the honey bee, Apis mellifera L. (Hymenoptera: Apidae) Part I. Chemical characterization. J. Chem. Ecol. 6(2): 425-434.

(46) Sanes, J.R., and Hildebrand, J.G. 1976. Structure and development of antennae in the moth Manduca sexta. Developmental Biology 51: 282-299.

(47) Sanes, J.R.; Hildebrand, J.G.; and Prescott, D.J. 1976. Differentiation of insect sensory neurons in the absence of their normal synaptic targets. Developmental Biology 52: 121-127.

(48) Schäfer, S., and Bicker, G. 1986. Distribution of GABA-like immunoreactivity in the brain of the honeybee. J. Comp. Neurol. 246: 287-300.

(49) Schneidermann, A.M., and Hildebrand, J.G. 1985. Sexually dimorphism development of the insect olfactory pathway. Trends in Neurosci. 8(11): 494-499.

(50) Schürmann, F.W. and Klemm, N. 1984. Serotonin-immunoreactive neurons in the brain of the honeybee. J. Comp. Neurol. 225: 570-580.

(51) Schweitzer, E.S.; Sanes, J.R.; and Hildebrand, J.G. 1976. Ontogeny of electroantennogram responses in the moth, Manduca sexta. J. Insect Physiol. 22: 955-960.

(52) Suzuki, H. 1975. Antennal movements induced by odour and central projection of the antennal neurones in the honey bee. J. Insect Physiol. 21: 831-847.

(53) Tolbert, L.P.; Matsumoto, S.G.; and Hildebrand, J.G. 1983. Development of synapses in the antennal lobes of the moth Manduca sexta during metamorphosis. J. Neurosci. 3(6): 1158-1175.

(54) Vareschi, E. 1971. Duftunterscheidung bei der Honigbiene. Einzelzellableitungen und Verhaltensreaktionen. Z. vergl. Physiol. 75: 143-173.

Learning and Memory

Flower-shape, Landmark, and Locale Memory in Honeybees

James L. Gould

Department of Biology, Princeton University, Princeton, New Jersey 08544, USA

Abstract. There are two main published models for flower-shape memory, for landmark memory, and for locale memory in honey bees. Recent experiments have shed light on the actual mechanisms in each of these cases. Both shape and landmark memory are pictorial, as opposed to parameter-based; they have different resolutions, and so are probably stored separately; neither is eidetic. Locale memory involves a cognitive map rather than just route-specific memory. One of the most interesting questions about learning is how information is processed and stored. This paper will review recent progress in the understanding of how honeybees store and use visual information gathered on foraging flights.

FLOWER LEARNING

Bees learn many things about food sources (rev. 15, 28), including the shape and pattern of the flowers they are visiting. Hertz (22, 23, 24) concluded that shape discrimination was quite crude, and based largely on spatial frequency - roughly, the ratio of edge to area of a figure, which is high for a dissected shape like a cross but low for a compact figure like a circle. Later investigators (1, 2, 3, 6, 9, 30, 31) found much better shape learning and discrimination, but still credited it to an ability to remember spatial frequency and certain other, less important "parameters" like color area, distribution of line angles, and the like. Wehner (35) initially concluded that shape memory was probably pictorial, but later (36) agreed with the parameter interpretation.

As Gould (15) pointed out, however, the experimental evidence for parameter-based flower learning is not conclusive. Implicit in most analyses is the assumption that pictorial memory must be eidetic (that is, have the same resolution as real-time vision), and that the neural processing of the memory for pictorial memory would emphasize and suppress features in much the same way it does in our nervous systems. Hence it would be possible for Anderson (1) to state that the inability of the bees to generalize from a solid triangular target to a triangular checker board - a generalization most humans readily make - argued against pictorial memory. Most experimental designs used only a single, horizontal target during training, an approach with at least two possible difficulties: bees may view horizontal figures from any angle as they circle, whereas vertical figures can be presented with no ambiguity as to what the bees see; and some animals, when trained with only one alternative (the rewarded stimulus, S^+) or in the presence of a second, unrewarded stimulus (S^-) very different from the S^+, learn only a single, diagnostic cue (a "part figure") and ignore the rest (26). On the other hand, if the S^+ and S^- are very similar, the same animals will remember the pattern pictorially.

To see whether bees can remember flowers pictorially rather than only on the basis of a list of parameters, Gould (16, 18) trained bees on vertical pairs of similar targets, reversing the left-right relationship of the S^+ and S^- after each visit. The parameters said to be most important - spatial frequency, color area, and line angles - were the same for both stimuli (Fig. 1); any possible spontaneous preference for particular stimuli was controlled for by reversing the roles of S^+ and S^- before repeating the experiment. Some patterns (Fig. 1 F, G) also took into account possible interactions with the background. Testing consisted of allowing the trained bee to choose between an unrewarded S^+ and S^-.

Bees were able to discriminate the rewarded and unrewarded shapes after only 10 training trials for patterns with up to 16 elements (Fig. 1), and for 24-element patterns after 20 training trials. When choosing between the more complex patterns, bees hovered in front of the "flowers" at a characteristic distance, and thus it was possible to calculate the number of ommatidia directed at each element, and hence the likely resolution of the memory: the value determined in these experiments was 8°. Since real-time visual resolution is said to be $1\text{-}2^o$ (12, 33), the memory is obviously not eidetic. Although the resolution is relatively low, an 8° memory would probably take only a fraction (0.06 - 0.02) of the "space" required by eidetic memory.

Gould (18) also demonstrated a role of conditioned inhibition (learning that the S^- is reliably associated with the absence of food) in flower learning. He also argues that it is worth keeping in mind that bees, like vertebrates, may use a less demanding part-figure or parameter strategy when circumstances permit; indeed, Gould and Marler (21) explicitly argue that parameters, part figures, and the sorts of simple cues ethologists in other contexts call sign stimuli are one in the same.

LANDMARK LEARNING

Honeybees are able to use nearby surronding landmarks to locate an inconspicuous food source (rev. 12; 25, 5; rev; 36; 7, 8; rev. 15). Anderson (5) found that bees trained to find food at a site surrounded by landmarks (Fig. 2a) and then tested with some of the landmarks removed would search too close to the remaining landmarks (Fig. 2b). He concluded that the bees could not be matching against a stored picture since the configuration seen from the new the new search point would not match a stored visual image. Instead, he proposed that that the bees simply remembered whether or not each of perhaps four 90° sectors in their

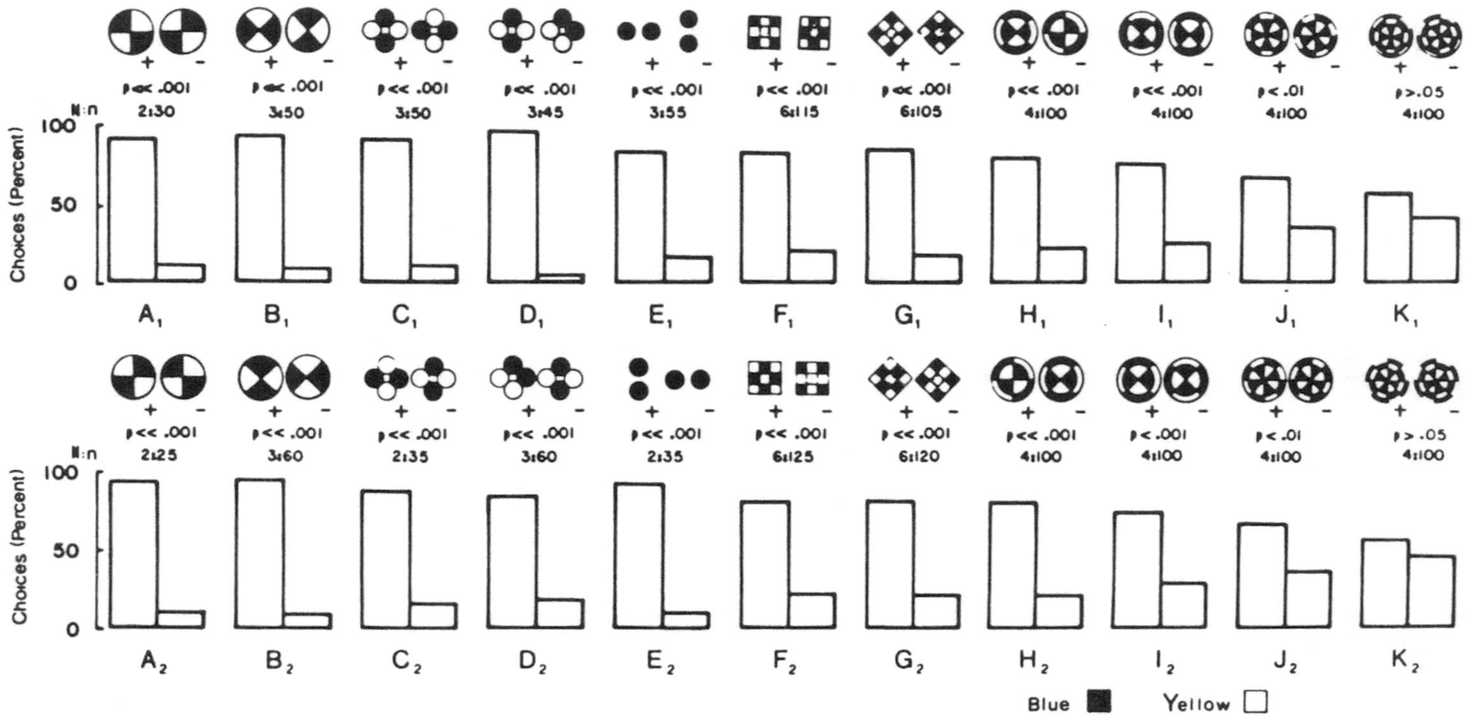

Fig. 1 - Bees were trained to find food at the center of the pattern marked "+". Number of bees tested (N) and number of landings (n) are indicated as N:n under the P values. The center squares in the patterns of experiments F and G were green, the same color as the background. The percentage of choices of the correct (+) and incorrect (-) patterns are indicated by the bar graphs under the alternative patterns.

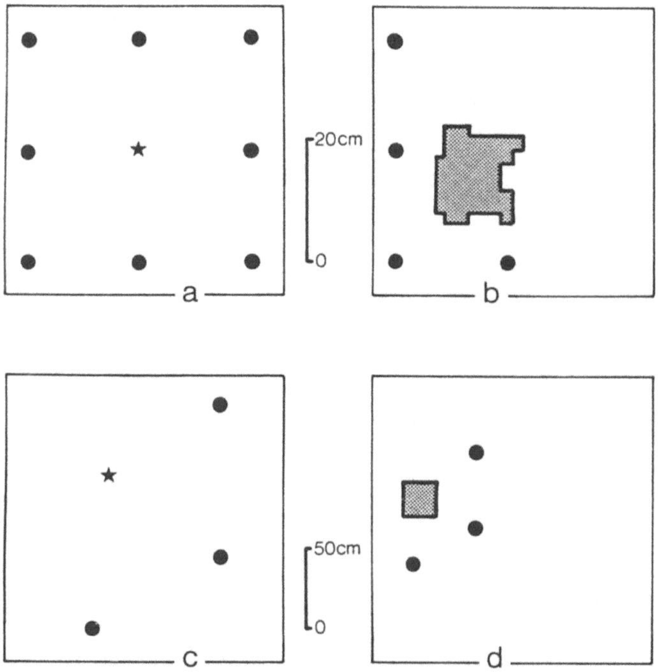

Fig. 2 - Anderson trained bees to find food in the center of a square array of 8 landmarks (a), and then recorded where returning bees searched when some of the landmarks were removed (hatched area in b). Cartwright and Collett, on the other hand, generally used only 3 landmarks positioned to one side (c). Alterations of the array usually left the landmarks in an arrangement such that returning bees could find a location from which the landmarks were all in the same azimiths as during training (d).

visual world as seen from the food source was occupied by a nearby landmark. Hence the removal of some of the landmarks would require bees to move closer to the remaining ones in order to "fill" the now-empty sectors. The precise number of sectors was never determined.

The "sector hypothesis" has a very low - perhaps a uselessly low - predicted resolution and, since all landmarks are basically equal (being encoded as either present or absent), is fraught with potential ambiguity. However, by analogy with the intriguing parameter hypothesis of shape memory discussed earlier, one could easily extend the sector theory to include memory of the parameters of the landmarks in each sector, and so greatly increase the system's theoretical precision without losing its low-storage-space advantage over a pictorial system. Alternatively, Anderson's data are also consistent with a very low resolution pictorial memory, or a medium-resolution system in which the bees simply confused some of the remaining landmarks for some that were missing.

Cartwright and Collett (7, 8) performed a series of experiments from which they concluded that bees have an eidetic memory of landmarks. The bees were usually trained with three landmarks (Fig. 1c) and then with an altered set. But unlike Anderson's protocol, Cartwright and Collett's experiments usually involved testing landmarks arranged so that there was a point in the array from which the landmarks would all appear to be at the same azimuth angles encountered during training (Fig. 1d). Their data and protocol, however, leave something to be desired (rev. 15). Most obviously, they never sought to determine the resolution of landmark memory, and it cannot be said to be eidetic without demonstrating that it has the same resolution as real-time vision. Nor, for that matter, do their experiments address the question of whether or not the memory is pictorial: Anderson's original sector hypothesis is not convincingly excluded (the original experiments were not repeated), nor is the possibility of a parameter-based system considered.

Gould (19) examined the landmark-memory system by training individual bees to find food between a pair of landmarks in one of 225 possible locations, the landmarks being moved after each visit. After 10 training visits to one pair (type A landmarks), the training pair and alternative pair of landmarks (B) were offered arranged in the form AABB, BBAA, or BAAB. Bees could land between an AA pair, an AB pair or a BB pair.

When tested between landmarks differing only in color, bees readily learned the discrimination; similarly, when tested between landmarks differing only in shape, bees were able to choose with good accuracy (Fig. 3). Neither of these tests excludes the parameter hypothesis. However, when tested between pairs with identical parameters of spatial frequency, color area, and line angles, the bees were still able to discriminate reliably, indicating that the memory is at least pictorial.

To see whether landmark memory is eidetic, its resolution must be measured. This was accomplished by determining the maximum visual angle necessary to a) respond to the presence of an object, and b) match a particular object to landmark memory. Response resolution was about 1.5°, while memory resolution was about 3.5° - about 5-6 times worse. (The resolution of flower memory, as discussed above, is about 8°.) This indicates not only that the memory is not eidetic, but that it is stored separately from flower memory (as all previous workers appear to have assumed) rather than as an all-purpose "panorama" including both flower and nearby landmarks. This may make good sense because bees can to some degree compensate for their relatively "grainy" memory of flower shape/pattern by flying closer, whereas they are necessarily constrained, during their attempts to triangulate flower location from the azimuths of nearby landmarks, to be near the food source rather than close to the landmarks.

Gould (19) also sought to discover why Anderson's results appear to support the sector rather than the pictorial hypothesis. He reasoned that Anderson's bees might have mistaken one or more of the remaining landmarks for missing ones - all of Anderson's landmarks were identical - and so moved too close in an attempt to match as many, widely separated landmarks as possible. Gould tested this idea by comparing the behavior of trained with identical landmarks (Fig. 4a) to those trained on a mixture of landmarks of two different colors (Fig. 4c); with the mixed set, the potential ambiguity between landmarks was not possible. In fact, bees under the latter conditions matched the remaining landmarks as predicted by the picture hypothesis (Fig. 4d).

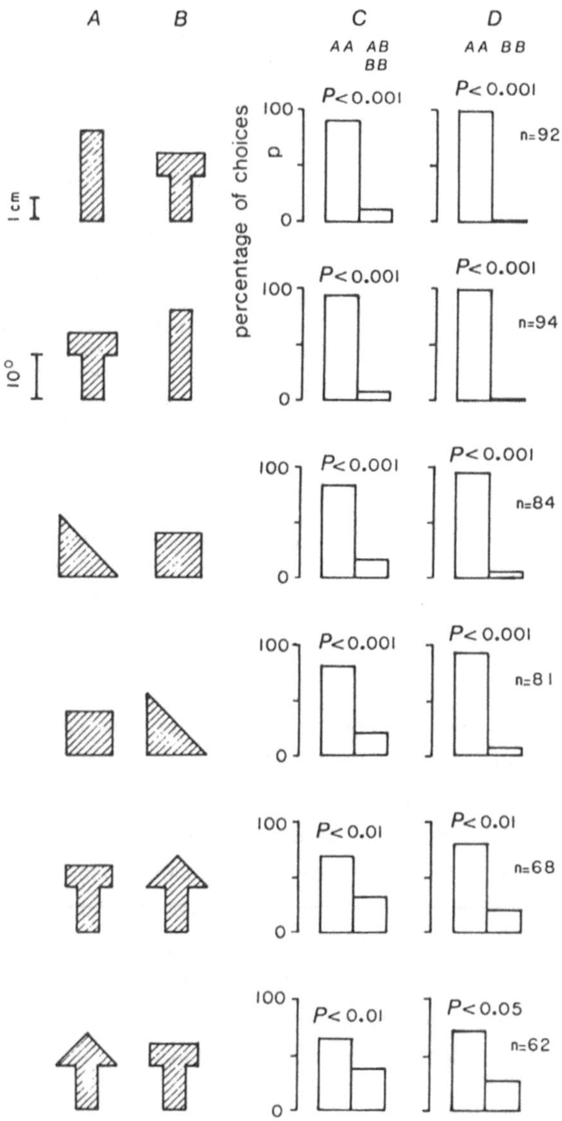

Fig. 3 - To determine whether honeybees can learn the shape of landmarks, bees were trained to find food between a pair of landmarks of the shape shown in the A column, and then tested in arrays offering a pair of A's, a pair of an alternative shape (B's), and a hybrid pair (AB), or an array with a pair of A's and two hybrid pairs. The B landmarks were the same color as A landmarks, and had the same visual area. The data in column C indicates the percentage of choices for the training pair (AA) versus the two alternatives (AB and BB), while the data in column D compares landings on AA versus BB. The sample sizes in column C are always 150; the sample sizes in column D, where AB landings are excluded from analysis, are shown.

COGNITIVE MAPS

Bees are well known for their ability to use celestial cues in navigating to unfamiliar food sources (rev. 12, 11). They are also able to use prominent landmarks, at least on the outward journey, as the route becomes familiar (13); indeed, the entire celestial reference system can come to depend on landmarks during overcast conditions (10).

There are two main possibilities for how bees might use prominent landmarks to navigate in their home range. The first, articulated most concisely by Wehner (36), suggests that bees remember the sequence of landmarks encountered on familiar foraging routes. A different

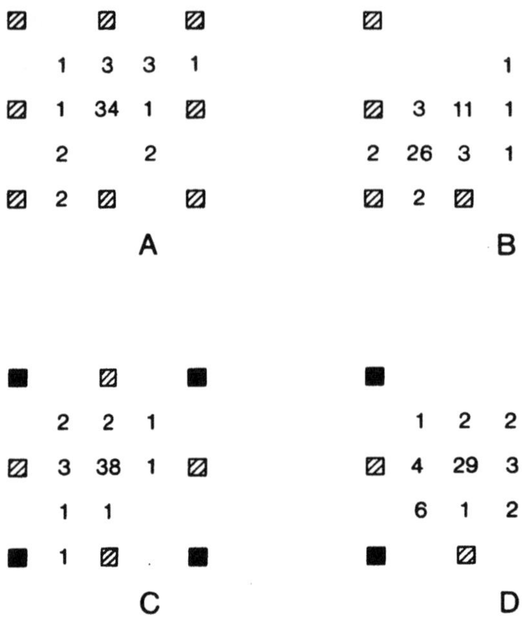

Fig. 4 - When bees were trained to find food in the middle of an array of 8 identical yellow landmarks and tested in the same array (A), they searched in the middle of the array; the landmarks are indicated by squares, and the number of landings at each location is indicated. When tested with 4 of the landmarks removed, bees searched closer to the remaining landmarks (B). Bees trained to find food in the middle of a hybrid set of landmarks (4 yellow and 4 blue, with the blue one in the corner of the array) searched accurately when tested either with an unaltered array (C) or with only 4 landmarks (D).

route-specific series would then be remembered for each other foraging route. This route-specific navigation hypothesis is essentially identical to early formulations of learning theory, in which animals were supposed to learn mazes in terms of a sequence of responses to landmarks and other cues encountered en route (rev. 32). In the case of rats, however, Tolman (34) demonstrated an ability to build up what he called a "cognitive map" of the maze; as a result, if the barriers are removed, the rat can take a novel direct route toward the (unseen) goal, independent of the usual circuitous route and its landmarks. The rats could also integrate and use information gathered during separate trips to different goals. This ability, also known as "latent learning", has since been analyzed in detail in rats (rev. 29) and chimpanzees (27); it is generally considered to represent a basic form of thinking.

Although there was no evidence of similar cognitive abilities in invertebrates, Gould and Gould (20) pointed out some data consistent with the idea that honeybees might have maps. Later Gould (15) argued that the evidence for route-specific navigation was not conclusive, and pointed out that the essential difference between the cognitive-map hypothesis ("locale map" in his terminology) and the route-specific hypothesis is that in the latter, bees only know about landmarks in relation to others along the same route; a cognitive map, on the other hand, would allow the animal to understand the spatial relationship between landmarks on separate routes - landmarks never encountered on the same flight.

Gould (17) tested the ability of bees to form and use cognitive maps by training a group of marked foragers from a hive to a food source 160 m or 350 m away. Later, while they were still making regular trips to the training site, these bees were captured individually and transported in the dark to a release site equally far away but 60° to the left or right of the training site (Fig. 5). Upon release, the transported bee circled and departed, its departure bearing being recorded. From measurements of the altitude at which orientated flight began, Gould confirmed that an intervening forested ridge blocked all view of the training site and its surrounding landmarks.

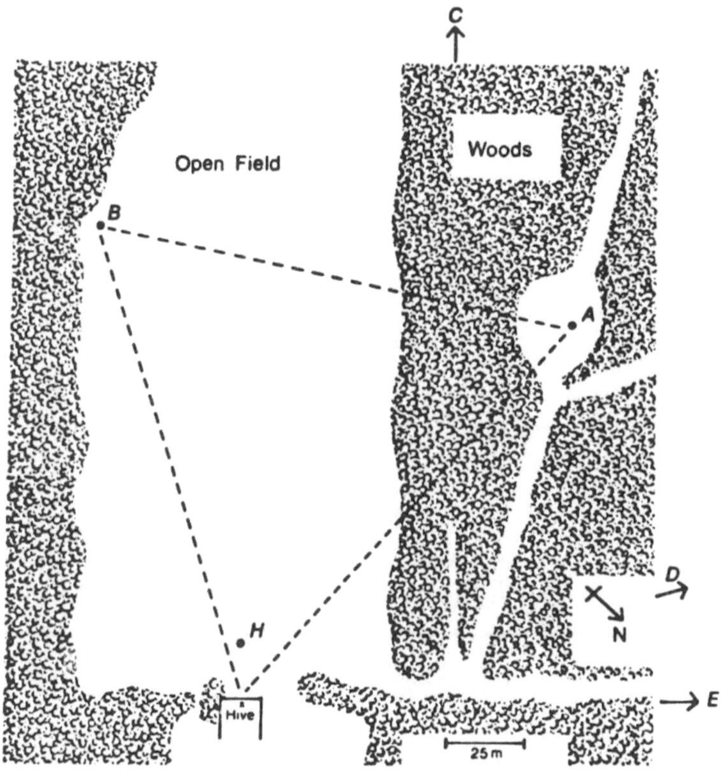

Fig. 5 - Bees from a hive (bottom center) were trained to either Site A, Site B (both 160 m from the hive), or (off the top of the map) Site C (350 m from the hive); on subsequent days these foragers and others were captured and transported to a different site and released -Site B for those trained to A, Site A for those trained to B, and Site D (350 m from the hive) or Site E (4425 m from the hive) for those trained to Site C. As a control, some trained foragers were realeased at Site H as well.

If bees were disorientated by this procedure, they might be expected to fly off randomly; if they failed to recognize that a displacement had occured, they might be expected to fly off in the direction normally adopted when leaving the hive for the food source; if dependent on route-specific information, they might (at best) recognize the release site as part of a familiar foraging route, use that information to set course for the hive, and then, perhaps, pick up the route-specific sequence leading to the food source. Gould performed controls to establish the distribution of bearings for each of these possibilities (Fig. 6a, b, c; the random-scatter prediction was measured only in the first test). Finally, if bees have cognitive maps, they ought to be able to use the landmarks at the release site to plan a novel route to the food source and depart in the correct direction, which is precisely what they did (Fig. 6a, b, c).

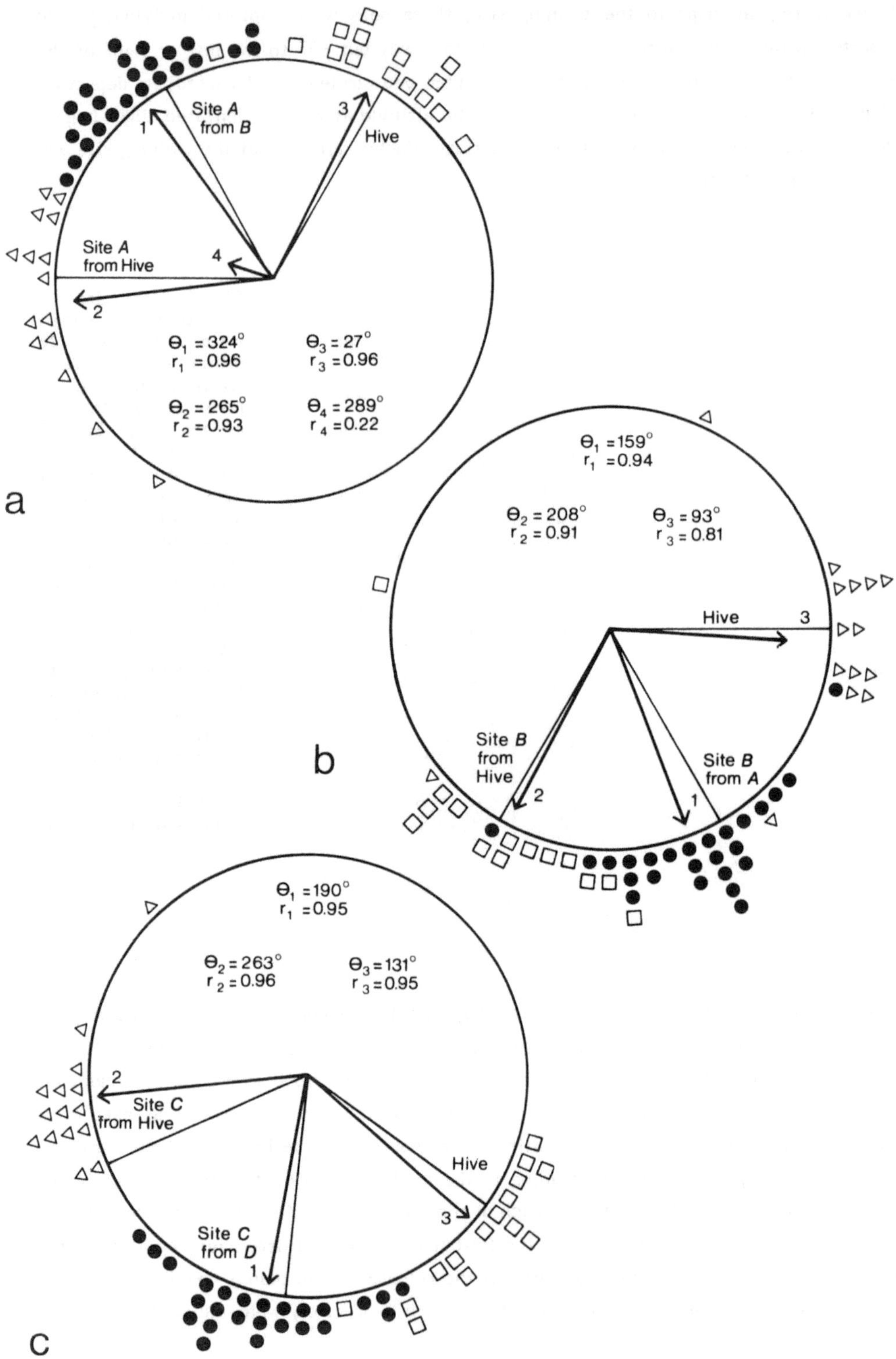
Site A from B
Hive
Site A from Hive
1
2
3
4
Θ1 = 324°
r1 = 0.96
Θ3 = 27°
r3 = 0.96
Θ2 = 265°
r2 = 0.93
Θ4 = 289°
r4 = 0.22
a
Θ1 = 159°
r1 = 0.94
Θ2 = 208°
r2 = 0.91
Θ3 = 93°
r3 = 0.81
Hive
3
Site B from Hive
2
Site B from A
1
b
Θ1 = 190°
r1 = 0.95
Θ2 = 263°
r2 = 0.96
Θ3 = 131°
r3 = 0.95
2
Site C from Hive
Hive
3
Site C from D
1
c

The discovery that bees can use cognitive maps adds new impetus to the question, posed by Gould and Gould (20), of whether recruit bees can "place" dance locations while still in the hive, perhaps by "calling to mind" the landmarks surrounding the advertized site. If so, it is possible that the dance language may have evolved from the bees' cognitive map rather than from some fortuitous combination of orientational artefacts as suggested by von Frisch (12).

The discovery also underscores the unanswered question of whether, fo experienced bees, celestial navigation or a cognitive map is the primary basis for navigation even to unfamiliar food sources. The traditional view of the primacy of celestial information, which may well be correct, is based in large part on two kinds of observations: orientation of horizontal dances in the hive depends on celestial cues, which, though interesting, is probably irrelevant to the use of prominent landmarks in this field; field orientation in the absence of familiar landmarks is clearly celestial, which appears equally irrelevant. We should keep in mind the possibility that familiar-landmark navigation is, when available, the primary system, and the better-known celestial system is the backup. If this were the case, we might imagine that bees use their knowledge of celestial movement to calibrate landmark information, much as pigeons use their sensitivity to magnetic fields to calibrate their sun-compass system, which then becomes the primary navigational tool for adult birds (rev. 14).

Finally, we should not assume that since adult bees can form and use a cognitive system map, they cannot use route specific information as well. Just as animals that can remember pictorially nevertheless use simple part figures when conditions allow, there is no reason to believe that the two navigational systems are mutually exclusive; indeed, they might well complement each other, and only further work can fully establish the ontogeny and the role of landmark use by bees.

Fig. 6 - The vanishing bearings of bees trained to one site - Site A in part a, Site B in part b, and Site C in part c - and then transported and released at another site at the same distance from the hive but in a different direction are indicated by the circles at the periphery of these circular distributions. The relative bearing of the feeding station is labelled "Site A from Site B" in part a, "Site B from Site A" in part b, and Site C fropm Site D" in part c. The mean vector - a measure of the average and degree of clustering - is shown, with the values for mean direction and vector length, O_1 and r_1 respectively, listed. The triangles represent the vanishing bearings for trained foragers released at Site H; the corresponding predicted bearing (labelled "Hive to Site"), mean vector, and associated values are also presented. The squares represent the vanishing bearings of incoming foragers transported to the release site. The predicted bearing (labelled "Site to Hive"), mean vector, and associated values are shown. All three of these mean vectors in all three distributions are significant at P 0.001 by the z test. The shorter mean vector in part a represents unmarked foragers captured as they left the hive and transported to the release site; there is no predicted bearing for these bees.

REFERENCES

(1) Anderson, A. M. 1972. The ability of honey bees to generalize visual stimuli. In Information Processing in the Visual System of Arthropods, ed. R. Wehner, pp. 207-212. Berlin: Springer-Verlag.

(2) Anderson, A. M. 1977a. Shape perception in the honey bee. Anim. Behav. 25: 67-79.

(3) Anderson, A. M. 1977b. Parameters determining the attractiveness of stripe patterns in the honey bee. Anim. Behav. 25: 67-79.

(4) Anderson, A. M. 1977c. The influence of pointed regions on the shape preference of honey bees. Anim. Behav. 25: 88-94.

(5) Anderson, A. M. 1977d. A model for landmark learning in the honey bee. J. comp. Physiol. 114: 335-355.

(6) Anderson, A. M. 1979. Visual scanning in the honey bee. J. comp. Physiol. 130: 173-182.

(7) Cartwright, B. A., and Collett, T. S. 1982. How honey bees use landmarks to guide their return to a food source. Nature 295: 560-564.

(8) Cartwright, B. A., and Collett, T. S. 1983. Landmark learning in bees. J. comp. Physiol. 151: 521-543.

(9) Cruse, H. 1972. A qualitative model for pattern discrimination in the honey bee. In: Information Processing in the Visual System of Arthropods, ed. R. Wehner, pp. 201-206. Berlin: Springer-Verlag.

(10) Dyer, F. C., and Gould, J. L. 1981. Honey bee orientation: a backup system for cloudy days. Science 214: 1041-1042.

(11) Dyer, F. C., and Gould, J. L. 1983. Honey bee navigation. Amer. Sci. 71: 587-597.

(12) Frisch, K. v. 1967. The Dance Language and Orientation of Bees. Harvard University Press, Cambridge, Mass.

(13) Frisch, K. v., and Lindauer, M. 1954. Himmel und Erde in Konkurrenz bei der Orientierung der Bienen. Naturwiss. 41: 245-253.

(14) Gould, J. L. 1982. The map sense of pigeons. Nature 296: 205-211.

(15) Gould, J. L. 1984. Natural history of honey bee learning. In: The Biology of Learning, eds. P. Marler and H. Terrace, pp.149-180. Berlin: Springer-Verlag.

(16) Gould, J. L. 1985. How bees remember flower shapes. Science 227: 1492-1494.

(17) Gould, J. L. 1986. The locale map of honey bees: do insects have cognitive maps? Science 232: 861-863.

(18) Gould, J. L. in press, a. Pattern learning by honey bees. Anim. Behav.

(19) Gould, J. L. in press, b. Landmark learning by honey bees. Anim. Behav.

(20) Gould, J. L., and Gould, C. G. 1982. The insect mind: physics or metaphysics? In: Animal Mind - Human Mind, ed. D. R. Griffen, pp. 269-298. Berlin: Springer-Verlag.

(21) Gould, J. L., and Marler, P. 1984. Ethology and the natural history of learning. In: The Biology of Learning, eds. P. Marler and H. Terrace, pp. 47-74. Berlin: Springer-Verlag.

(22) Hertz, M. 1929. Die Organisation des optischen Feldes bei der Biene, I. Z. vergl. Physiol. 8: 693-748.

(23) Hertz, M. 1930. Die Organisation des optischen Feldes bei der Beine, II. Z. vergl. Physiol. 11: 107-145.

(24) Hertz, M. 1931. Die Organisation des optischen Feldes bei der Beine, III. Z. vergl. Physiol. 14: 629-674.

(25) Hoefer, I. and Lindauer, M. 1976. Der Schatten als Hilfsmarke bei der Orientierung der Honigbeine. J. comp. Physiol. 122: 5-18.

(26) Lashley, K. 1938. Conditioned reactions in the rat. J. Psychol. 6: 311-324.

(27) Menzel, E. W. 1984. Spatial cognition and memory in captive chimpanzees. In: The Biology of Learning, eds. P. Marler and H. Terrace, pp. 509-301.

(28) Menzel, R. 1984. Learning in honey bees in an ecological and behavioral context. Fort. Zool. 31: 55-74.

(29) Olton, D. S. 1979. Maps, memories, and mazes. Amer. Psychol. 34: 583-596.

(30) Ronacher, B. 1979. Beitrag einzelner Parameter zum wahrnehmungsgemassen Unterschied von zusammengesetzen Reizen bei der Honigbiene. Biol Cybernetics 32: 7-83.

(31) Schetter, B. 1972. Experiments on pattern discrimination in honey bees. In: Information Processing in the Visual System of Arthropods, ed. R. Wehner, pp. 195-200. Berlin: Springer-Verlag.

(32) Schwartz, B. 1984. Psychology of Learning and Behavior. New York: Nortons.

(33) Seidl, R., and Kaiser, W. 1982. Visual field size, binocular domain, and the ommatidial array of the compound eyes in worker honey bees.

(34) Tolman, E. C. 1948. Cognitive maps in rats and men. Psychol. Rev. 55: 189-208.

(35) Wehner, R. 1972. Pattern modulation and pattern detection in the visual system of Hymenoptera. In: Information Processing in the Visual System of Arthropods, ed. R. Wehner, pp. 183-194. Berlin: Springer-Verlag.

(36) Wehner, R. 1981. Spatial vision in arthropods. In: Handbook of Sensory Physiology, ed. H. Autrum, pp. 287-616, Berlin: Springer-Verlag.

Memory Traces in Honeybees

Randolf Menzel

Institut für Tierphysiologie, Neurobiologie, Freie Universität Berlin, Königin-Luise-Str. 28–30, D-1000 Berlin 33, FRG

Abstract. Bees learn quickly and effectively the signals which mark a nectar source. The memory for these signals (colors, odors) is characterized by behavioral experiments. Four sequential memory stages - called working memory, early, late and permanent memory - are found, which differ with respect to their sensitivities to unrewarded choices, to new learning trials, and to amnestic treatments. The neuropiles in the brain are differentially involved in the respective memory traces for odor signals. It is concluded that the primary afferent structure, the antennal lobe, participate only in the working memory phase. The most important neuropiles for memory formation are the mushroom bodies. The content of the early and late memory differs for a floral odor, but not for an attractive pheromone component. Genetic selection for low learning performance reveals bees, which lack the late memory but are unaffected in the early memory. The results are discussed in relation to the adaptations of the memory stages to the particular search behaviour of bees at floral patches.

INTRODUCTION

Honeybees collect nectar and pollen from flowers, not randomly, but with a systematic search strategy. The most important component of this strategy is the learning behavior of the individual bee, and the long lasting memory which results from a fast and effective learning process. If one follows marked bees on their way from one flower to another, it becomes obvious that the individual bee sticks to one kind of flower, although other species of flowers in the same area offer nectar at the same time and are visited by other bees (23, 25, 34). Flower constancy - as this behavior is called - has been known for a long time, and is well documented. One easily accessible document of this is the pollen load carried on the hind legs of every pollen collecting bee. Inspection indicates that in nearly all bees the pollen comes from one plant species only (8). Bees observed carrying pollen from 2 - 3 different species of flowers were later found to sample pollen from only one of these flower species, and were thus observed initially at that moment when they switched from one plant species to the next.

Flower constancy requires that the bee not only recognizes the species - specific signals of the flowers but also has the ability to store the signals in a memory which guides the choice behavior in the future. We know from Karl von Frischś early training experiments (9) that this memory is the result of a learning process in which the flower signals are associated with food reward (19). The learning process follows basic rules of associative learning (1, 15). In addition, associative predispositions and selective associations guide the learning behavior - aspects which shall not be elaborated on here (see 10, 18). The memory is stable and can last for a lifetime, even after a short period of learning. The first report on the stability of memory in bees comes from Lindauer (14), who found that a group of bees searched at the same feeding place after more than 3 months of winter rest. Similarly, I observed that the summer bees did not forget a color signal for 2 weeks, even after only 3 rewards on that color (15).

The aim of this paper is to characterize the memory trace for food signals in honeybees with behavioral experiments. I shall start with observations of the natural, undisturbed choice behavior, and finish with experiments which are designed to locate and manipulate the memory traces in the bee brain. The concept behind these experiments is that an associative learning trial triggers a sequence of automatic memory processes, the neural properties of which are reflected, at least partially, in behavioral and physiological measurements.

The idea of a central nervous automatic memory processor has its roots in the ethological concept that the continuous flow of behavior can be partitioned into components which reflect the operation of elementary mental processes. Such elementary processes are relatively close to the neural mechanics of the brain. Their separation and characterization may tell us something about the neural machinery involved, and thus, may help us to identify more precisely the underlying neuronal mechanisms.

Memory traces are needed at two distinct temporal windows

Under natural conditions bees fly out from the hive many times during a day and visit many flowers during one foraging bout. The time interval between foraging bouts is in the range of several minutes, and the frequency of landings on flowers lies in the range of a few seconds. Examples are given in Fig. 1. Fig. 1a plots the frequency of intervals between bees returning to the hive and successive arrivals at an artificial feeding place about 100 m from the hive. Fig 1b gives a frequency histogram of intervals between successive choices at four different plants, whose flowers appear in patches. These were the leopardś-bane Doronicum, the orange tree Citrus, the crested lark Corydalis, and the willow Salix. The measurements from the four different plant species have been cumulated because no great differences between species were observed, even though the average distance between the flowers was quite different and the quantity and kind of food (nectar, pollen) offered at each species was also different. It appears from these observations that the memory from former experience is needed at two distinct temporal windows, immediately after a choice (time interval in the range of seconds), and when the animal returns from the hive (time interval in the range of several to many minutes). Furthermore, a stable, long lasting memory is needed for choice behavior after long intervals (days, weeks and months).

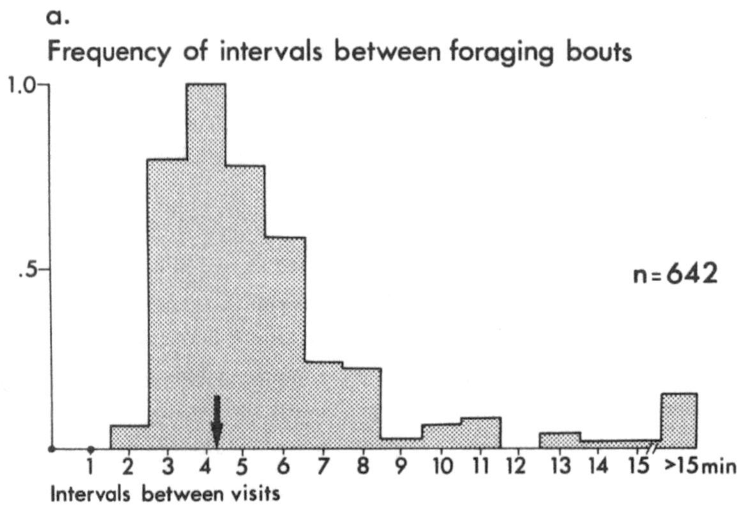

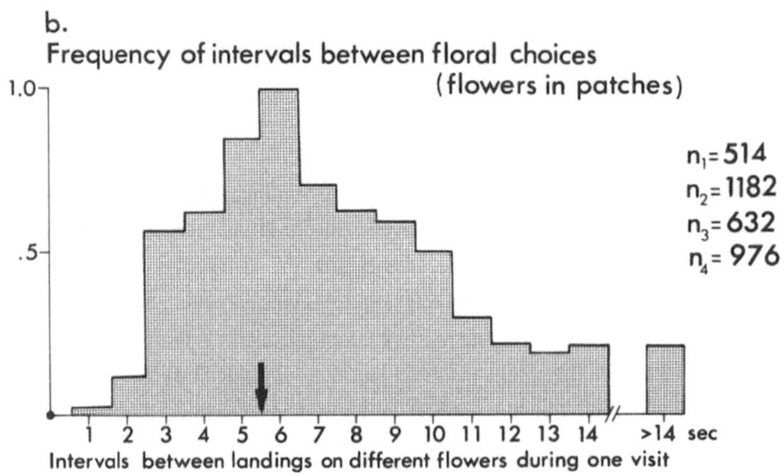

Fig. 1 - Temporal windows for the choice behavior of honeybees. a. Frequency of intervals between arrivals at an artificial feeding place 100 m from the hive. Data were collected over 1 week during late summer. b. Frequency of intervals between approaches of flowers in a patch. Individual bees were followed from flower to flower, and intervals between successive landings on flowers were recorded. The flower patches were: Doronicum (1), Citrus (2), Corydalis (3) and Salix (4). n: number of choices at respective flowers (1-4).

The temporal dynamics of the memory trace

When we tried to test the question whether bees apply different kinds of memory for the second, minute and day range, we ran into the problem that the bees learned too fast: after only three learning trials on a blue feeding place a very high proportion of the bees chose blue (80 % corrrect in a dual choice situation). They retain the memory at the same high level for their life time. Odor trained animals are even more precise: three learning trials change the behavior to 100 % correct choices. However, when free flying bees were trained in only one learning trial to a color signal or fixed bees conditioned by one trial to an odor, we found the following temporal dynamics in a free running recall test: Immediately (up to 2 min) after the learning trial the proportion of correct choices is very high, then it decreases and reaches a minimum at about 3 min, and then learned perfomance rises again after 4 min, Fig. 2 a, b). In this experiment each bee was tested only once at a particular time after the one - trial learning. The time course is the same for free flying bees trained to a color signal and fixed bees conditioned to an odor signal. The improvement of the memory with time without additional learning experience reminds us of memory consolidation in mammals and man (4, 26).

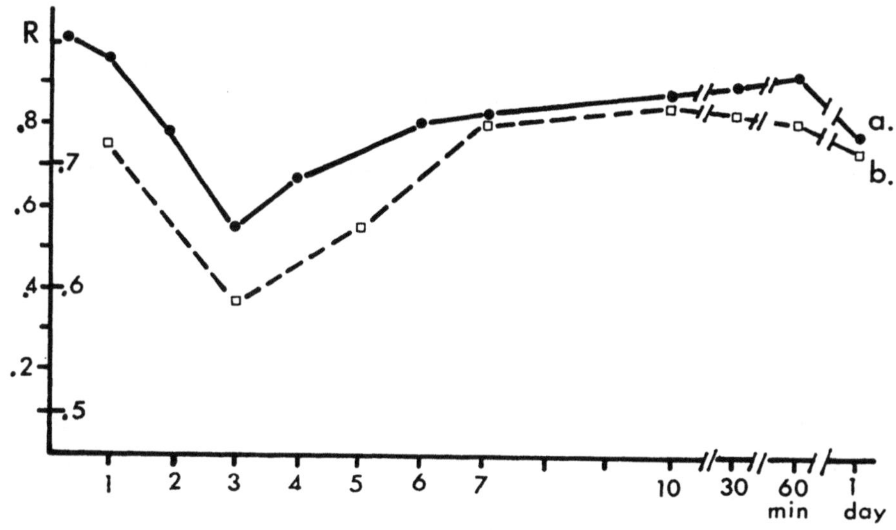

Fig. 2 - Temporal dependence of choice behavior (a) and of conditioned responding (b) in a free running recall experiment. In (a), the freely flying bees were trained by one trial to blue and tested at various intervals in a dual forced choice test between blue and yellow. The inner scale of the ordinate gives the percentage of choices for blue. (.5 refers to the spontaneous choice level at 50%, 1.0 to 100 % correct choices of blue), (n = 7.852). In (b), the fixed bees were conditioned with one trial to geraniol and tested for conditioned responses at various intervals. Each of the 240 bees were tested only once. The outer scale of the ordinate gives the percentage of conditioned responses. No bee responded before conditioning (.0). (curve a after Ref. 14, curve b after Ref. 21)

After consolidation, memory decays over several days following a one-trial learning. As mentioned above, no memory decay was found when bees were trained in three trials and were not allowed to make any new experience.

A corresponding temporal dynamic of the memory trace can also be seen in other memory tests. Two such tests shall be considered here: (1) sensitivity to a new learning experience, and (2) sensitivity to amnestic treatments.

(1) If free flying bees are trained first to blue and then, after various intervals, to the alternative color yellow, the bees are more resistant to reversal with shorter and longer intervals between the training sessions than with intermediate intervals (Fig. 3a). With very short intervals (less than 1 min) bees reverse to the second color signal also very efficiently. However, this latter effect depends on the duration of the reward: it is not apparent with longer reward durations. Bees conditioned to two odors in succession at intervals of 1 min, 3 min or 10 min, respond to the odor conditioned first equally frequently, but differently to the odor conditioned second: the response is highest at an interval of 3 min, and lower at 1 and 10 min intervals, although the memory tests have been performed 30 min and 90 min after conditioning. Both series of experiments indicate a weak memory trace for the signal learned first at 3 min after the single learning trial, just at the time when the learned behavior is less well under the control of the memory trace (compare Fig. 2 and 3).

As mentioned above, the memory trace immediately after the learning trial (up to 1 min) depends on the reward duration (Fig. 3a), indicating a particular weak memory trace shortly after a small reward. This conclusion is supported by the finding that extinction trials following a one-trial learning of a color signal, weaken the learned behavior more after short rewards than after long rewards (Fig. 4).

(2) The memory trace following a single learning trial also has temporal dynamics with respect to experimental procedures like narcosis, cooling and electric stimulation of the brain (EBS). Erber (5) demonstrated that these procedures cause retrograde amnesia if applied shortly after the learning trial. After the memory trace has been consolidated (more than 5 min after the single learning trial) it is no longer susceptible to interference. Massed learning trials facilitate the consolidation process. If 2, 3 or 4 learning trials follow each other quickly and well within the period of high susceptibility after one trial (within 1 min after the learning trial), only the contribution of one learning trial is erased with e. g. EBS.

The same temporal and event processes are found in odor conditioned bees (Fig. 5a) (7, 19, 20). A particularly quick repetition of conditioning trials make the memory trace immune against amnestic treatments. The obvious questions that arise from these findings are: (1) what protects the early memory trace from the amnestic effect - the additional CS (conditioned stimulus) or US (unconditioned stimulus) alone or the pairing of CS and US (an

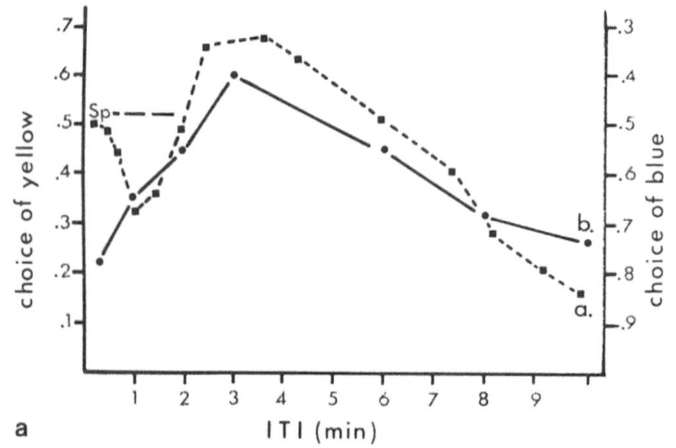

a

Fig. 3a - Two trial reversal learning experiment. Individual free flying bees were trained by one trial to a blue target and then after various intervals (intertrial interval ITI, abscissa) to a yellow target by one additional trial. The two colors (blue and yellow) were were presented 15 - 30 min later, and the choice behavior of each bee was tested for 4 min. Before training the bees chose the two alternatives nearly equally frequently (dotted line sp). The choice behavior after the two trial reversal learning depends on ITI. Short (5 sec, curve a) and long (15 sec, curve b) reward durations result in different time courses for ITI ś of up to 1 min. The two ordinates give the percentage of choices for the yellow target (left side) and for the blue target (right side) in the dual forced choice test. (curve a: number of animals N = 57, number of choices 1.493; curve b: N = 14, n = 278) (After Ref. 15)

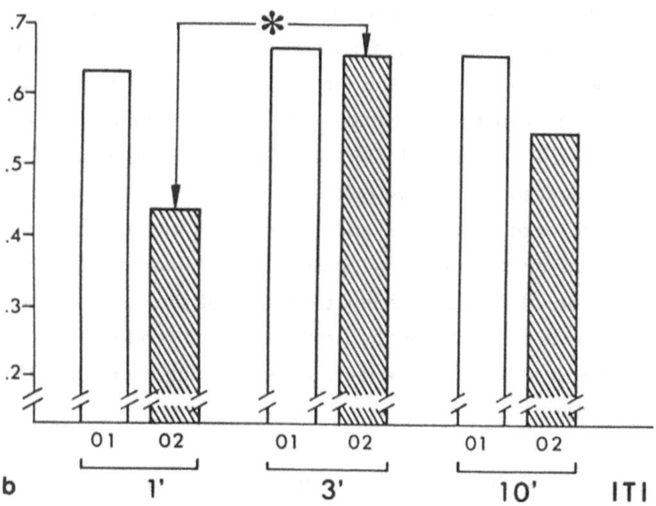

b

Fig. 3b - Two trial reversal conditioning experiment. The bees were first conditioned by one trial to either carnation or geraniol (O1) and after 1, 3 or 10 min ITI by one trial to geraniol or carnation (O2). The response to geraniol and carnation was tested 30 min later. The sequence of the odors during the tests was balanced by two subgroups each, and the results pooled. Since the kind of odor conditioned (carnation or geraniol) did not matter the groups were pooled. Thus the response value to O1 or O2 includes both odors. The conditioned response to O1 is independent of the subsequent conditioning to O2, but the conditioned response to O2 depends on ITI.

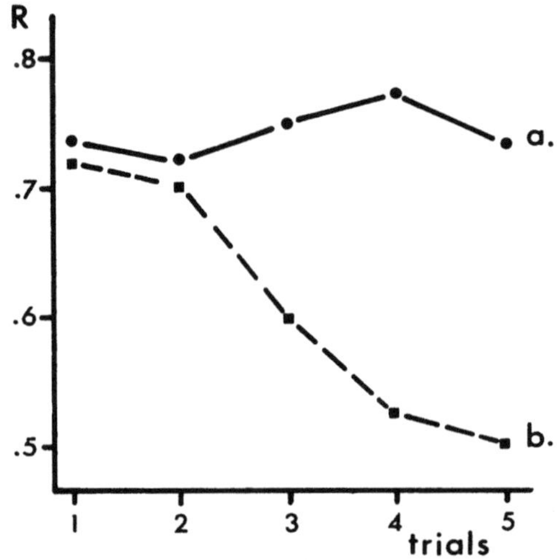

Fig. 4 - The effect of extinction (unrewarded choices) after one long reward (curve a, 15 sec) and after one short reward (curve b, 5 sec). Free flying bees were trained by one reward to a blue target and tested 15 - 30 min later in a dual forced choice test (blue - yellow). (After Ref. 14)

associative trial), (2) is the memory trace of the first learning trial shifted to a stable form more quickly, or does the memory trace of the second learning trial reach the stable form immediately? We found that an additional exposure to the CS or the US alone, prior to EBS or cooling, does not protect the memory trace, but an additional learning trial does protect it, even if a different odor is used in the second learning trial (19). This finding gives us the unique oppurtunity to address the question of whether the memory trace of the first or the second learning trial reaches the stable memory more quickly. In our experiments, the two different odors (O1 and O2) were carnation and geraniol. Since both odors were used as a first or a second odor, and the data are pooled, in Fig 5b, we refer to the odors as first or second trained odor (O1 and O2). O1 and O2 were trained in quick succession, and the EBS was applied immediately thereafter (within 30 sec). As Fig. 5b shows, the amnestic effect is restricted to O2. The response level for O1 is not different from that of the control group. (The response level of the control group is different for the first and second conditioned odor. This indicates a so called recency effect, which is well known in the learning literature. This effect shall not be discussed further here.)

We can conclude from these experiments that the memory trace has dynamic properties which depend on time and on associative events. The establishment of a stable memory form is faster with repetitions of associative events (but not just US or CS). After a single associative event the memory requires a much longer time to reach the same stable form. The correction by a new learning trial is more effective within the first minute after the learning trial if the duration of the reward is short, and less effective if it is long. The behavioral consequence of this is that after one learning trial the time period for corrections within the labile memory form is considerably extended and reward dependent, whereas after

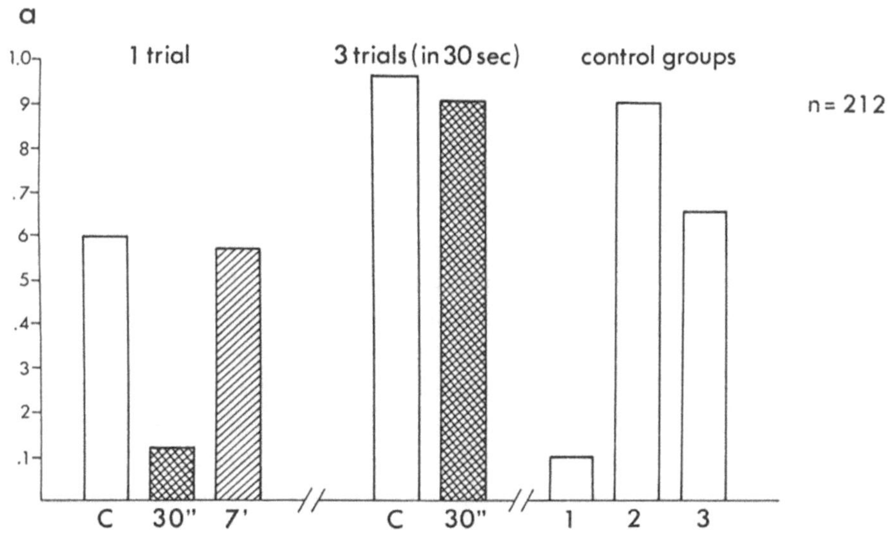

Fig. 5a - The effect of EBS on memory consolidation. 1 trial: 3 groups of animals (40 in each) were conditioned by one trial to carnation and tested 30 min later. The control group C was sham treated, the 30 sec group was shocked 30 sec after the learning trial, and the 7 min group was shocked 7 min after the learning trial. 3 trials (in 30 sec):two groups of animals (C: 14 animals, 30": 17 animals) were conditioned by 3 trials within 30 sec. The control group (C) was sham treated, the 30 sec group shocked 30 sec after the last learning trial. The animals were tested 30 min later. Control groups: 1 : odor paired with EBS. The response level to the odor is not different from untreated animals (n = 14) 2: EBS treatment 10 min prior to conditioning (n = 32) (3 trials). (Compare with the control group of the 3 trials experiment).

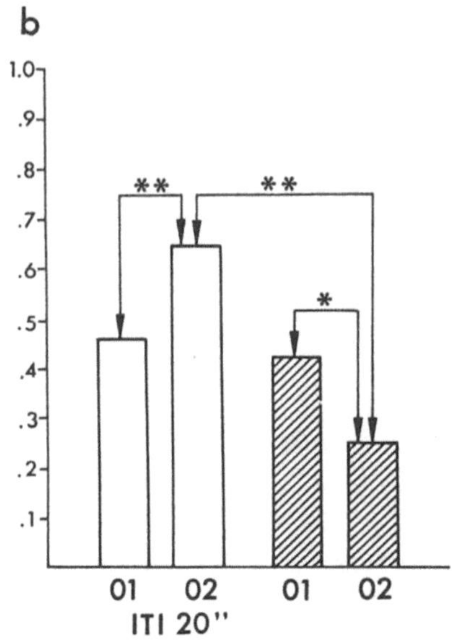

Fig. 5b - Dual odor conditioning and the effect of EBS. Two groups of bees were conditioned first to odor 1 (O1, carnation or geraniol) and then to odor 2 (O2, geraniol or carnation) by one trial each in quick succession (within 20 sec). The control groups were sham treated (open bars), the experimental groups treated immediately by ECS (hatched bars). The response to the conditioned stimuli O1 and O2 were tested 30 min later. Half the bees of each group were tested first to O1, the other half to O2, and the results pooled. One star (*) indicates significant differences on the level of p 0.05, two stars (**) of p 0.01. (see text). (Courtesy of M. Sugawa).

several learning trials, the response reaches asymptote quickly, is independent of reward duration, and the memory trace is strong and stabile.

Selection for good and bad learners reveals differences in the dynamics of the memory trace

Recently, Brandes (2) selected bees for their learning ability using the olfactory conditioning paradigm. He isolated good and bad learners and bred them first parthenogenetically and later sexually by internal crosses (see Moritz and Brandes, this vol.). We tested the two lines after 3 generations of separation, in a free running recall test, and found the well known biphasic time course in the good learners with a somewhat speeded-up early memory phase, and a very different time course in the bad learners (Fig. 6). Initially, the bad learners respond equally well to the CS than the good learners, but the memory in the bad learners deteriorates more quickly. Furthermore, the early dynamic properties are reversed in the bad learners, although this effect is not statistically significant in a point to to point comparison. These results remind us of the Drosophila memory mutants dunce, rutabaga and amnesiac (22), which are affected in their ability to establish a long-term memory. Other than in Drosophila, we do not know how many genes are involved and which enzymatic processes are damaged, but we can conclude from these results that the dynamics of the memory trace, following a single learning trial, are under the control of the genome and thus reflect an inherent property of the underlying neural network.

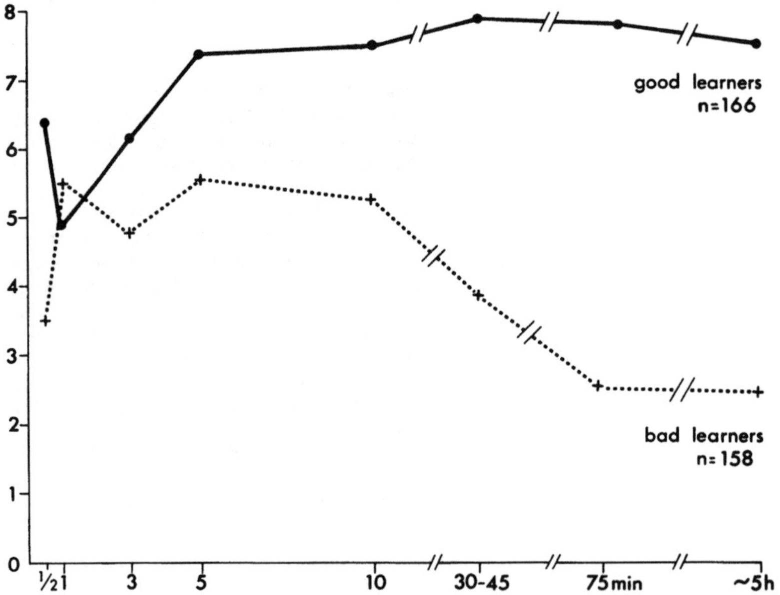

Fig. 6 - The time course of recall after one trial odor conditioning in bees selected for good and bad learning behavior. Each of the two groups of bees (n: number of bees) was conditioned once to geraniol and tested once only at varing intervals after conditioning (abscissa).

The content of the early and late memory trace

So far, we have tried to characterize the conditions which are necessary to establish a stable, long-term memory. Now we want to ask whether the content of the early and late memory trace is the same or different. Again we can approach this question only with indirect behavioral methods. One way is to determine whether the generalization gradient is the same at different times after one learning trial (Fig.7).

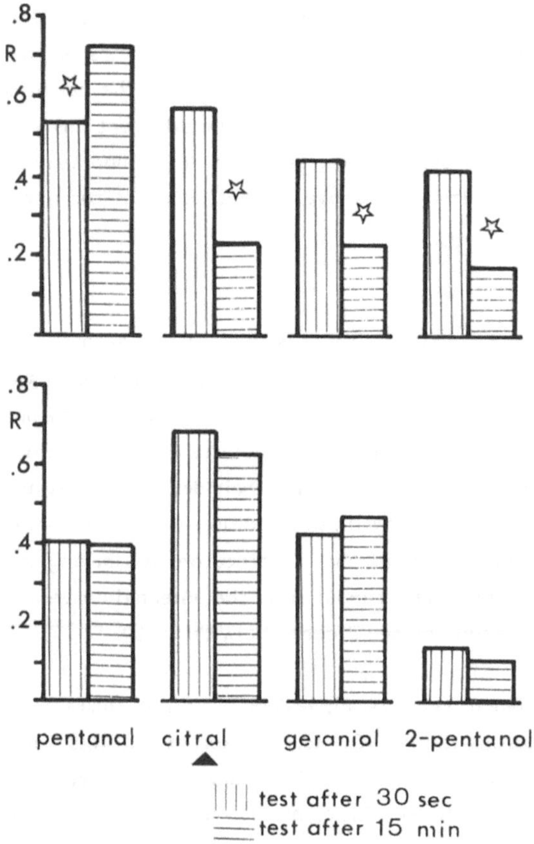

Fig. 7 - Generalization gradient during the early and late memory. Groups of bees trained to pentanal (upper part of the figure, total n = 235, each group: n = 25 or more) or citral (lower part of the figure, total n = 245, each group: n = 30 or more) by one trial. 30 sec (vertical stripes) or 15 min (horizontal stripes) after the conditioning trial the bees were tested by presenting one of four different odors (pentanal, citral, geraniol, 2 - pentanol). (See text) (Courtesy of B. Smith).

A group of bees is trained to either pentanal or citral in one conditioning trial, and then tested by 1 of 4 different odors either 30 sec or 15 min after conditioning. It is established beforehand that all 4 odors are well descriminated by the bees if they are differentially conditioned in several trials. After one trial the bees also partially respond to the non-reinforced odors, demonstrating a profile of generalization. It turns out that if the floral odor pentanal is conditioned this profile is significantly different for the early and the late memory trace. This is not so, if the pheromone component citral is conditioned. In the case of pentanal, the neural processing underlying the transfer from an early to a late memory trace makes the profile sharper, and thus increases discrimination by some process that we might call "mountain climbing", in analogy to the properties of an associative matrix (24).

"Mountain climbing" might be seen as a process which changes the content of the memory trace by some internal control mechanism (e. g. an autocorrelation of the neural excitation subserving the early memory trace). Such a mechanism may be involved in the consolidation of an unspecified stimulus like a floral odor, which can be one out of very many kinds of odors. In the case of a specified or labelled stimulus, like the component of the Nasanov secretion citral, the final memory content may be reached immediately because the neural structures for such an appetitive association may exist already in a highly prepared form. Learning of labelled stimuli may thus follow the scheme of an alpha-conditioning as discussed by Gould (10), whereas unlabelled stimuli may require a much more flexible and unspecified network with higher self-organizing properties. It is tempting to speculate that the patterns of connections in the brain for prepared associations are the same for the different memory phases, but different for the open or unspecified associations. However, it is important to notice that the time and event dependencies as described above are not different for floral odors and pheromone components.

An attempt to localize the memory trace

The bee brain may be relatively large by insect standards, but it is small -1 mm across - for the coarse methods which are available for a search for neural correlates of the proposed memory traces. Many of the 950,000 neurons are located in the visual system, which may not concern us in the context of olfactory learning. The prominent structures of the olfactory system are the two antennal lobes, the two mushroom bodies with their double calyces and single alpha and beta-lobes, and the fibre tracts connecting these structures (see Masson, this vol.). The suboesophageal ganglion (SOG), which contains the motorneurons subserving the motor-program of the proboscis extension, recieves direct input from the antennal nerve and descending neurons from the deuto- and protocerebrum (see Bicker et al., this vol.).

Recordings have been made from the AGT-neurons (13), alpha-lobe extrinsic fibres (11), Kenyon cells (6), motor- and pre-motor neurons in the SOG (see Bicker et al., this vol.). Unfortunately, no clear correlations between neural activity and learning or memory, other than relatively long lasting stimulus after effects (6, see Erber and Homberg this vol.) have been found so far. The search for the memory trace, therefore, is still restricted to the identification of neuropiles possibly involved in the storage process.

In our first attempt we used cold needles (tip diameter 150 um) to reversibly block neural activity for a few sec at various intervals after one-trial learning (7, 17, 19). Different courses for the retrograde amnestic effect were found for different regions in the brain. If only one antenna was stimulated during conditioning and either the ipsi- or the contralateral neuropile cooled, the participation of the ipsi- or contralateral structure could be observed. It appeared that there is no amnestic effect if the lateral protocerebrum was cooled, a very transient one if the antennal lobes were cooled, but longer lasting effects if the alpha lobes and the calyces were cooled. Although we can not firmly conclude from such experiments that the process of transfer to a stable memory trace resides in the mushroom bodies, these results indicate that the mushroom bodies are essential structures for the process involved in establishing a stable memory trace over several minutes. Furthermore, neither a reverberating circuit antennal lobe - calyces - lateral protocerebrum - antennal lobe, nor the antennal lobe or the lateral protocerbrum seperately are essential for the process. The antennal lobes are involved in the very first period (up to 1 min) after a learning trial. It is thus likely that the antennal lobes are involved in the very first and very sensitive period of the memory trace, but not in the consolidation of the memory.

To appreciate the results after unilateral olfactory stimulation of the antennae and the local cooling of the ipsi- or contralateral structures, a peculiar property of olfactory learning in bees has to be pointed out. If only one antenna is exposed to the odor during conditioning, the bee will respond to that odor only if it is presented to the same antenna and not, if the other antenna is stimulated (19). Does that mean that the memory trace is restricted to the ipsilateral side of the brain? Indeed, no contra-lateral cooling effects are seen in the antennal lobes, but the contra-lateral mushroom bodies, particularly the calyces, are involved. Also, the contra-lateral alpha lobe appears to participate in the memory trace, because bi-lateral cooling is much more effective than ipsi-lateral cooling alone. However, contra-lateral cooling in the alpha lobe alone had very little effect in our first experiments (7, 19). We studied this question again with better temporal resolution and higher spatial selectivity (Fig. 8).

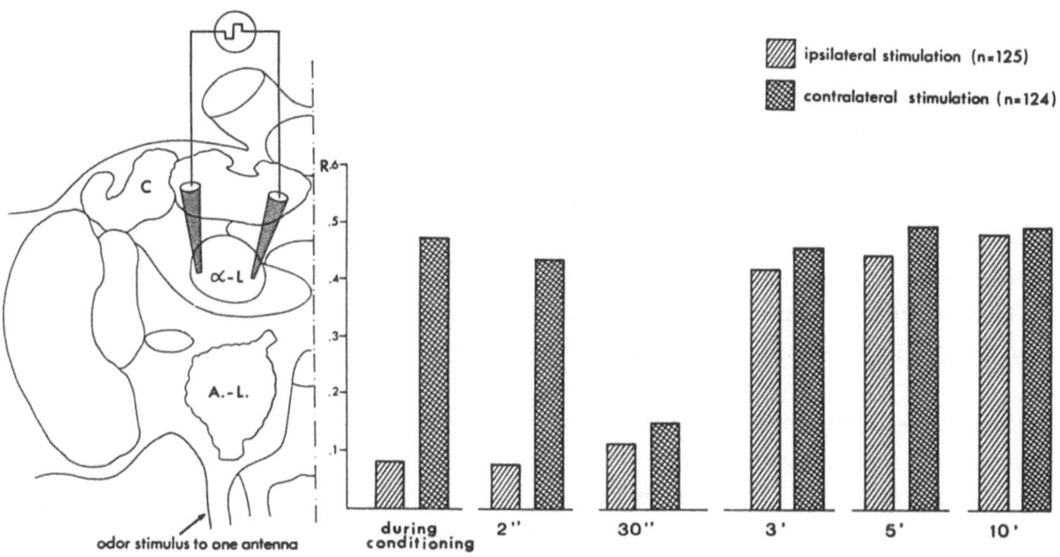

Fig. 8 - The amnestic effect of electric stimulation of the alpha - lobe. The bees were conditioned once to geraniol by stimulating only one antenna with the odor. EBS was applied to the ipsi- or contralateral alpha-lobe immediately during conditioning, or after intervals of 2 sec, 30 sec, 3 min, 5 min or 10 min. The conditioned response was tested 30 min after the EBS application by stimulating the same antenna with the odor as was done during conditioning. (The bees never responded to the stimulation of the other antenna). (Courtesy M. Sugawa).

In this experiment the amnestic treatment is a weak electric stimulus (ac 100uA, 50 Hz, pulse duration 1 ms, for 2 sec) applied differentially through 2 microcapillaries at the median and lateral margin of the ipsi- or contra-lateral alpha lobe. There is a normal retrograde amnestic function if the ipsi-lateral lobe is treated. But if the contra-lateral lobe is stimulated we find a bi-phasic function with no amnestic effect during and shortly after the learning trial. It should be emphasized that the tests for an amnestic effect are carried out 30 min after the treatment, and the CS is presented to the same antenna as during the conditioning trial. (If the CS is presented to the other antenna there is never a conditioned response as mentioned above).

It thus appears that localized amnestic treatments focuses our attention on the mushroom bodies as being potential structures subserving the inherent self-organizing process for the establishment of a permanent memory trace.

CONCLUSION

A few associative learning trials can change the behavior of an animal like the honeybee for its life time, a single learning trial for many hours or even days. The learning trial is a very short event. In the honeybee it may last just 3 sec including the full length of the exposure to the CS and US. The changes executed in the brain by such a short event develop over time and under the influence of additional learning trials. The engram or memory trace must, therefore, result from an inherent automatic machinery that is specifically triggered by the associative event and involves internal, self-organizing neural processes. Hebb (12) has used the term "cell assemblies" for these self-organizing, self-instructing groups of neurons, which are assembled temporarily or permanently by the process of learning. It is very likely that a "cell assembly" is in reality composed of many neurons, and that its crucial functions are only incompletely reflected in single members of the group, or the synaptic connection between two members. Cellular neurobiology may have limited access to these crucial functions. We have relied heavily, therefore, on behavioral methods in our attempt to characterize these automatic memory processes. It is obvious, however, that behavioral methods give only indirect and - at the best - suggestive evidence. Neurophysiological approaches are needed for more direct tests of these hypotheses, and these approaches have to built on the cellular neurobiological methods that are used so successfully in learning studies with molluscs.

Our results are consistent with a model that assumes a time and event dependent sequential structure of memory stages. These memory stages are characterized by their time course in free running recall tests, their differential control of choice behavior, their sensitivities towards associative events and retrograde amnestic treatments, their distribution in the brain and their separation by genetic selection. Furthermore, the memory content may be different in the early and late memory stages.

Nothing is known so far about the neural and cellular mechanisms underlying the memory phases. The enormous speed-up by additional associative events indicates that the slow process of consolidation after a single learning trial may not be limited by metabolic restraints, but is rather an actively retarded process that exposes the recently learned information to additional controls before a permanent trace is established. It is conceivable that the same critical substance (e.g. a second messenger like cAMP) is synthesized very slowly after a single trial and very rapidly after massed trials, and that the consolidation into a late and permanent memory may depend on the concentration of just this substance at critical locations within the "neural assembly".

The experiments reported here suggest a sequence of 4 memory stages following a single associative learning trial:

(1) a working memory lasting up to 1 min, which controls learned behavior very well, is sensitive to reward duration, to extinction trials, to reversal learning, to amnestic treatments, and which resides in the ipsi-lateral brain including the antennal lobe; (2) an early memory, which initially controls learned behavior very well, but also looses this ability quickly (within 2 -3 min), is less sensitive to extinction, reward duration and reversal learning. It can be erased by amnestic treatments. Bees genetically selected for low learning performance are not effected in the early memory. The mushroom bodies in both sides of the brain take part in this memory trace. (3) A late memory, which develops over time after 4 min following the learning trial, gains increasing control over learned behavior with time (consolidation) and becomes more resistant to reversal learning. Late memory deteriorates after more than 12 hours. It is insensitive to amnestic treatment, and is absent in animals selected for low learning performance. The localization of the late memory trace in the brain is unknown, but most likely involves both mushroom bodies. (4) a permanent memory, which is established only after more than one learning trial, is stable for the life time of the animal and is changed only by new learning trials.

A multiple memory trace system is not a unique feature of the bee brain. However, the actual temporal dynamics and the particular qualitative and quantitative properties are adaptations of the species to the general pattern of food encounters under natural conditions. The sequence of the memory phases after one learning trial ensures that the initially stored information is transferred to a lasting memory only if it is reinforced by additional learning trials, or by an extended period of undisturbed consolidation time. This period can be the happy flight back to the hive. In any case, when the bee returns to the floral patch, she has a firmly established and well structured memory at her disposal.

(Supported by DFG grant ME 365 / 11 - 3)

REFERENCES

(1) Bitterman, M. E.; Menzel, R.; Fietz, A.; Schäfer, S. 1983. Classical conditioning of proboscis-extension in honeybees. J. Comp. Physiol. Psychol. 97: 107 - 119.

(2) Brandes, H. in press. Genetic differences in learning behaviour in honeybees, Apis mellifera capensis. Anim. Behav.

(3) Darwin, C. R. 1877. The effects of cross and self-fertilisation in the vegetable kingdom. New York: Appleton.

(4) Ebbinghaus, M. 1885. Über das Gedächtnis. Leipzig: K. Bühler.

(5) Erber, J. 1975. The dynamics of learning in the honeybee, Apis mellifica carnica. J. Comp. Physiol. 99: 231 - 242.

(6) Erber, J. 1983. Neural correlates of learning in the honeybee. T. I. N. S. 4: 270 - 273.

(7) Erber, J.; Masuhr, T.; Menzel, R. 1980. Localization of short-term memory in the brain of the honeybee, Apis mellifera. Physiol. Entomol. 5: 343 - 358.

(8) Free, J. B. 1963. The flower constancy of honeybees. J. Anim. Ecol. 32: 119 - 131.

(9) Frisch, K. von. 1914. Der Farbesinn und Formensinn der Bienen. Zool. J. (Physiol) 35: 1 - 188.

(10) Gould, J. L. 1984. Natural history of honeybee learning. In The Biology of Learning, eds. P. Marler and H. S. Terrace, pp. 149 - 180. Berlin - Heidelberg - New York - Tokyo: Springer Verlag.

(11) Gronenberg, W. 1984. Das Protocerebrum der Honigbiene im Bereich des Pilzkörpers - eine neurophysiologisch-anatomische Charakterisierung. Dissertation, Freie Universität Berlin.

(12) Hebb, D. O. 1949. The organization of behavior. New York: Wiley.

(13) Homberg, H. 1984. Processing of antennal information in extrinsic mushroom body neurons in the bee brain. J. Comp. Physiol. 154: 825 - 836.

(14) Lindauer, M. 1963. Allgemeine Sinnesphysiologie, Orientierung im Raum. Fortschr. Zool. 16: 58 -140.

(15) Menzel, R. 1968. Das Gedächtnis der Honigbiene für Spektralfarben. I. Kurzzeitiges und langzeitiges Behalten. Z. vergl. Physiol. 60: 82 - 102.

(16) Menzel, R. 1979. Behavioural access to short-term memory in bees. Nature. 281: 368 - 369.

(17) Menzel, R. 1984. Short-term memory in bees. In: Primary Neural Substrate of Learning and Behavioural Change, eds. D. L. Alkon and J. Farley. Cambridge University Press.

(18) Menzel, R. 1985. Learning in honeybees in an ecological and behavioural context. In: Experimental Behavioural Ecology, eds. B. Hölldobler and M. Lindauer, pp. 55 - 74. Stuttgart - New York: G. Fischer.

(19) Menzel, R.; Erber, J.; Masuhr, T. 1974. Learning and memory in the honeybee. In: Experimental Analysis of Insect Behaviour, eds. L. Barton - Brown, pp. 195 - 217. New York: Springer Verlag.

(20) Menzel, R and Sugawa,M. in press. Time course of short-term memory depends on associative events. Naturwiss.

(21) Mercer, A. R.; Menzel, R. 1982. The effect of biogenic amines on conditioned and unconditioned responses to olfactory stimuli in the honeybee, Apis mellifera. J. Comp. Physiol. 145: 363 - 368.

(22) Quinn, W. G. 1984. Work in invertebrates on the mechanisms underlying learning. In: The Biology of Learning, eds. P. Marker and H. S. Terrace, pp.197 - 248. Berlin - Heidelberg - New York - Tokyo: Springer Verlag.

(23) Ribbands, C. R. 1949. The foraging method of individual honeybees. J. Anim. Ecol. 18: 47 - 66.

(24) Rolls, E. T. in press. Information representation, processing, and storage in the brain: analysis at the single neuron level. In: Neural and molecular basis of learning, eds. J. P. Changeux and M. Konishi. Berlin - Heidelberg - New York - Tokyo: Springer Verlag.

(25) Wells, H. and Wells, P. H. 1983. Honeybee foraging ecology: optimal diet, minimal uncertainty or individual constancy? J. Anim. Ecol. 52: 829 - 836.

(26) Weiskrantz, L. 1970. A long-term view of short-term memory in psychology. In: Short-term changes in neural activity and behaviour, eds. G. Horn and R. A. Hinde, pp. 63 - 74. London: Cambridge University Press.

Subject Index

Acetylcholine 281

Achromatic vision 173

After effects 253-263

Age (see also Castes) 14, 71, 266-276, 282-285

Amacrine (cell) 130-139, 144-156, 212, 213, 257

Amnestic treatment 310-325

Antagonistic color coding 172-188

Antenna(e) 25, 96-100, 112-119, 202-221, 244, 250, 253-263, 280-292, 320-322

Antennal lobe 192, 202-221, 226, 235-242, 244-250, 253-263, 280-292, 310, 320-323

Aorta (see also Heart) 106-109

Apis

- cerana 8-19, 54-64
- dorsata 8-19, 54-64
- florea 10-14, 54-64

Associative predispositions 311

Axon bundle 130-139, 147, 191

Bad learners 310-325

Bee

- Africanized 121-127
- Asian 54-64
- bumble 72, 73, 102-109
- carpenter 107
- drone 4, 22-27, 96-100, 102-109, 139, 237, 280-285
- Italian 62, 121-127
- queen 4, 21-29, 97, 139, 266-276, 280-292,
- receiver 38-51
- recruit 38-51, 54-64, 68, 270, 307

Behavior

- -al development 266-276
- colonial 267
- defensive 28, 273
- learning 21-29, 260, 314-323
- foraging 270, 272
- stinging 121-127, 269

Biogenic amines, see Dopamine, Serotonine, Octopamine

Blood (circulation of) 102-109

Body temperature 102-109, 112-119

Cacoon 97
Calliphora erythrocephala 169
Calyx (Calyses) 142, 160, 198, 205, 210, 226-231, 239, 246, 247, 258
Cartridge 130-139, 144
Cast (Castes)(see also Age) 42, 66-74
Celestial cues (orientation to) 5, 6, 54-64, 76-92, 303, 307
Cell wall (texture of) 97
Central body, (see also Central complex) 141-156, 202-221, 226, 228, 235-242, 245, 247, 257-262
Central complex, (see also Central body) 155, 192,203. 205, 217, 241, 253-263
Centrifugal (fiber, neuron) 131-139, 144, 156, 212
Cervical (connective, nerve) 159-170, 204-221
Chiasma 130-139, 142-144, 206-213
Chromatic diagram 174-185
Circadian rhythm 112, 118
Classical conditioning 313-323
Cognition 51
Cognitive map 298-307
Color 15, 66-74, 84, 134, 139, 147-156, 172-188, 298-307
  biased behavior 187,188
  brightness of 172-184
  catagories 184-188
  code 144, 147, 156
  constancy 172-188
  contrast 141-156, 172-188
  mixing 187
  opponency 298-303
  opponent cell 134, 135, 141-156, 172-188
  opponent model 172-188
  receptor (s) 130-139, 141-156, 172-188, 191-199
  space 167, 172-188
Comb 4, 5, 46, 54-61
Commissure (-al fibers) 141-156
Communication (see also Dance behavior) 2, 5, 12, 14, 38, 49, 56-64
Compound eye 3, 5, 33-35, 62, 76-92, 130-139, 144-156, 158-170, 180, 191-199, 207, 253, 260
Consolidation (of memory) 310-325
Cooling (see also Thermoregulation) 102-109
Cooperation 46, 48-51
Corpora allata 267, 268
Corpora cardiaca 207, 226
Corpora pendunculata 205, 226,
Critical period 288, 290
Crystalline cone 131

Dance (language, behavior) 3-14, 38-51, 54-64, 68-71, 81-90, 105, 307
Dark adaptation 134
Decision making 40-49, 66-74
Descending interneurons 138, 141-156, 158-170, 191-199, 202-221, 227, 258-263, 320

Deutocerebrum 158-170, 202-221, 238,
244-250, 254, 280-292
Development (of neurons) 202, 218, 280-292
Dichroism 77
Directional selectivity 141-156, 158-170
Division of labor 269, 273, 274
Dopamine 225, 228, 231, 235, 241, 245,
246, 249
Dorsal lobe 203, 204, 209, 214
Double opponent (neuron) 145-149, 152, 153,
183, 184
Drosophila 21-29

Electrical coupling 134, 135, 156
Electroantennogram (EAG) 273-276, 286
Electromyogram (EMG) 117
Electroretinogram (ERG) 14
Electrical stimulation of the brain (EBS),
(and memory) 314-322
Elementary mental processes 311
Endothermy 102, 104
Energetics 43, 66, 71
Engram, see Memory trace
Enkephaline 121-127
Eumine (wasps) 97
Evaporation 109
E-vector sensitivity,
see Polarization sensitivity
Evolutionary models (of foraging) 54-64,
67, 74
Exocrine glands 266-276
Extinction trials 314, 316, 323

Fiber tract (See also axon bundle)
130, 141-154, 159, 161, 198, 203, 207, 209,
210, 232-242, 254-263, 284-292, 320
Flight 4, 6, 15, 22, 68-73, 99, 102-109,
298, 304, 305, 323
control of 139, 149, 158, 164, 165, 170,
173, 199
direction 54-64
Flight (ctd)
foraging 269, 270, 272
nuptial 4, 6, 116
Floral choice 72, 298-307, 310-325
Flower
constancy 72, 310-325
shape, learning of 298-307
Food collection 14, 15, 25, 38-51, 54-64
Food transfer 14, 44, 45
Foraging
behavior 2, 4, 38-51, 54-64, 96-98,
105-109, 122-127, 266-276, 290,298-307
costs 66-74
decisions 66, 67, 72
mechanisms 38-51, 66-74
models 67, 96-98

GABA 202-221, 225-233, 236, 240. 241, 257, 258, 281
GAD 202, 221, 281
Gap junction 135
Gastrin/CCK 235-242
Generalization 298, 319
Generalist system of olfactory neurons) 281
Glomeruli (of antennal lobe) 202-221, 238-242, 245, 248, 254, 280-292
Good Learners 310-325
Grooming 112-119

Head movement 158-170
Heart 106, 108
Heat loss 102-109, 113
2-Heptanone 268, 269, 273
Horizontal fiber 130-139, 150, 151, 158-170, 207, 219
Hormone-mediated (behavior) 271
5-HT (5-hydroxytryptamine), see Serotonine
Hypopharyngeal glands 268

Information processing 38-51, 54-64, 66-74 79-82, 202-221, 225-233, 253, 254, 280, 281, 298, 310-325
Information sharing 38-51
Intake(s) 39-51, 66-74
Intensity dependence 134, 135, 178, 184
Intracellular staining 184, 191
Intrinsic fiber (cell, neuron), (see also Amacrine cell) 148, 149, 205, 216, 217, 225-233, 237, 246, 254, 261, 284, 287
Isopentyl acetate 269, 270, 273
Ionotophoretic staining, see Intracellular staining

Juvenile hormone (JH) 266-276
JND (Just noticable differences) 176, 177, 178, 187

Kenyon cells 205, 226-233, 320

L-glutamic acid decarboxylase, see GAD
L-neuron (fiber) 131-139, 191-199, 203, 214, 238
Lamina 130-139, 141-156,202-221, 226, 237, 238, 246
Landmarks
  orientation to 5, 6, 54-64, 298-307
  learning of 298-307
Learning of, see
  associative behavior
  behavior
  celestial cues
  color
  flower shape
  landmarks

polarization patterns
rules of
textures
Light adaptation 134, 135
Lobula 130-139, 141-156, 159-170, 184, 192-198, 202-221, 226, 235, 237, 238, 248, 254, 260, 261
Lobula plate 138, 164, 194

Mandibular
glands 268
nerve 204, 210, 211, 219
Map learning 298-307
Mating (behavior) 21-29
Mechanoreceptive Hairs 155, 170
Mechanoreceptors 155, 170
Mechanosensitivity 96-100
Mechanosensory information 167, 169, 170 205, 260
Medulla 130-138, 141-156, 184, 192, 197, 204-221, 226, 237, 238, 248-250, 261
Memory
early 310-325
eidetic 298-307
flowershape 298-307
landmark 298-307
late 310-325
locale 298-307
of colors 173, 188
permanent 310-325
pictorial 298-307
route specific 298-307
stages of (phases) 310-325
traces 310-325
working 310-325
Mesometathoracic ganglion 158, 159, 167, 170, 192
Metabolic rate 23, 24, 27, 68, 105, 109, 323
Metamorphosis 286, 287
Methoprene 266-276
Microvilli (photoreceptor) 77, 82, 83, 89, 130
Morphine 121-127
Motoneurons 158, 167, 169, 170, 202-221, 253, 260, 261, 320
Multimodal(ity) 154, 156, 196, 197, 254, 255, 260-263
Muscle contraction 102-109, 112-119
Muscle tone 112-119
Mushroom bodies (MB) 142, 147, 149, 153, 158, 160, 192, 202-221, 225-233,236-242, 244-250, 253-263, 281, 285, 287, 310, 320, 321, 322, 323

Naloxone 121-127
Navigation 303, 304, 307
Neck muscle 169, 170
Neuroblast 287
Nectar guides 96, 98
Neuropeptide(s) 236, 242
Nocturnal dances 57, 58, 62

Ocellar
function 167, 242
interneuron 167, 191, 194, 214
158, 159, 168, 170, 191, 241
neuropile 215
system 191, 192, 199, 209, 214
tract 159, 161, 203, 214, 235, 238, 242, 282
Octopamine 216, 228, 241, 245, 246, 260, 261, 262
Olfactory
cells 280, 281
coding 281
conditioning 280, 318
glomeruli 245, 248
Olfactory (ctd)
information 205
inputs 249, 260
interneurons 249
learning 249, 320, 321
memory 253
neurons 286, 287
orientated behavior 241
plasticity 280, 282
processing 280
receptor 280, 214
stimulation 249, 253, 254, 257
system 280, 288-290, 320
Ommatidium (-tidia), (see also Retinula cell) 82, 83, 85, 90, 130-139, 143, 144, 156, 175, 299
One trial learning 290, 292, 310-325
Opiates 121, 127
Optical cartridge, see Cartridge
Optic ganglion, see Lamina, Medulla, Lobula
Optic lobe, see Lamina, Medulla, Lobula
Optic neuropil 257
Optic tubercle 142, 148, 149, 154, 204, 207, 226, 238, 254, 260, 262
Optimal foraging 42, 66-74
Optomotor response (system) 151, 164, 173
Osmia 97
Outer chiasma, see chiasma
Overheating 44, 45, 46, 102-109, 113

Pain 121, 127
Paravespula vulgaris 167, 168
PCT, see Protocerebro-calycal tract
Pendunculus, see Mushroom bodies
Perceptual dimensions (of color vision) 172-188
Petals (texture of) 96, 98, 99
Pheromone 266-276, 281, 310, 319, 320
Photoreceptor (s), (see also Visual cells) 77-90, 130-139, 141-143, 151, 156, 172-188, 191-196, 201-221
Phototaxis 63, 64, 173
Pitch 158, 161, 164, 167
Plasticity 260, 280-292
Polarized light
detection of 76-92,147

orientation to 76-92
pattern of 5, 76-92
sensitivity to 54, 76.92, 135
Pollen 15, 38, 57, 66, 68, 109, 310, 311
Polyethism (see also Age and Castes) 22, 266-276
Prothoracic ganglion 159, 253
Protocerebral bridge 147, 155, 160, 203-205, 209
Protocerebro-calycal tract (PCT) 202-221, 231, 257, 258
Protocerebrum 130, 138, 141-156, 159, 202-221, 235, 238, 239, 245-246, 253-263, 280-292, 320, 321
Pupation 288

Receptive field (of visual neurons), (see also Visual field) 144-156, 169, 181, 182
Response intensity (R/I function), (see also Intensity dependence) 194-195
Resting state 68, 311
Resting site 96, 104, 112-119
Retinula cells (see also Photoreceptors) 130-132, 141
Rhabdom 130-132
Roll 158, 161, 164, 165, 167
Rules of associative learning 310-325

Selective associations 310-325
Sensilla placodea 280, 282, 287
Sensilla trichodea 96-100
Serial homologues 202, 218-221
Serotonine 202-221, 225-228, 235-241, 244, 245, 260-262
Sexual dimorphism 139
Sleep 112-119
Small field (visual neurons) 138, 144-156, 175
Specialist system (of olfactory neurons) 281
Spectrally broad band neurons 134, 135, 144, 153, 158, 169
Spectrally narrow band neurons 134, 144
Spectral discrimination 177
Spectrally opponent cell, (see also Color opponent cell and Color opponency) 135, 145, 146, 153, 172, 184, 187
Spectral receptor (type) 78, 172
Spectral sensitivity 132, 134, 141, 143, 144, 172, 175, 178, 187, 195, 196
Spiking response 148, 166, 191-199
Stinging behavior 121-127
(see also Defensive behavior)
Suboesophagael ganglion 142, 156, 159, 162, 169, 170, 202-221, 260, 282, 320
Sunflower 98
Synapse 134, 136, 203, 205, 217, 225-233, 237, 280, 288, 290

Tangential (fiber, cell) 130-139, 146, 164, 211, 212, 213, 257, 258

Texture discrimination 96-99

Textures, learning of 96-100

Thermoregulation 68, 72, 102-109

Thoracic temperature 102-109, 112-119

Threshold adjustment 38-51, 70

Transmitter binding sites 253-263

Tritocerebrum 159, 162, 170, 202-221, 238

Velocity sensitivity 158-170

Visual fiber 130-135

Visual field, (see also receptive field) 135, 138, 149, 155, 159, 161, 169, 181, 182, 184

Visual interneurons 112, 118, 173, 181, 184, 198

Visual stabilization 158, 167, 170

Waggle dance, see Dance

Warm-up 102, 103, 106

Wasp(s), (see also Paravespula) 97, 106

Water collection 44-46, 68, 107-109

Weather conditions 38, 40, 46, 47, 49, 51, 64

Wide field (visual neurons), (see also Receptive field) 135, 138, 141-156, 158-170

Wind 167, 170

Xylorhiza wrightii 98

Y-cell 130-139

Yaw 161

MIX
Papier aus verantwortungsvollen Quellen
Paper from responsible sources
FSC® C105338

If you have any concerns about our products,
you can contact us on
ProductSafety@springernature.com

In case Publisher is established outside the EU,
the EU authorized representative is:
Springer Nature Customer Service Center GmbH
Europaplatz 3, 69115 Heidelberg, Germany

Printed by Libri Plureos GmbH
in Hamburg, Germany